IMMUNOLOGICAL ASPECTS OF TRANSPLANTATION SURGERY

IMMUNOLOGICAL ASPECTS OF TRANSPLANTATION SURGERY

Edited by
PROFESSOR ROY CALNE

MTP
MEDICAL AND TECHNICAL
PUBLISHING CO LTD
1973

Published by

MTP
Medical and Technical Publishing Co. Ltd
St Leonard's House
St Leonardgate
Lancaster, England.

Softcover reprint of the hardcover 1st edition 1973

Thanet Press, Margate

ISBN-13: 978-94-011-6602-7 e-ISBN-13:978-94-011-6600-3
DOI: 10.1007/978-94-011-6600-3

LIST OF CONTRIBUTORS

MARILYN L. BACH, PH.D.
Departments of Medical Genetics, Surgery, Pediatrics and Pharmacology
University of Wisconsin
Madison, Wisconsin 53706, USA

FRITZ H. BACH, M.D.
Departments of Medical Genetics, Surgery, Pediatrics and Pharmacology
University of Wisconsin
Madison, Wisconsin 53706, USA

PROFESSOR L. BRENT
Department of Immunology
Wright-Fleming Institute
St Mary's Hospital Medical School
London W2 1PG, England

PROFESSOR ROY Y. CALNE
Department of Surgery
University of Cambridge
Tennis Court Road
Cambridge, England

ROBERT J. CORRY, M.D.
Harvard Medical School
Massachusetts General Hospital
Boston, Massachusetts 02114, USA

D. A. L. DAVIES, M.A., PH.D., D.SC.
Department of Immunology
Research Division
G. D. Searle and Son
Lane End Road, High Wycombe
Bucks HP12 4HL, England

ERWIN DIENER, PH.D.
MRC Transplantation Unit
University of Alberta
Edmonton 7, Alberta, Canada

DR. WILLIAM L. FORD
Department of Pathology
University of Edinburgh
Medical Buildings
Teviot Place, Edinburgh, Scotland

DR. BASIL M. HERBERTSON
Department of Pathology
University of Cambridge
Tennis Court Road
Cambridge, England

DENNIS W. JIRSCH, M.D.
MRC Transplantation Unit
Provincial Laboratory
University of Alberta
Edmonton 7, Alberta, Canada

THOMAS L. MARCHIORO, M.D.
School of Medicine
University of Washington
Seattle, Washington, USA

GERHARD OPELZ, M.D.
School of Medicine
University of California
Los Angeles, California, USA

L. G. QUADRACCI, M.D.
School of Medicine
University of Washington
Seattle, Washington, USA

PROFESSOR PAUL S. RUSSELL, M.D.
Harvard Medical School
Massachusetts General Hospital
Boston, Massachusetts 02114, USA

DR. ELIZABETH SIMPSON
Immunology Branch
National Cancer Institute
National Institutes of Health
Bethesda, Maryland, USA

GARY E. STRIKER, M.D.
School of Medicine
University of Washington
Seattle, Washington, USA

PROFESSOR FRANK P. STUART
Department of Surgery
University of Chicago
950 East 59th Street
Chicago, Illinois 60637, USA

PAUL I. TERASAKI, PH.D.
School of Medicine
University of California
Los Angeles, California, USA

ALAN TING, PH.D.
School of Medicine
University of California
Los Angeles, California, USA

DR. E. WHITE
Department of Endodentics
School of Dentistry
University of South Carolina
Charleston, South Carolina 29401, USA

CONTENTS

Introduction

R. Y. Calne

Surgeons are transplanting kidneys in ever increasing numbers—more than 10000 renal allografts have now been reported to the Transplant Registry. With related donors 75% of grafted kidneys continued to function after 2 years, compared with 50% when the donors were unrelated. The therapeutic value is obvious, but the management is largely empirical and results have improved little in the past 5 years. The basic sciences related to tissue transplantation have advanced rapidly. New serological and tissue culture techniques and chemical analysis of antigens and antibodies have produced complicated data that is almost incomprehensible to the non-specialist. Mathematical treatment of genetic probabilities and of immunological kinetics are similarly difficult to follow for those not especially trained.

There has always been a gulf between the practical clinician whose patients do not behave like inbred rodents and the biologist who likes carefully controlled experiments with easily observed results. Both realize, however, that predictable and safe control of rejection must involve close collaboration and co-operation between the laboratory and the clinic. Unfortunately, the different nature of the work and the workers has widened the gap between them. The clinicians tend to improve their techniques and patient care, whilst the biologists seek clearer and more precisely defined experiments which lead them to use increasingly artificial experimental models.

A simple basic dogma of tissue transplantation has become established. Thus, tolerance in the foetus is produced by antigen. Antibody can either destroy grafts, or enhance their survival. Histocompatibility antigens defined serologically determine the fate of grafted tissue. None of these axioms however seems to have much practical relevance. Classical fetal tolerance is of great academic biological interest, but cannot be applied directly. Our inability to differentiate between destructive and enhancing antibodies makes the clinician suspicious of all antibodies. The obvious lack of close correlation between HLA antigens and the fate of unrelated renal allografts has undermined major schemes of national and international organ sharing. It would seem nevertheless to be clear that further understanding of the biology of rejection and donor specific immunosuppression is of fundamental importance if there is to be clinical progress.

Perhaps the potentially most fruitful lines of investigation are the established anomalies. The 'rule breakers' which stick out of the official dogma like sore thumbs—

for example, how is it that patients can retain renal allografts for years with excellent function on modest doses of immunosuppressive drugs despite their being 'full house' mismatches of HLA antigens between donors and recipients? How can a patient with no detectable cytotoxic antibodies reject a kidney from an HLA identical and MLC negative sibling despite immunosuppressive drug treatment? (Dick *et al.*, 1972a; 1972b). How can 25 mg of azathioprine twice a week hold in check a potentially strong allograft reaction 5 years after transplantation (Woodruff, personal communication)? Why is it that a patient with a high titre of cytotoxic antibody, capable of killing 100% of donor leukocytes, can, nevertheless, accept a liver graft from that donor (our own observations)? Why do patients who have received multiple blood transfusions without producing cytotoxic antibodies accept badly matched cadaver kidney allografts more readily than untransfused recipients (Terasaki *et al*, Chapter 4)? What is the mechanism whereby rats, mice and pigs reject violently allografted skin from a given donor source, yet may accept indefinitely organ allografts from the same or similar donors?

The clinician is interested in safe immunosuppression that has a prolonged effect in terms of the life of the organism. Slight prolongation of survival requiring a '*p* value' for its substantiation is likely to be of limited value. Rejection of grafted tissue is a dynamic process in which the dimension of time is often ignored. Biological factors probably play differing rôles in the course of rejection and these may be complicated favourably or unfavourably by attempts at immunosuppressive treatment. Thus, maximal non specific immunosuppression may prevent the development of enhancement. The survival of organ allografts from isologous donors varies greatly in identically treated recipients from highly inbred rodent strains (Brent and Pinto, Chapter 13). This lack of predictability in a controlled laboratory situation points to caution in expecting consistent results in humans receiving allografts from unrelated donors. It is likely that when the relevant factors are known and can be measured, individual repeated titrations will be required in manipulating immunosuppressive regimens for each donor recipient combination.

This volume is not intended to be a comprehensive review, but is a collection of essays aimed at narrowing the gap between basic immunology and experimental organ allografting. The authors have been requested to point out what is factual and what is speculation. Their help has been specifically sought on an analysis of phenomena that do *not* fit in with established theories in the hope that these 'sore thumbs' may point the way, no matter how inelegantly, to new concepts relevant to organ grafting.

Several authors have introduced their subject with remarks on classical experiments and their interpretation. Inevitably, similar ground has been covered by a number of authors and I considered cutting such repetitive material from the definitive text. On reflection, however, I felt it would be of interest to readers to see how the same investigators and their concepts were interpreted by different contributors to this volume, so that the reader could determine for himself where there was a consensus of agreement and where there was controversy. I would not imply that widespread agreement on a phenomenon indicates that it is probably true, rather it points to current acceptance of a given explanation. A variety of different views on the same experimental findings, however, would indicate uncertainty and ignorance of the mechanisms involved.

It is hoped that the book will be of interest to surgeons working in organ transplantation and also to immunologists who might feel that the immunological aspects of transplantation surgery are worthy of more intensive research.

References

Dick, Heather M., Briggs, J. D., Wood, R. F. M. and Bell, P. R. F. (1972a). Severe rejection of an HL-A identical sibling renal transplant. *Tissue Antigens*, **2**, 345

Dick, Heather M., Boyd, Gillian A., Briggs, J. D., Wood, R. F. M. and Bell, P. R. F. (1972b). Severe rejection of an HL-A identical sibling renal transplant. Results of MLC test. *Tissue Antigens*, **2**, 480

1
The Morphology of Allograft Reactions

B. M. Herbertson

INTRODUCTION

The behaviour of transplanted organs and tissues and the morphological changes developing in them are closely inter-related and depend on various controlling factors. The principal circumstances affecting the fate of a graft include the genetic relationship between the donor and recipient, the species to which they belong, the nature of the grafted tissue, the anatomical position of the graft, the condition of the recipient's immune system and the strength and kind of the allergic response it is capable of mounting. With so many factors affecting transplants it is not surprising that their behavior is extremely variable. On the one hand, as a result of tolerance or enhancement, an allograft may be accepted as if it were an autograft and remain normal for an indefinite period. At the other extreme, if the recipient has been previously sensitized to donor antigens, the allograft may be rejected in a rapid and violent fashion. Yet a third possibility is the development of a graft-versus-host reaction causing debility or death of the recipient. If this is to occur, the allograft must contain sufficient immunologically competent cells capable of responding to host histocompatibility antigens and these donor cells must themselves be secure against successful attack by the recipient's immune system. This situation arises when cells of parental strain lymphatic tissue are introduced into F_1 hybrid recipients. These simple examples illustrate the wide diversity of response after grafting between dissimilar members of the same species and emphasize the need for defining the circumstances of any reaction being described.

The purpose of this chapter is to provide a general account of the morphology of allograft reactions and to prepare the ground for the more advanced and specialized topics considered by other contributors. First, a brief outline is given of the events occurring during the rejection of organ and tissue allografts, and this is followed by a more detailed treatment of certain outstanding features, such as mononuclear cell infiltration, vascular lesions, changes in the graft parenchyma, and the response of host lymphatic tissue.

GENERAL OUTLINE OF ALLOGRAFT REJECTION

As is well known, most organ and tissue allografts transplanted to normal recipients behave for a few days like autografts similarly transplanted. For example, a first-set allograft of skin heals in place in the same fashion as a patch of the animal's own skin transplanted in the same way. Likewise, first-set renal allografts produce urine and hepatic allografts provide the vital metabolic functions of normal liver and secrete bile. On the other hand, when an organ or tissue graft is transplanted to an individual already sensitized to donor tissue, the reaction may be dramatic and result in rapid death of all the grafted tissue. For instance, with an organ graft in which anastomoses are formed and there is full interplay between recipient blood and donor endothelium, the reaction may be virtually immediate. In the more violent forms of 'hyperacute' rejection a renal allograft becomes flaccid and cyanosed within minutes of re-establishing blood flow and perishes during the next few hours. However, with a free graft of skin a reaction of comparable severity only becomes apparent after 2 or 3 days when the graft fails to vascularize in the usual way (the 'white graft' reaction). These examples illustrate the substantial variation in the time interval between grafting and the first macroscopic evidences of rejection.

The course of allograft rejection may also differ in other respects. Although allograft rejection unmodified by treatment is usually regarded as a progressive process which continues uninterruptedly until the transplanted tissue is destroyed, there are circumstances in which a more delicate immune balance spontaneously develops between the recipient and the grafted tissue. For instance, in certain experimental systems rejection of renal allografts may be a distinctly intermittent process with phases of allergic injury alternating with periods of partial recovery. This is most often seen when the antigenic disparity between donor and recipient is relatively slight and a transplant may then survive for long periods, despite occasional episodes of rejection. A rather different and more extreme example of an altered type of relationship is the long-term survival of hepatic allografts between strains of pig which regularly reject skin and renal allografts (Calne *et al.*, 1967). In such animals a relatively slight short-lived allograft reaction is sometimes observed in the liver during the first month or so after transplantation but the recipient later becomes unresponsive to the graft and the reaction completely subsides. Complete or partial suppression of allograft rejection can, of course, be achieved by the various immunosuppressive measures used in clinical practice but the natural variation in the pattern of allograft reactions in the unmodified animal has perhaps been insufficiently appreciated.

Macroscopic features

In organ and tissue allografts the macroscopic features of rejection consist of a mixture of appearances due to circulatory disturbances, cellular infiltration, edema and parenchymal destruction. The manifestations of vascular change include pallor, congestion, swelling, cyanosis and hemorrhage and the cellular infiltration and edema contribute to the enlargement and pallor of the graft. The kind of parenchymal damage and its effect on the appearance of a graft depend on the form and intensity of the rejection process and on the organ or tissue involved. If rejection occurs rapidly, necrosis of the parenchyma is a major feature and, if not dominated by the deep colors of congestion or hemorrhage, the affected parts will usually appear pale and rather opaque. On the other hand, if rejection occurs much more gradually, atrophy of the specialized tissue with increasing fibrosis may be the major feature. In these circumstances the involved tissue tends to be rather shrunken, greyish-white and may become somewhat tougher than normal. The distribution of these destructive changes varies. Sometimes there seems to be no particular pattern but often, particularly in organ grafts, the lesions have a pronounced vascular arrangement with the development of clearly defined infarcts or wedge-shaped atrophic and fibrotic lesions.

The appearance of an allograft also depends in great measure on the stage which the rejection process has reached. Obviously the changes in orthotopic skin and other superficially placed allografts can be readily seen as the reaction develops but with organ allografts the progress of rejection is less readily observed and a number of similar transplants may have to be examined at intervals before the pattern of the macroscopic features is adequately known. Similarly, the extent to which it is possible for rejection of certain transplants to progress also needs to be considered. For example, if an animal depends for continuing life on a transplanted heart, liver or kidney, the structural changes can develop to a certain degree only before function fails and death ensues. On the other hand, if the animal is not so dependent on the function of the graft, the rejection process can run its complete course. In this event the graft may become completely necrotic and then either slough, or be resorbed or organized. Equally with a slower form of rejection it may be destroyed by a more gradual process but nevertheless ultimately become a fibrous remnant.

Despite the wide variations in the macroscopic appearance of allografts during rejection, for most organs and tissues certain broad groups can be distinguished. For example, with renal allografts there are several common forms. First, there is the large pale kidney, up to three times its original weight, with an edematous bulging cut surface (Figure 1.1). Sometimes such kidneys have a blotchy appearance with ill-defined congested patches irregularly scattered in their otherwise pale fawn to

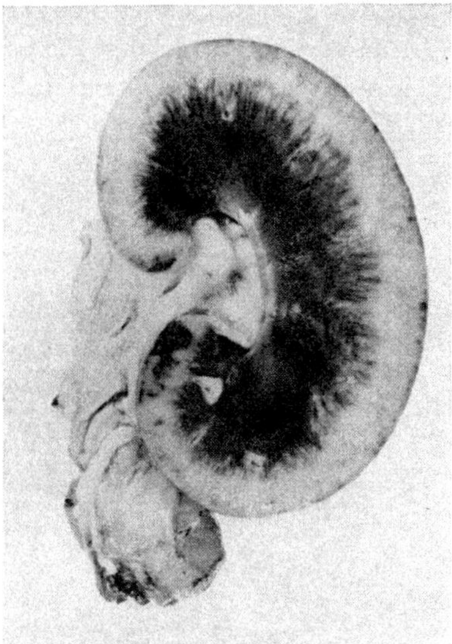

Figure 1.1 *Dog renal allograft (first-set) 17 days after transplantation. No immunosuppression. A considerably enlarged kidney with a moist pale greyish-white cortex and congested medulla. A few small hemorrhages in cortex. Microscopically: intense mononuclear cell infiltration, considerable edema, acute arterial lesions and focal parenchymal necrosis. Half natural size*

whitish-grey substance (Figure 1.2). A second group comprises the massive deep reddish-purple kidneys, even five times their original weight, with hemorrhages distributed throughout their substance and in the wall of the edematous and congested pelvis and ureter (Figure 1.3). In addition there may be some irregular pale opaque necrotic patches in the cortex or typical well-defined infarcts. A third group consists of the renal allografts which as a result of rejection are totally or mostly necrotic. These kidneys vary considerably in their other features some being large and rather hemorrhagic, others being of about normal size and having a uniform opaque brownish cut surface. In a fourth group the kidneys are of about normal size or somewhat smaller, have an uneven rather coarsely scarred and pitted pale outer surface and irregularly narrowed rather tough fibrotic cortex (Figure 1.4). However, although these divisions serve some purpose in helping description, it would be a mistake to believe that they are more than parts of a broad spectrum which merge imperceptibly with one another. It should also be emphasized that the macroscopic features of an allograft depend on the pattern of rejection in the particular individual concerned. For instance, during the early stages the kidney may become large, pale and edematous; later it may become intensely congested and hemorrhagic, and

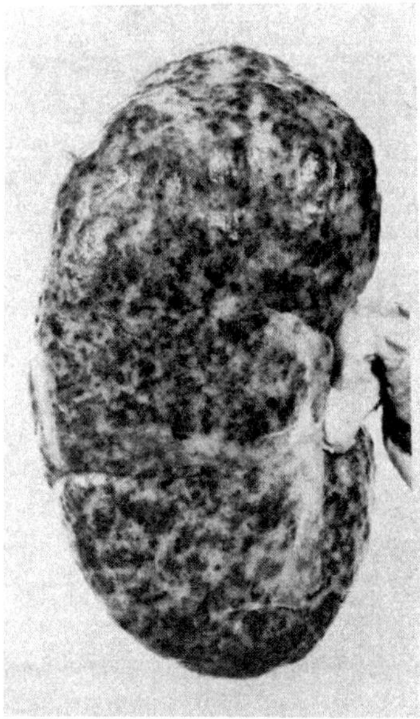

Figure 1.2 *Human renal allograft (first) 121 days after transplantation. Immunosuppression with steroids and azathioprine. A slightly enlarged kidney (180 g) with a blotchy appearance. Microscopically: atrophy and fibrosis and recent necrosis of cortex, fibrinoid necrosis of arteries and arterioles and slight mononuclear cell infiltration and edema. Half natural size*

finally, especially if the recipient is not dependent on the function of the allograft, it may become completely necrotic. Of course, a renal transplant could become completely necrotic by a rather more direct route, for example, as a result of hyperacute rejection. The macroscopic features would then usually be rather different from the necrotic and hemorrhagic kidney seen as the final stage of the sequence described above.

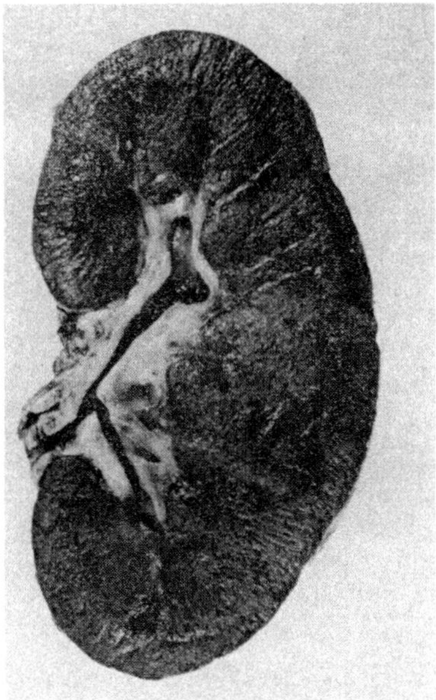

Figure 1.3 *Human renal allograft (first) 29 days after transplantation. Immunosuppression with steroids and azathioprine. A greatly enlarged deep purple-red kidney (610 g). Main renal artery and vein free from thrombus. Microscopically: extensive recent parenchymal necrosis, fibrinoid necrosis and thrombosis of intrarenal arteries and arterioles. Substantial edema and interstitial hemorrhage and only slight mononuclear cell infiltration.*
Two-fifths natural size

Microscopic features

The principal microscopic changes developing during allograft rejection include mononuclear cell infiltration, edema, vascular lesions and destruction of the parenchyma of the graft. However, the precise character, timing and severity of the lesions in individual grafts depend, like the other features, on the various donor and host factors already mentioned.

Mononuclear cell infiltration is the first morphological change during rejection of most first-set grafts and usually begins a day or two before there is any macroscopic evidence of an allograft reaction. The tissue soon becomes slightly edematous. As the mononuclear cell infiltration increases, vascular lesions develop but their type and time sequence vary considerably from graft to graft. In some transplants the

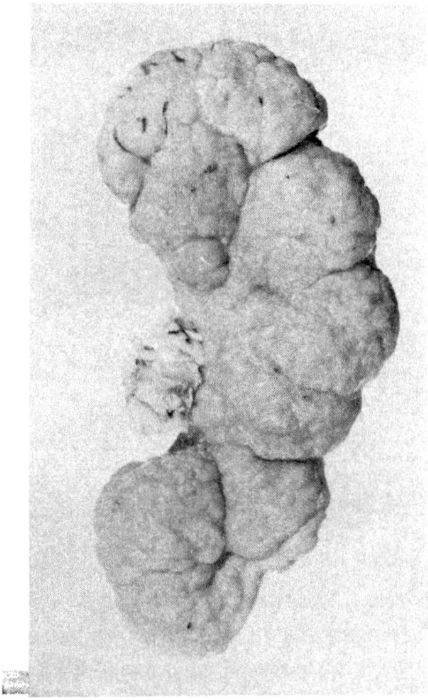

Figure 1.4 *Pig renal allograft (first-set) 483 days after transplantation. No conventional immunosuppression but given 1 litre donor blood during transplantation. A small coarsely scarred and fissured fibrotic kidney. Microscopically: focal parenchymal atrophy and fibrosis with intimal thickening of related arteries. No evidence of pyelonephritis.*
Half natural size

capillaries, venules and veins are principally involved but in others arterial changes become prominent. Sometimes the arterial lesions are of a proliferative kind but on other occasions fibrinoid necrosis of arteries and arterioles occurs and platelet–fibrin thrombi may develop. In many first-set grafts the parenchyma and other components of the graft undergo necrosis but if the recipient's reaction is less vigorous atrophy and fibrosis gradually occur.

The accelerated rejections of allografts by sensitized recipients may take various forms. If the recipient is only moderately sensitive the reaction may have the same general characteristics as a first-set response but develop more rapidly and be more intense. For example, with second-set skin allografts mononuclear cell infiltration is often the predominant feature in the initial stages of the reaction but the cells tend to be concentrated in the graft bed near the interface between host tissue and the transplant rather than in the substance of the graft itself.

With highly sensitized recipients the reaction may be virtually immediate, primarily vascular and involve very little mononuclear cell infiltration. For example, with renal allografts the major initial change is vascular obstruction due to severe endothelial cell injury and the development of occluding thrombi consisting of varying proportions of platelets, leukocytes, fibrin and red cells. Sometimes these vascular lesions take several hours to form but even then there is little mononuclear cell infiltration in the graft. Necrosis of the parenchyma and other components of the graft inevitably follows.

Despite the differences in these various types of reaction, the histological features of graft rejection, like the macroscopic appearances, undoubtedly form a continuous series. Although, if the extremes are compared, the lesions seem rather diverse, a thorough examination of experimental and human transplant material soon demonstrates their essential continuity. This does not, of course, exclude the possibility that various types of allergic mechanism are responsible for the lesions and that among other factors the pattern depends on their relative strengths.

CELLULAR INFILTRATION

Mononuclear cell infiltration

Timing—Mononuclear cell infiltration is a prominent feature of virtually all first-set allograft reactions and is usually the first morphological difference between comparable allografts and autografts. In the early stages the mononuclear cells tend to be clustered around capillaries, venules and veins but later they extend widely throughout the graft. Although the time interval between transplantation and the appearance of mononuclear cells varies, the infiltration in organ grafts frequently begins within 2 or 3 days. For example, after transplanting (Lewis $\times$ BN) F_1 rat kidneys to unmodified Lewis recipients Guttmann *et al.* (1967) observed collections of mononuclear cells in the interstitial tissue around cortical blood vessels 2 days after transplantation (Day 2). Similarly, in rat liver transplant experiments Lee and Edgington (1968), using Sprague–Dawley donors and Lewis recipients, found that mononuclear cell infiltration began abruptly on Day 3. There are also numerous reports of similar time intervals in experimental renal, hepatic, cardiac and pulmonary allografts in other species. Even in the presence of immunosuppressive treatment mononuclear cell infiltration has been observed on Day 3 in a first-set human renal allograft (Figure 1.5). In a few instances, mononuclear cell infiltration of organ allografts has

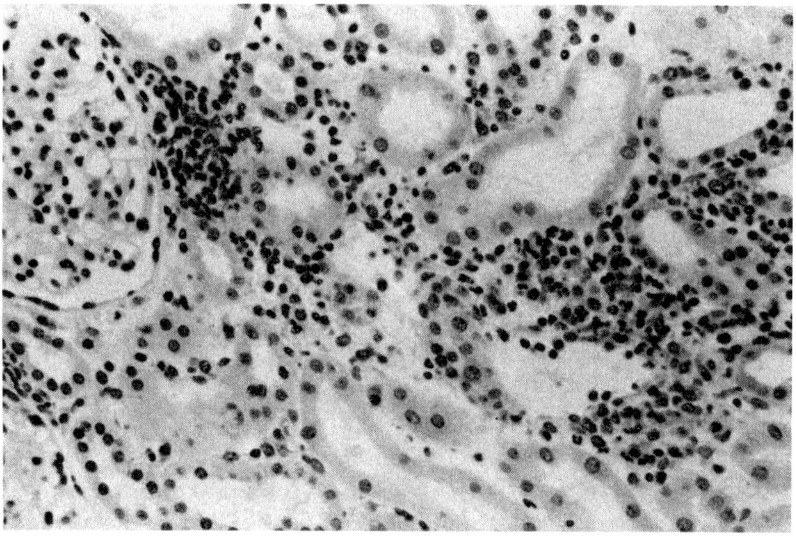

Figure 1.5 *Human renal allograft (first): biopsy 3 days after transplantation. Immunosuppression with steroids and azathioprine. Focal mononuclear cell infiltration in edematous interstitial tissue between tubules and near glomerulus. Very few neutrophil polymorphs. Well preserved tubules.*
H. & E. × 270

been noticed after a much shorter time. For example, Chiba *et al.* (1962) described perivascular collections of lymphocytes and other mononuclear cells in canine heart homografts 5 hours after transplantation but this has not been regular experience with most types of organ allograft. In their informative studies on the behavior of sheep renal transplants, Pedersen and Morris (1970) found that the total number of mononuclear cells in the lymph leaving allografts was beginning to rise significantly about 24 hours after transplantation. Although this does not necessarily mean that there were increased numbers of mononuclear cells in the substance of the allograft at that time it does suggest that this may be so. Relatively slight increases in a particular type of cell are not readily detected by conventional histological methods and these cell counts of efferent lymph may well be a more sensitive indicator of the mononuclear cell content of renal transplants. While this may seem a relatively small matter, the timing of mononuclear cell infiltrations is of considerable significance particularly in relation to the role of host lymphatic tissue in graft rejection.

In most species the mononuclear cell infiltration of a first-set skin allograft usually begins 1 or 2 days later than in organ grafts between comparable donors and recipients. For example, in genetically heterogeneous rabbits mononuclear cell infiltration of orthotopic, full-thickness, first-set skin allografts usually begins to appear 4 to 6 days after transplantation compared with about 3 to 4 days for renal allografts between similar animals. Although several factors probably contribute to this difference, the contrasting circumstances of a free graft of skin in which fresh vascular connections form naturally over a period of 2 days or more and of an organ graft in which vascular anastomoses are created at the time of transplantation must surely be important. The investigations by Hall (1967) of the lymph draining the sites of skin allografts in the sheep are of considerable interest. Contrary to the observations of Pedersen and Morris (1970) on the lymph from sheep renal allografts, Hall found comparatively little increase in the cell content of the lymph leaving skin allografts in the same species, even while the graft was being actively rejected. This apparent difference deserves further investigation.

Type of cells—Most morphologists would agree about the difficulty of distinguishing different kinds of mononuclear cells in sections of tissue, particularly when the population consists of a mixture of transforming cell types. In a study of the mononuclear cell response in delayed hypersensitivity in the guinea pig, Turk *et al.* (1966) express this problem clearly and their comments apply with equal force to recognizing the various forms of mononuclear cell in graft reactions. In many species the most impressive point is the substantial morphological heterogeneity of the mononuclear cell infiltrate. With ordinary light microscopy the variations in size, shape and structure of the infiltrating mononuclear cells are readily seen and using simple staining procedures on sections or smears many observers would recognize three kinds, namely, small lymphocytes, plasma cells and a group of larger mononuclear cells. In this third category some morphologists have considered it possible to distinguish lymphocytes of larger size, monocytes, histiocytes, and blast cells, and possibly other kinds also. However, others would regard it as rather naive to suppose that such cells can be individually identified with certainty by such elementary morphological means. During recent years the nature of individual mononuclear cells in allografts and similar reactions has been further investigated by a variety of techniques. These include the pyronin–methyl green method for RNA, acid phosphatase techniques for lysosome content, immunofluorescence methods for immunoglobulins and electron microscopy for fine structure. In most investigations of this kind four major categories of mononuclear cell have been distinguished:

(1) lymphocytes (small and large)
(2) blast cells
(3) plasma cells (immature and mature)
(4) macrophages.

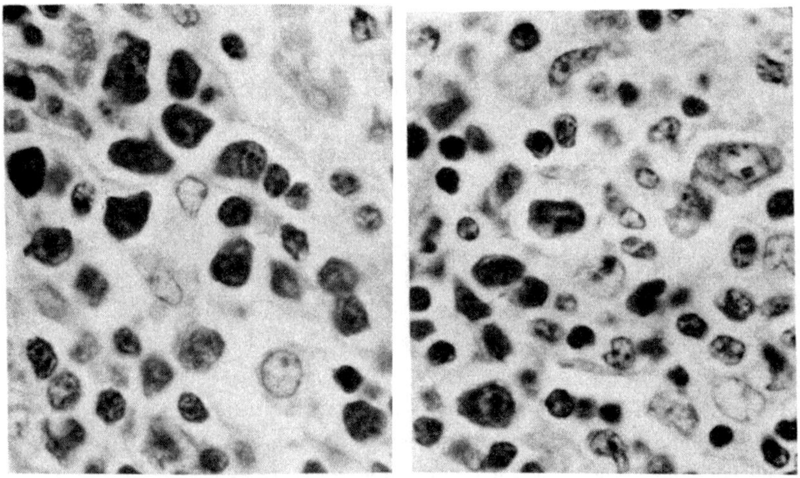

Figure 1.6 *Rhesus monkey renal allograft (first-set) 25 days after transplantation. High power light microscope photograph of mononuclear cells infiltrating interstitial tissue of cortex. Considerable cellular pleomorphism. Pyroninophilic cells have dark cytoplasm. Pyronin–Methyl green. × 970*

These cell types are illustrated in Figures 1.6–1.9 and their distinguishing features are outlined in Table 1.1. However, while recognizing typical cells in each of these categories is a relatively simple task, many of the mononuclear cells in actively developing allograft reactions are not sufficiently characteristic to enable them to be identified with confidence.

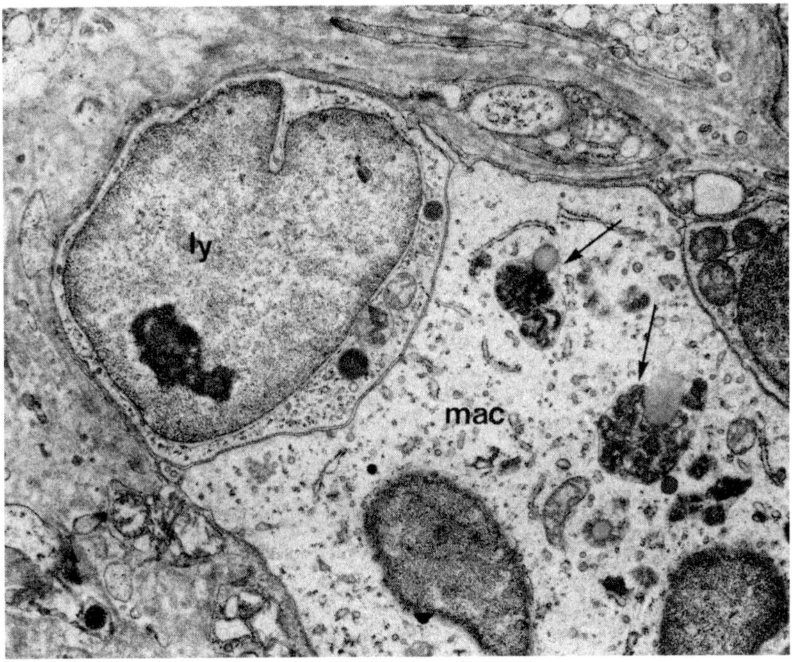

Figure 1.7 *Human renal allograft (second) 838 days after transplantation. An electron micrograph of cells in interstitial tissue. A small lymphocyte (ly) and part of a macrophage (mac) with phagocytic vacuoles (arrows). Osmium, epon and lead citrate.* × *8810*

In their investigations of allograft rejection of rat kidneys, Lindquist *et al.* (1971) examined the fine structure of the infiltrating mononuclear cells. They described three types of mononuclear cell in addition to mature lymphocytes. Their first type appears to correspond with the blast cell mentioned previously. Morphologically, their second kind resemble the cells usually regarded as belonging to the plasma cell series but they suggest that many of these cells may be collagen-forming. The reasons for this interpretation are first, the absence of demonstrable immunoglobulins in these cells at the appropriate time and second, the presence of bundles of collagen

Table 1.1 *Mononuclear cells in allografts: some cytoplasmic characteristics of the major cell types*

Cell type	*Synonyms*	*Light microscopy*		*Electron microscopy*					*Immunofluorescence*
		Cytoplasmic pyroninophilia	*Lysosomes**	*RER‡*	*Free polyribosomes*	*SER†*	*Golgi complex*	*Lysosomes**	*Immunoglobulins*
Lymphocytes		o to +	o to +	o to +	o to +	+	+	o to +	o
Blast cells	Immunoblasts Large pyroninophilic cells Lymphoblasts Lymphoid blast cells Transforming blast cells	+ to +++	o to +	o to +	++ to ++++	+	+ to ++	o to +	o
Plasma cells									
(a) immature	Plasmablasts	++ to +++	o to +	+ to +++	+ to ++	+	++	o to +	+ to ++
(b) mature		++ to ++++	o to +	+++ to ++++	+	+	++ to +++	o to +	++ to ++++
Macrophages		o to +	++ to ++++	+ to ++	o to ++	+ to ++	++ to +++	++ to ++++	o

*Lysosomes = intracytoplasmic bodies containing acid phosphatase
‡Ribosome-bearing endoplasmic reticulum
†Smooth-surfaced endoplasmic reticulum

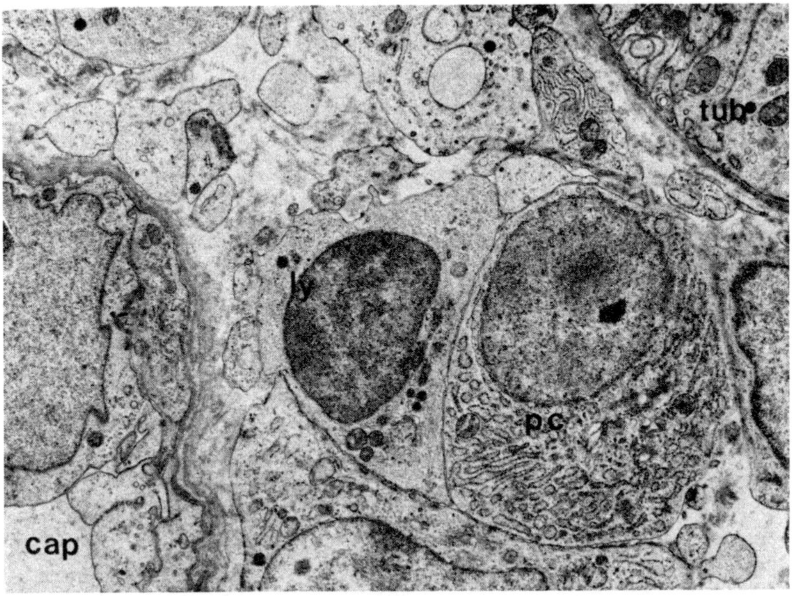

Figure 1.8 *Rabbit renal allograft (first-set): biopsy 5 days after transplantation. An electron micrograph of a large blast cell (bl) with numerous free polyribosomes in cytoplasm The cell lies in lumen of intertubular capillary (end = endothelial cell) and similar blast cells were in mitosis. From work of D. C. Dunn.*
Osmium, epon and lead citrate. × 4940

fibrils in close proximity to them. Their third kind of cell appear to resemble conventional fibroblasts and these became the commonest form of interstitial mononuclear cell at about 7 days. Their investigation was concentrated on the first 7 days after transplantation and they saw no typical plasma cells during this period but, as they remark, typical plasma cells containing demonstrable IgG do appear slightly later. Lindquist and his colleagues emphasized that there was an uninterrupted series of intermediate cells between mature lymphocytes and their first type of cell and between the extremes of their first and second types. Most morphologists who have investigated the fine structure of allograft reactions in rats and other species would agree with these comments.

Origin of cells—The origin of the mononuclear cells infiltrating allografts has been fairly thoroughly investigated and there can be no doubt that the majority are recipient cells which are carried to the graft by the bloodstream and then invade the transplanted tissue. The reader will be familiar with the entirely reasonable proposals of Dempster (1953) and Simonsen (1953) that the cells might be of donor origin and represent a graft-versus-host reaction. However, the studies of Porter and Calne (1960) and others using labeling techniques clearly demonstrated that most are derived from the recipient. Nevertheless, there remains the distinct possibility that a minority of the mononuclear cells may be of donor origin. This may be of some significance in determining the cellular events within an allograft and is undoubtedly worth further investigation.

Mechanism of infiltration—There are several rather perplexing and as yet unsolved problems about the mechanisms by which the recipient's cells enter the graft. Various experimental studies have shown that with a first-set allograft a reaction soon occurs

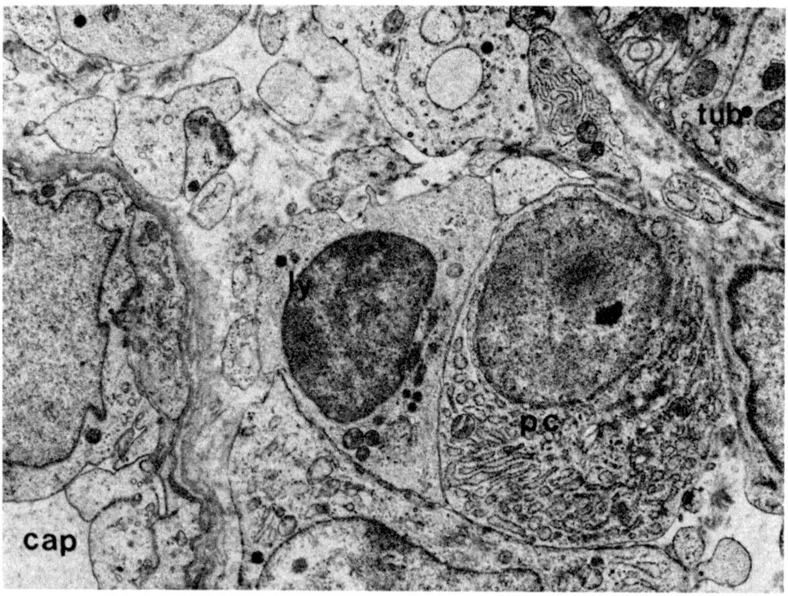

Figure 1.9 *Human renal allograft (first): biopsy 11 days after transplantation. An electron micrograph illustrating a small lymphocyte (ly) and a plasma cell (pc) in interstitial tissue between a capillary (cap) and a tubule (tub).*
Osmium, epon and lead citrate. × *4300*

in the recipient's lymphatic tissue and a newly formed population of specifically modified or activated lymphocytes is produced. At first it was assumed that many of these newly produced reactive cells entered the bloodstream and when by chance they happened to pass through the graft they became specifically attached to the surface of the allogeneic endothelial cells. Subsequently, perhaps due to chemotaxis, the altered lymphocytes migrate through the vessel wall into the interstitial tissue of the graft. However, Najarian and Feldman (1962), Prendergast (1964) and Hall (1967) have shown that in mouse, rabbit and sheep skin allografts there is either little or no selection of specifically sensitized donor lymphocytes. Investigations by Turk (1962) and others on the characteristics of mononuclear cell infiltration in delayed hypersensitivity reactions had provided similar equally surprising results and fresh explanations for this phenomenon in allograft and related delayed hypersensitivity reactions must be sought. As a considerable proportion of the infiltrating cells are macrophages, the mechanism responsible for their adherence to the endothelium and emigration has also to be considered. It seemed at one time that cytophilic antibody bound to monocyte plasma membranes might be responsible for their becoming attached to the endothelium but it was also thought that specific selection and emigration of appropriately altered lymphocytes could in some way provide a suitable, if non-specific, method of introducing macrophages.

In most organ allografts mononuclear cells begin to adhere to the endothelium of capillaries, venules and veins, and less frequently of arteries, 2 to 4 days after transplantation. Shortly afterwards some of them begin to emigrate through the vessel walls into the surrounding interstitial tissue. One impressive feature is the focal quality of this process, at least in the earlier phases. In most allografts the mononuclear cells are initially found in and around only a small proportion of the capillaries, venules and veins and there seldom seems to be any particular anatomical pattern or convincing physiological explanation. Why only some vessels are involved at this stage remains obscure. However, this problem of localization of lesions is a common aspect of cardiovascular pathology and, like the arterial lesions in graft rejection, the explanation probably depends on hemodynamic and other functional features rather than on special immunological factors. As the mononuclear cell infiltrate seems not to be a highly selected population of cells with specific reactive functions, it is unlikely that the adherence of the cells is due to specific reaction with antigenic sites on endothelial cells. Even if this were the mechanism of cell adherence, it seems unlikely that the focal distribution of cells could be explained by a significantly higher concentration of histocompatibility antigens on certain groups of endothelial cells.

Fine structure studies of mononuclear cells adhering to the endothelium have provided little evidence about the nature of this process. Like the pavementing of neutrophil leukocytes in acute inflammation, the plasma membranes of the lymphocytes and endothelial cells are usually distinct and, in electron micrographs, appear to be separated by a narrow undulating but regular gap which contains no obvious cementing material. It seems certain, however, that although the plasma membranes usually remain intact the external glycoprotein coats of the opposing cell surfaces are in intimate contact and are linked to one another by bonds of some kind. Some investigators believe that, while a mononuclear cell is adhering to the endothelium,

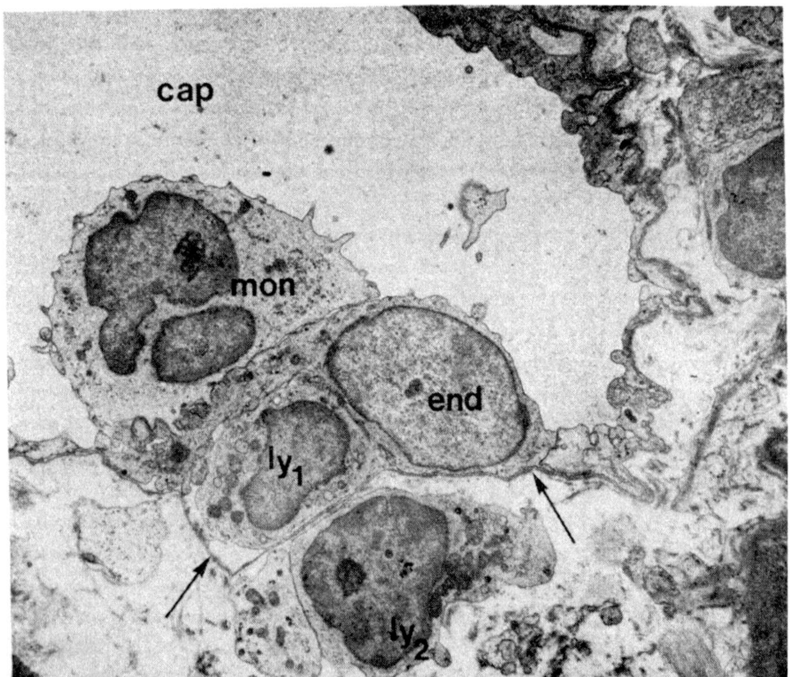

Figure 1.10 *Human renal allograft (first): biopsy 11 days after transplantation. Same specimen as Figure 1.9. An electron micrograph showing a lymphocyte* (ly_1) *migrating through wall of capillary (cap) and lying between an endothelial cell (end) and the capillary basement membrane (arrows). However, this does not help to reveal precise route of emigration. A second lymphocyte* (ly_2) *in interstitial tissue and another mononuclear cell (mon) adherent to endothelium.*
Osmium, epon and lead citrate. × *3520*

corresponding parts of the plasma membrane of the two cells sometimes disappear and their cytoplasm becomes continuous. Although this may occur, tangential sectioning can cause confusing appearances and this feature requires further investigation.

The pathway which the lymphocytes and monocytes follow during their migration through the vessel walls is another point of interest (Figure 1.10). There is general agreement that inflammatory cells usually migrate from blood vessels by passing between endothelial cells but, at least in the post-capillary venules of lymph nodes, lymphocytes appear to migrate by moving through the cytoplasm of the rather tall endothelial cells. The route of emigration of lymphocytes in allograft reactions remains uncertain. In some investigations electron micrographs have been interpreted as supporting an inter-cellular pathway. On the other hand, Astrom *et al.* (1968), in their study of experimental allergic neuritis, believed that most lymphocytes emigrated by passing through the substance of the cytoplasm of endothelial cells. As this response seems to be fundamentally similar to allograft reactions these observations are manifestly relevant. Despite this uncertainty about lymphocytes, it seems fairly certain that monocytes emigrate by passing between endothelial cells and, as with neutrophil polymorphs in acute inflammation, there may be no permanent lesions after they have passed into the perivascular tissues.

Proliferation and transformation—Proliferation of the infiltrating mononuclear cells is a prominent component of most allograft reactions and can be readily detected by conventional histological methods and by labeling techniques. In organ grafts, mitoses can be found among the mononuclear cells almost as soon as cell infiltration begins. For example, in their studies of rat renal allografts Guttmann *et al.* (1967) observed frequent mitoses from Day 3 onwards. Similarly Porter *et al.* (1964) found that, 4 days after transplantation, about 4 per cent of the mononuclear cells infiltrating dog renal allografts incorporated tritiated thymidine within 30 minutes. Most of the dividing cells are present in the interstitial tissue of the grafts but mitoses are also seen among the mononuclear cells still within the blood vessels.

The morphological heterogeneity of the infiltrating mononuclear cells has already been emphasized and a brief account of the continuous range of intermediate cells between mature lymphocytes, blast cells and cells of the plasma cell series has already been given. There is increasing evidence that the morphological and functional changes within the mononuclear cell population of many allografts are very similar to and may be identical with the reactive changes which occur in the lymphatic tissue of allograft-bearing recipients. The investigations of Pedersen and Morris (1970) and Lindquist *et al.* (1971), in particular, have provided considerable support for the growing belief that in some circumstances a significant part of the allergic response providing the capacity to destroy the foreign tissue may actually develop within the graft itself. The morphological features of many first-set allografts are in keeping with this concept. Certainly there is a striking similarity between the cell content of a rejecting first-set allograft and of a lymph node draining such a graft and, by analogy with general observations about the transformation of lymphocytes after exposure to antigen and other agents, it seems likely that the blast cells and the immature and mature plasma cells found in allografts are in many instances formed within the graft from infiltrating blood-borne lymphocytes. A beginning has been made with population studies of the mononuclear cells in allografts and there is now need of much more quantitative and qualitative information about the cells entering grafts, about their multiplication, transformation and function within grafts and about the numbers and quality of the cells leaving them.

Polymorphonuclear leukocytes

Polymorphonuclear leukocytes are usually regarded as playing a subsidiary role in allograft reactions but there are certain features about their behavior in transplanted tissue which deserve comment. In the majority of autografts and allografts some cell injury, caused by ischemia or mechanical damage, occurs at the time of transplantation. A brief acute inflammatory response, including some emigration of neutrophil polymorphs, is therefore a common accompaniment of many transplant procedures. This initial neutrophil polymorph infiltration is usually slight and of little consequence but it must be appreciated for what is is and not regarded as being due to an acute allergic reaction, or to infection, without adequate evidence. Similarly, neutrophil polymorph infiltration frequently occurs in the final stages of graft rejection. In this instance it also tends to be a response to tissue necrosis caused by the allergic process itself or by the accompanying ischemia but other possible factors, including infection, have again to be considered.

In addition to these commonplace circumstances neutrophil polymorphs may play a significant role during hyperacute allograft rejection and xenograft reactions. In these instances circulating neutrophil polymorphs tend to aggregate with platelets and fibrin within the blood vessels and help to form occluding thrombi. At one time it was suggested that lysosomal enzymes liberated from polymorphs might play some part in graft destruction but recently Palutke *et al.* (1972) observed no degranulation of neutrophil polymorphs and concluded that such a mechanism did not contribute to tissue injury in hyperacute rejection of their pig-to-dog heterografts. In other circumstances, however, it seems likely that lysosomal enzymes derived from polymorphs may be a factor in damaging tissue. For instance, breaks in the internal elastic lamina of arteries frequently develop in organ allografts and if the natural history of such lesions is examined it appears that neutrophil polymorphs probably take a part in destroying the elastic tissue.

An excess of neutrophil polymorphs is sometimes seen in glomerular tufts in biopsy specimens of human renal allografts taken towards the end of a transplant operation. In some instances the increased numbers have been related to the presence in the recipient's plasma of cytotoxic antibodies directed against donor cells and the allograft has been rejected either immediately or within a short period. Kincaid-Smith *et al.* (1968) found that the number of neutrophil polymorphs in the glomeruli in such biopsy specimens gave a reasonable indication of the future behavior of the transplant, increased numbers presaging a stormy course. In our experience such counts have not proved a reliable guide.

As well as neutrophil leukocytes, eosinophil polymorphs sometimes infiltrate grafts. For example, Rogers *et al.* (1953) described considerable infiltrations of eosinophil leukocytes in human skin allografts and not infrequently they are found in moderate numbers among the mononuclear cell infiltrate during rejection of human renal allografts. The significance of these observations remains uncertain but in clinical renal transplantation the degree of eosinophil infiltration does not appear to be related to the severity of allograft reactions.

EDEMA

Slight to moderate edema develops in almost all organ grafts during the first day or so following transplantation. At this early stage autografts and allografts are equally affected and the edema is presumably due to the combined effects of increased tissue fluid formation associated with tissue injury and temporarily diminished lymph drainage as a result of severing the organ's main lymphatic connections. After 24 hours or so this initial edema subsides and in the absence of complications does not recur in autografts. On the other hand, edema is an exceptionally common component of allograft reaction, and with first-set organ grafts usually develops shortly after the mononuclear cell infiltration begins. For example, in a renal allograft in which mononuclear cell infiltration appears 3 days after transplantation, slight but definite edema can usually be detected the following day. Pedersen and Morris (1970) found that the volume of lymph draining from sheep renal allografts begins to rise above control autograft levels at about 48 hours and if a similar pattern occurs in other species it is likely that lymph flow is slightly raised a day or two before the edema is histologically recognizable. This is, of course, what might be expected. The degree of edema at subsequent phases varies greatly but in dogs it often develops to and continues at a moderate level until the later stages of the rejection process. For example, in their investigations of first-set canine renal allografts Williams *et al.* (1964) found that the dry weight/wet weight ratios did not alter greatly until oliguria occurred. At this stage the water content of the kidney increased dramatically. However, as they point out, the interpretation of dry weight/wet weight ratios is often complicated by a considerable increase in total dry weight due to the mononuclear cell infiltration. In some circumstances compensatory renal enlargement would add to the total dry weight and make such ratios even more difficult to evaluate. Suffice to say, edema is often substantial in the later stages of rejection, may be more prominent in some parts of an allograft than others and may be complicated by interstitial hemorrhages. Of course, the amount of edema fluid in a tissue or organ depends essentially on the quantity of tissue fluid formed and the amount draining away as lymph; the degree of edema therefore by itself gives little information about the volumes of fluid involved. In the sheep, Pedersen and Morris (1970) found that lymph flow from renal allografts rose to as much as 60 ml/hour compared with a maximum of 3.2 ml/hour for similarly transplanted autografts. In the same experiments they measured the protein content of the lymph and found that as the volume of lymph increased the total protein content per hour also increased but the protein concentration fell slightly from about 5 g/100 ml to a more normal level of 3–4 g/100 ml. These measurements are probably a fairly accurate indication of the flow of fluid through the interstitial tissues in the graft and of the protein concentration of the edema fluid within the kidney. They may also provide some indirect guidance about the possible mechanisms of edema development but the precise method remains uncertain. In acute inflammation, gaps develop between endothelial cells of the finer vessels, especially of venules, and these are believed to provide the pathway by which most of the increased quantity of fluid escapes into the interstitial tissue. Such gaps have not been regularly found in allografts but a similar mechanism may be at least partly responsible. Of course the vascular endothelium of the graft is likely to suffer mounting allergic injury with degeneration and necrosis of its cells and this may by itself be sufficient to cause edema. Venous thrombosis due to allergic injury of veins may also be a contributory factor in the development of edema.

VASCULAR LESIONS

With the interface between donor endothelium and recipient blood being the major functional area of contact between a graft and its host it is not surprising that the blood vessels of transplanted organs and tissues are directly involved in virtually all

allograft reactions. In most grafts substantial vascular lesions develop but their time of onset, type and severity vary greatly. In first-set organ allografts the adherence of mononuclear cells to the endothelium, particularly of capillaries and venules, is the earliest vascular change. Although this has been observed in certain canine renal allografts within a few hours of transplantation (Porter, 1966) mononuclear cell adherence with subsequent emigration into the interstitial tissues only becomes a regular histological feature after 2 or 3 days. This phase in the relationship between the allogeneic blood vessels and host mononuclear cells has already been described. Initially, the recipient mononuclear cells appear to exert only a trivial effect on the foreign endothelium which is in keeping with the concept that many infiltrating cells are not at first specifically active against the allogeneic cells. Subsequently, however, as the allergic response mounts against the graft, the morphological features strongly suggest that host mononuclear cells are able to cause necrosis of endothelial and other cells in the vessel walls and play a major role in the development of the vascular lesions. At one time cell-mediated allergic injury was believed to be the only significant specific immune mechanism causing graft rejection but most workers now accept that humoral immunoglobulins and plasma co-factors are also very important. Indeed present evidence about allergic destruction of allogeneic cells suggests that endothelial cells, smooth muscle cells and other cellular components of vessel walls in allografts may be damaged or killed by various specific mechanisms, including (1) the direct action of immune lymphocytes, (2) the interaction of cell surface antigens, free immunoglobulins and complement, (3) the reaction of antibody with cell antigens and subsequent killing by normal non-immune lymphocytes and (4) the action of macrophages bearing specific cytophilic antibodies. Moreoever, it is almost certain that more than one mechanism may be responsible for allergic vascular damage during rejection of a particular allograft but much further investigation, especially combined *in vivo* and *in vitro* studies, is necessary. Although for descriptive purposes it is convenient to consider the arterial, fine vessel and venous changes separately, there seem to be no fundamental causative differences between them. Similarly, while the morphological features of the lesions as they develop in vessels of different calibre and structure may appear remarkably diverse, there can be little doubt that they are expressions of the same process.

Arteries

A very wide range of arterial lesions may be found in allografts. At one extreme there is rapidly developing fibrinoid necrosis with destruction of the whole arterial wall (Figure 1.11) and often accompanied by thrombosis. At the other end of the scale there are chronic obliterative changes (Figure 1.12) which develop more slowly.

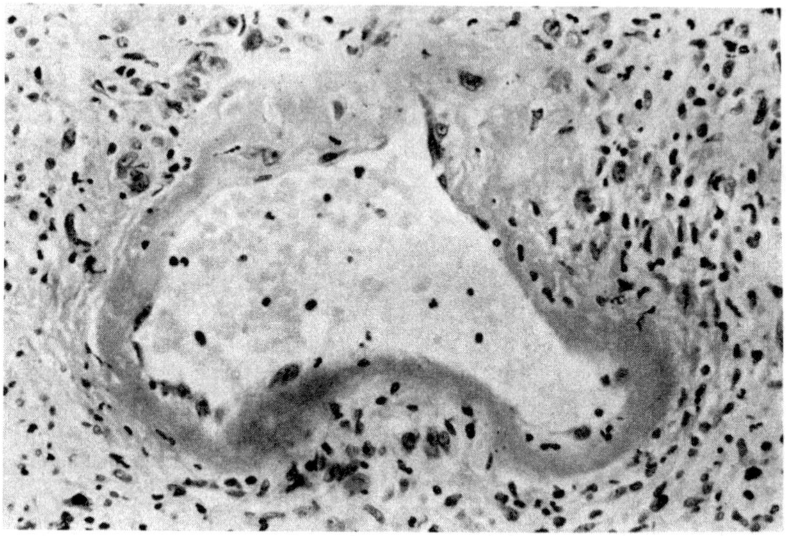

Figure 1.11 *Human renal allograft (first) 38 days after transplantation. Immunosuppression with steroids and azathioprine. Fibrinoid necrosis of a small arcuate artery. H. & E. × 270*

The type of arterial lesions occurring in a particular graft almost certainly reflects the effective antigenic disparity between donor and recipient and the force and kind of the recipient's allergic response. Morphologically the lesions are very similar to the vascular changes found in various naturally occurring human disorders, particularly polyarteritis nodosa and allied diseases, and there are certain experimental models, for example the allergic arteritis developing in foreign protein treated rabbits, which also provide a close structural counterpart. Although the morphological resemblance of these lesions must be partly due to similarity of cause, it is probably also a product of the similarity of reactions of damaged arterial tissue, whatever the cause of injury. A full review of these arterial lesions is outside the scope of this chapter and only certain points of particular interest such as the mechanisms of the arterial injury, and the position of the lesions will be considered here.

While other factors may modify the arterial and arteriolar lesions in allografts, allergic injury of cells comprising the vessel wall is undoubtedly their prime cause. The available evidence suggests that both cellular and humoral forms of allergy are responsible for the arterial damage. Sometimes there is focal mononuclear cell infiltration of the vessel walls with degeneration and necrosis of smooth muscle and neighboring cells. In the absence of demonstrable immunoglobulins and complement components in such lesions it seems probable that the vascular damage is cell-mediated. These lesions give the impression of being of the more slowly developing kind. In other lesions, particularly when extensive vascular necrosis is developing, there may be no recognizable mononuclear cells in the vessel wall. On the other hand, immunoglobulin and complement fractions have been demonstrated in such lesions and most investigators believe that, here, a humoral mechanism is responsible for the injury. Although mononuclear cells tend to be very few in these circumstances, some neutrophil polymorphs are often present but whether this is directly associated with the allergic reaction or is merely a non-specific response to tissue necrosis is not known. If one accepts that this particular group of arterial lesions is mediated by antibody and serum co-factors, the specificity of the immunoglobulins and the type of allergic reaction must be considered. Earlier the resemblance between these acute necrotic arterial lesions and those in foreign protein treated rabbits was mentioned. These latter

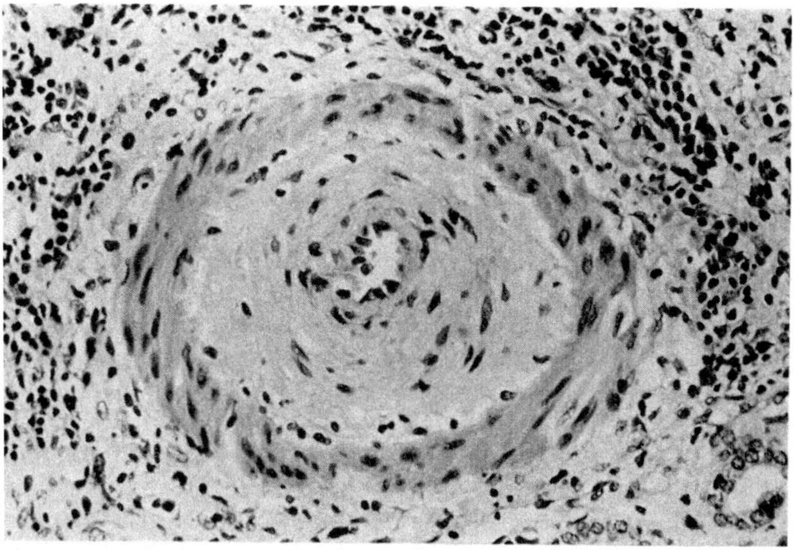

Figure 1.12 *Human renal allograft (second) 1010 days after transplantation. Immunosuppression with steroids and azathioprine. Substantial fibrous intimal thickening of small arcuate artery causing profound narrowing of lumen.*
H. & E. × 270

lesions are generally thought to result from the deposition of immune complexes, and, like Arthus reactions, are believed to be typical examples of a Type III reaction of Coombs and Gell (1968). While the pathogenesis of these arterial lesions in allografts may sometimes be similar, it seems more likely that they are produced by a specific reaction between antibody and antigens on the surface of the allogeneic cells, i.e. a Type IIa reaction of the Coombs and Gell classification. Although this may seem a trivial matter it is of some consequence in understanding the pathogenesis of the lesions. If the lesions were really of the Arthus kind, there would be various interesting implications, one being the probable role of neutrophil polymorphs in causing cell injury. Although there are usually fewer neutrophil polymorphs in the allograft arterial lesions than at comparable stages in the arterial lesions in foreign protein treated rabbits, this difference is not sufficiently clear cut to be decisive.

The peculiarly focal distribution of the vascular and other lesions has already been referred to during discussion about mononuclear cell infiltration but it is such a prominent aspect of the arterial lesions that it deserves further comment. Arterial lesions develop in the vast majority of organ allografts during rejection and are scattered in a seemingly random fashion in the donor vascular tree. Even when rejection is advanced and severe arterial lesions are present, structurally normal arteries or parts of arteries can usually be found somewhere in the graft. Although many forms of naturally occurring arterial disease, whatever their cause, have a patchy distribution, the focal pattern of these lesions in organ allografts is somewhat surprising and the factors determining the site of the lesions must be sought. While it is possible that specific factors, such as local variation in antigen concentrations on the surfaces of allogeneic cells, may be concerned, it seems much more likely that non-specific factors are responsible. In various morphological studies of allografts the bifurcation of arteries and the origin of branches have been found to be especially common sites for lesions. This is in keeping with the position of lesions in various naturally occurring arterial disorders, including polyarteritis nodosa. However, although mechanical factors are almost certainly significant, the precise mechanisms have still to be determined. Moreover, while it is easy to understand that the lesions at such sites may be especially severe it is remarkable that patches of morphologically normal artery are present in allografts which are otherwise being savagely rejected.

The effects of the arterial and other vascular lesions on the rest of the allograft are fairly predictable and are in large measure determined by the degree of interference with blood flow and by the sensitivity to ischemia of the parenchymal cells of the allograft. If the arterial lesions develop rapidly and significant occlusion is swiftly produced, infarcts or other forms of ischemic necrosis are virtually certain to occur. Subsequently, if the recipient survives, organization of the dead tissue may take place and scar tissue will replace the parenchyma. In chronic obliterative lesions the parenchyma is replaced by fibrous connective tissue but the process is gradual and consists of atrophy and replacement fibrosis rather than necrosis and organisation. The detailed effects obviously depend on the organ or tissue involved.

Capillaries and venules

In addition to mononuclear cell adherence and emigration, the major structural changes in the finer vessels are enlargement and proliferation of endothelial cells, necrosis of endothelial cells with disruption of the vessel walls and thrombosis. Endothelial cell hypertrophy with a conspicuous increase of endoplasmic reticulum frequently occurs and is usually most prominent in vessels in which host mononuclear cells are numerous. This change fairly often develops before there is any apparent necrosis of donor endothelium and may possibly be a response by donor cells to cells which they regard as foreign. Enlargement and multiplication of donor endothelial cells are also common following endothelial cell damage but at this stage these changes are perhaps more readily explained as being part of an attempt at healing.

Necrosis of vascular endothelium frequently occurs during rejection and morphological evidence suggests that cell injury may be mediated by cellular or humoral mechanisms. Sometimes lymphocytes and monocytes are seen closely adherent to the surface of endothelial cells and are undergoing necrosis, and it seems likely that the mononuclear cells have had a direct cytotoxic effect on the dying endothelium. As mentioned previously, some workers have described the disappearance of adjoining parts of the plasma membranes of endothelial and mononuclear cells but, although these lesions may be the structural expression of cytotoxicity, not nearly enough is known about the morphological aspects of cell-mediated cell destruction and much more information is needed. It seems probable that in certain circumstances humoral mechanisms are an important factor in causing endothelial cell destruction. This belief is based on the demonstration of immunoglobulins and complement components on and around damaged and necrotic endothelial cells which is well illustrated in the studies of Busch *et al.* (1971) on the role of vascular injury in early failure of human renal allografts.

In first-set allografts, adhering mononuclear cells are usually the earliest cause of capillary and vascular obstruction, and thrombosis, if it occurs, does not develop until later. Thrombi, consisting of varying proportions of platelets, fibrin, leukocytes and red cells, are particularly common in graft reactions in previously sensitized recipients and are also frequently found in severe acute rejection of human renal allografts (Figure 1.13). In hyperacute rejection of allografts and heterografts, thrombi may begin to form within minutes of revascularization. For example, in experiments

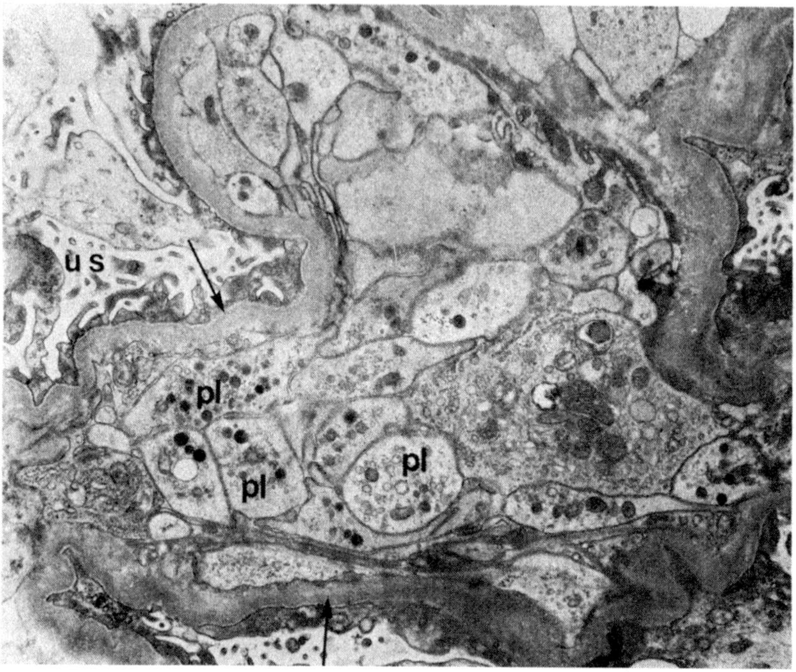

Figure 1.13 *Human renal allograft (first): biopsy 13 days after transplantation. An electron micrograph of a glomerular capillary occluded by platelets (pl). The endothelium is necrotic in places and some platelets are in direct contact with the basement membrane (arrows); us = urinary space.*
Osmium, epon and lead citrate. × *6900*

in which renal allografts were transplanted to previously sensitized dogs Claes *et al.* (1973) found that platelets were accumulating in intertubular capillaries and other vessels within 15 minutes of revascularization. At this stage the platelets were adhering to the endothelium and to each other and in certain places intercellular junctions between endothelial cells had separated and platelet pseudopodia were in contact with the underlying capillary basement membrane. An hour or two later there was severe endothelial cell injury and many more platelets had aggregated. Among the platelets there were some neutrophil polymorphs and deposits of fibrin had also formed. The behavior of platelets in allograft reactions of this kind is of great significance and is undoubtedly the cause of much of the ischemic necrosis occurring in acute rejection. The diminished blood flow appears to be mostly due to mechanical obstruction of the blood vessels but vasoconstriction caused by the release of vasoactive amines from the aggregated platelets may also be a contributing factor. Several mechanisms may be responsible for the initial platelet aggregation but antibody-mediated injury of endothelial cells or the local formation of antigen–antibody complexes are the most likely factors. Subsequently, if the capillary basement membrane and associated collagen fibrils are exposed by destruction of parts of the endothelium, this will stimulate further platelet aggregation. Because of the profoundly damaging effects of thrombosis in rejection there has been great interest in the possibility of preventing platelet aggregation and of dispersing any aggregates already formed. Despite encouraging experimental work using platelet de-aggregating agents, such as aspirin (MacDonald *et al.*, 1970), dextrans and cyproheptadine (Claes, 1973), there is as yet little evidence that this approach will prove practically useful in clinical organ transplantation. Similarly, heparin administration and other measures to prevent fibrin deposition have so far proved rather ineffective.

Veins

The principal venous lesions consist of mononuclear cell infiltration of the vessel walls, and mural and occlusive thrombosis. In longer surviving allografts fibrous connective tissue thickening of the intima with narrowing of the lumen frequently develops. These changes are fundamentally similar to those developing in other parts of the vascular tree of the allograft.

Origin of vascular endothelium in allografts

In recent years the idea that host cells might gradually replace donor endothelium has been suggested as an explanation of the tendency of allograft reactions to occur less frequently and to be less severe in longer lived grafts. Appropriate transplants between the sexes have been examined and the proportion of cells bearing the sex chromatin body has been used to indicate if the endothelium lining the graft vessels was derived from the donor or the recipient. Recent investigations have provided strong evidence that, at least in human renal allografts, the donor endothelium usually persists. For example, Sinclair (1972) examined material from 45 human renal allografts surviving up to $6\frac{1}{2}$ years and found that the sex chromatin counts were not significantly different from normal donor levels in 37 of 40 grafts between the sexes. However, in three allografts transplanted from male donors to female recipients the sex chromatin counts had increased in the intertubular capillaries and veins from the normal male control level of about 1 per cent (range 0.3–2 per cent) to between 31 and 38 per cent, the control count for female endothelium in the series being 52 per cent (range 47–54 per cent). These three allografts were more severely damaged than any of the other kidneys and their function was very slight. Sinclair concluded that, although donor endothelium usually persists, it may become partly repopulated with recipient cells if the graft is severely injured. As he points out, the adaptation shown by long lived transplants cannot be explained on the basis of the replacement of donor by host endothelium. In his study of the endothelial cells of the larger vessels of renal allografts De Bono (1972) reached the same conclusion and similar results were gained by Bieber *et al.* (1970) in their investigation of the larger vessels in cardiac allografts.

Parenchymal changes

During graft rejection the principal structural changes affecting the parenchyma are necrosis or atrophy of the specialized cells and their replacement by fibrous connective tissue. The relative significance of direct allergic destruction and of ischemic injury in causing these lesions is often difficult to assess and there are few examples of allograft rejection in which an adequate understanding has yet been achieved. Nevertheless there are various elementary morphological observations which undoubtedly help such an analysis.

In most grafts the relationship between the presence of mononuclear cells and the destruction of allogeneic cells is extremely variable and rather different from the impression often given. For example, considerable numbers of lymphocytes and other mononuclear cells may be present in organ allografts, both in untreated experimental animals and in immunosuppressed human recipients, without any evidence of parenchymal cell necrosis in the vicinity of the invading cells. For morphologists this is a commonplace observation, hardly worthy of note, but it does carry the clear implication that many of the mononuclear cells are not highly aggressive 'killer' cells. Moreover, in fine structure studies many investigators have noticed that even when mononuclear cells are present in considerable numbers there is often no direct contact between the infiltrating host cells and the parenchymal cells and therefore little evidence of cell-mediated cytodestruction, as it is usually envisaged. For example, although Lindquist *et al.* (1971) observed close association and even cytoplasmic continuity between recipient lymphoid cells during rejection of rat renal allografts, they found no evidence of intimate contact between the infiltrating mononuclear cells and the allogeneic parenchymal cells. Necrosis of parenchymal cells also often occurs in the comparative absence of host mononuclear cells. Sometimes immunoglobulin and complement can be detected on such cells and it then seems likely that humoral factors were responsible for damaging the cells. However, although the blood vessels often appear to be injured by such a mechanism, antibody-mediated destruction of parenchymal cells seems to occur much less frequently and in many instances ischemia resulting from allergic vascular damage is the probable cause of the tissue necrosis.

In their pioneer studies Dempster (1953) and Simonsen *et al.* (1953) considered the role of ischemia in rejection, and a fall in blood flow through organ allografts and heterografts during rejection has now been amply demonstrated. The reduction in blood flow is seen in its most sudden and dramatic form in hyperacute rejection (Rosenberg *et al.*, 1971) but it also appears to be a regular feature of the rejection process in virtually all organ and tissue allografts. It could be claimed that the fall in blood flow in rejecting grafts is a consequence of tissue damage rather than its cause, but the evidence as a whole strongly favors the idea that ischemia is responsible for much of the parenchymal injury. One significant morphological feature supporting this view is the similarity between the patterns of parenchymal damage in graft rejection and in disorders known to have a vascular basis and in which ischemia has been clearly shown to be a dominant factor in the underlying mechanism.

As previously mentioned, under certain circumstances rejection may become an intermittent process or cease altogether. The eventual structure and function of such grafts depends on various factors including the amount of tissue destroyed during rejection episodes, the natural capacity of the specialized parenchymal cells to regenerate, and the extent of any obliterative vascular lesions. As might be expected, the healing potential of a particular organ or tissue is fundamentally similar whether the injury has been caused by rejection or produced in other ways. Surviving liver cells and renal tubular cells, with their substantial capacity for proliferation, are usually able to restore liver cell columns and renal tubules, provided the appropriate framework has been preserved. On the other hand, the complex structure of glomeruli cannot be reproduced, nor can cardiac muscle fibres proliferate. Moreover, the extent to which an organ can recover depends greatly on the maintenance of an adequate blood supply. If severe obliterative vascular lesions of a permanent kind have developed, the parenchyma cannot be satisfactorily restored, whatever its innate potential. Similarly, if organization has occurred and much scar tissue produced, opportunities for recovery will be substantially impaired.

CHANGES IN RECIPIENT LYMPHATIC TISSUE

Scothorne and McGregor (1955) provided one of the first detailed accounts of the morphological changes in lymphatic tissue accompanying reactions against allografts. They examined the lymph nodes and spleen of rabbits with skin allografts transplanted to the ear and found that the ipsilateral cervical lymph node nearest to the graft was much enlarged 4–5 days after grafting and there was also a significant but much slighter enlargement of the spleen. Morphological changes were detected in the affected lymph nodes 2 days after transplantation but these were much more dramatic by Day 4. At this time the deeper part of the cortex (the so-called tertiary nodules or tertiary cortex), now known to be thymus dependent, was packed with large lymphoid cells. These cells, often 15–20 μm in diameter, had a single large pale nucleus, one or more nucleoli and strongly pyroninophilic, slightly vacuolated cytoplasm and seem to correspond with the large pyroninophilic blast cells seen in organ allografts. The germinal centers were normal and the large cells were thought to have developed *in situ* from the cells in the tertiary cortex. Despite the slight enlargement of the spleen no significant histological changes were discovered. Another interesting feature was the comparative lack of cellular response in the second lymph node in the cervical chain on the ipsilateral side. This suggests that the response to skin allografts is concentrated in the lymph node nearest to the graft to a greater extent than might have been expected. In a similar study in the rabbit André *et al.* (1962) examined the response of lymphatic tissue to first- and second-set skin grafts. Their results on first-set grafts were in general agreement with those of Scothorne and McGregor but differed in two respects. First, they believed that the initial cell proliferation leading to the formation of the large pyroninophilic cells (which they called 'hemocytoblasts') occurred initially in the primary follicles and germinal centers. Second, they discovered that while these changes were most prominent in the lymph node immediately proximal to the allograft, they also developed in distant lymph nodes and in the spleen. With second-set grafts, they found that the reaction occurred more quickly and was more intense and they understandably suggested that it had the features of an anamnestic response.

There have been fewer detailed morphological studies of the changes in lymphatic tissue after organ allografts than the subject deserves. In their investigation of renal allografts in dogs Simonsen *et al.* (1953) described an increase in pyroninophilic cells in the spleen of about half of their animals and noted that they were localized 'perifollicularly' and in relation to the trabeculae and vessels of the red pulp. Later, Porter *et al.* (1964) made an extensive morphological examination of the lymph nodes and spleen of dogs given renal allografts. In the spleen the earlier changes predominantly affected the periarteriolar sheath. At 2 days the number of large lymphocytes with slightly pyroninophilic cytoplasm and large pale nuclei was increased and at 3 days there were numerous similar large cells but with deeply pyroninophilic cytoplasm. These cells were especially prominent at the periphery of the sheath and some were extending out into the red pulp. Many of these cells were dividing and, later, there was a steady increase in the number of plasma cells. The lymph node changes were much more conspicuous in the nodes in the general vicinity of the graft. The minor differences between these observations and those of Scothorne and McGregor probably reflect the variations between dog and rabbit lymphatic tissue. Porter and his colleagues agreed that the germinal centers of the follicles appeared to be little involved.

There have been numerous experimental studies of the relationship of lymphocytes, lymphatic tissue and grafts during the development of transplantation immunity. In these investigations attempts have been made to follow the migration, localization, transformation, proliferation and other features of mononuclear cells concerned in allograft reactions. Work of this kind has provided much valuable information about allograft rejection and has helped to develop a coherent concept of the role of lymphatic tissue.

Another important unifying aspect of the changes in the lymphatic system after transplantation is their similarity to the response seen during the development of delayed hypersensitivity. This is to be expected as cellular immunity (Type IV reaction of Coombs and Gell) is the essential feature of delayed hypersensitivity responses and clearly plays a vital role in the rejection of most allografts. However, it would be unrealistic to believe that allograft rejection is solely mediated by immune lymphocytes and, as with many allergic phenomena, one can expect mixtures of various kinds of response, even if one type tends to predominate. This will doubtless be reflected in the morphological changes in lymphatic tissue and variations of account can therefore be expected.

ACKNOWLEDGEMENTS

The author wishes to thank members of the histological and photographic staff of the University Department of Pathology and Addenbrooke's Hospital, Cambridge, for help with preparing the illustrations, particularly Mrs J. Wardle for the electron micrographs and Miss J. Fendick for the photographs of the gross specimens.

References

André, J. A., Schwartz, R. S., Mitus, W. J., and Dameshek, W. (1962). The morphologic response of the lymphoid system to homografts. I. First and second-set responses in normal rabbits. *Blood*, **19**, 313

Astrom, K. E., Webster, H. de F., and Arnason, B. F. (1968). The initial lesion in experimental allergic neuritis: a phase and electron microscope study. *J. Exp. Med.*, **128,** 469

Bieber, C. P., Stinson, E. B., Shumway, N. E., Payne, R., and Kosek, J. (1970). Cardiac transplantation in man. VII. Cardiac allograft pathology. *Circulation*, **41,** 753

Busch, G. J., Reynolds, E. S., Galvanek, E. G., Braun, W. E., and Dammin, G. J. (1971). Human renal allografts: the role of vascular injury in early graft failure. *Medicine*, **50,** 29

Calne, R. Y., White, H. J. O., Yoffa, D. E., Binns, R. M., Maginn, R. R., Herbertson, B. M., Millard, P. R., Molina, V. P., and Davis, D. R. (1967). Prolonged survival of liver transplants in the pig. *Brit. med. J.*, **iv,** 645

Chiba, C., Wolf, P. L., Gudbjarnason, S., Chrysohoa, A., Ramos, H., Person, B., and Bing, R. J. (1962). Studies on the transplanted heart: its metabolism and histology. *J. Exp. Med.*, **115,** 853

Claes, G. (1973). The effect of platelet deaggregating substances on renal allograft rejection in sensitized dogs. *Acta Chir. Scand.*, **139,** 127

Claes, G., Svalander, C., and Bergentz, S. E. (1973). The accumulation and distribution of platelets and fibrin in rejecting dog kidneys. *Acta Chir. Scand.*, **139,** 91

Coombs, R. R. A., and Gell, P. G. H. (1968). Classification of allergic reactions responsible for clinical hypersensitivity and disease. In *Clinical Aspects of Immunology*. 2nd ed, p. 575 (P. G. H. Gell and R. R. A. Coombs, editors)

De Bono, D. P. (1972). Host repopulation of endothelium in human kidney transplants. *Transplantation*, **14,** 438

Dempster, W. J. (1953). Kidney homotransplantation. *Brit. J. Surg.*, **40,** 447

Guttmann, R. D., Lindquist, R. R., Parker, R. M., Carpenter C. B., and Merrill, J. P. (1967). Renal transplantation in the inbred rat. I. Morphologic, immunologic, and functional alterations during acute rejection. *Transplantation*, **5,** 668

Hall, J. G. (1967). Studies of the cells in the afferent and efferent lymph of lymph nodes draining the sites of skin homografts. *J. Exp. Med.*, **125,** 737

Kincaid-Smith, P., Morris, P. J., Saker, B. M., Ting, A., and Marshall, V. C. (1968). Immediate renal-graft biopsy and subsequent rejection. *Lancet*, **2,** 748

Lee, S., and Edgington, T. S. (1968). Heterotopic liver transplantation utilizing inbred rat strains. I. Characterization of allogeneic graft rejection and the effects of biliary obstruction and portal vein circulation on liver regeneration. *Amer. J. Path.*, **52,** 649

Lindquist, R. R., Guttmann, R. D., and Merrill, J. P. (1971). Renal transplantation in the inbred rat. VI. Electron microscopic study of the mononuclear cells accumulating in rejecting renal allografts. *Transplantation*, **12,** 1

MacDonald, A., Busch, G. J., Alexander, J. L., Pheteplace, E. A., Menzoian, J., and Murray, J. E. (1970). Heparin and aspirin in the treatment of hyperacute rejection of renal allografts in presensitized dogs. *Transplantation*, **9**, 1

Najarian, J. S., and Feldman, J. D. (1962). Passive transfer of transplantation immunity. I. Tritiated lymphoid cells. II. Lymphoid cells in millipore chambers. *J. Exp. Med.*, **115**, 1083

Palutke, M., Kihn, R., Perry, M., Riddle, J., Rector, F., and Rosenberg, J. C. (1972). Role of leucocytes and lysosomal enzymes in antibody-mediated (hyperacute) rejection of renal heterografts. *Lab. Invest.*, **27**, 287

Pedersen, N. C., and Morris, B. (1970). The role of the lymphatic system in the rejection of homografts: a study of lymph from renal transplants. *J. Exp. Med.*, **131**, 936

Porter, K. A. (1966). Renal Transplantation. In *Pathology of the Kidney*, p. 604 (R. H. Heptinstall, editor) (London: Churchill)

Porter, K. A., and Calne, R. Y. (1960). The origin of the infiltrating cells in skin and kidney homografts. *Transplant. Bull.*, **26**, 458

Porter, K. A., Joseph, N. H., Rendell, J. M., Stolinski, C., Hoehn, R. J., and Calne, R. Y. (1964). The role of lymphocytes in the rejection of canine renal homotransplants. *Lab. Invest.*, **13**, 1080

Prendergast, R. A. (1964). Cellular specificity in the homograft reaction. *J. Exp. Med.*, **119**, 377

Rogers, B. O., Converse, J. M., Taylor, A. C., and Campbell, R. M. (1953). Eosinophile in human skin homografting. *Proc. Soc. Exp. Biol. Med.*, **82**, 523

Rosenberg, J. C., Hawkins, E., and Rector, F. (1971). Mechanisms of immunological injury during antibody-mediated hyperacute rejection of renal heterografts. *Transplantation*, **11**, 151

Scothorne, R. J., and McGregor, I. A. (1955). Cellular changes in lymph nodes and spleen following skin homografting in the rabbit. *J. Anat.* (*Lond.*), **89**, 283

Simonsen, M. (1953). Biological incompatibility in kidney transplantation in dogs. II. Serological investigations. *Acta Path. Microbiol. Scand.*, **32**, 36

Simonsen, M., Buemann, J., Gammeltoft, A., Jensen, F., and Jørgensen, K. (1953). Biological incompatibility in kidney transplantation in dogs. I. Experimental and morphological investigations. *Acta Path. Microbiol. Scand.*, **32**, 1

Sinclair, R. A. (1972). Origin of endothelium in human renal allografts. *Brit. Med. J.*, **3**, 15

Turk, J. L. (1962). The passive transfer of delayed hypersensitivity in guinea pigs by the transfusion of isotopically-labelled lymphoid cells. *Immunology*, **5**, 478

Turk, J. L., Heather, C. J., and Diengdoh, J. V. (1966). A histochemical analysis of

mononuclear cell infiltrates of the skin with particular reference to delayed hypersensitivity in the guinea pig. *Int. Arch. Allergy*, **29**, 278
Williams, M. A., Morton, M., Tyler, H. M., and Dempster, W. J. (1964). A biochemical approach to the study of rejection of canine renal homotransplants. II. Chemical analysis of kidney homogenates. *Brit. J. Exp. Pathol.*, **45**, 235

2
Lymphoid Cell Kinetics in Graft-versus-Host Reactions and Allograft Rejection

W. L. Ford

INTRODUCTION

Some types of graft, e.g. allogeneic bone marrow cells, are vulnerable to an antibody response by the host but this chapter is concerned with those allografts which are rejected by a cell-mediated response. Most attention is directed towards the rejection of skin grafts exchanged between inbred strains of mice or rats because much of the experimentation on the lymphocyte response to allografts has used these species. Small rodents have also been most favored for graft-versus-host studies. Several aspects of the lymphocytic response to allografts in regional lymph-nodes and in the spleen were investigated many years ago and these have been lucidly reviewed by Gowans and McGregor (1965) and by Wilson and Billingham (1967). In the past few years important progress has been made in consolidating areas which have been doubtful or speculative. This chapter is intended to set some of these advances within a matrix of long-established information.

GRAFT-VERSUS-HOST REACTIONS

Graft-versus-host (GVH) reactions have proved to be an invaluable tool for the study of the reaction of lymphoid cells to transplantation antigens *in vivo*. A series of experiments devised by Gowans was responsible for three significant advances by proving that—

(a) small lymphocytes alone can initiate a GVH reaction,

(b) after encountering alloantigen a minority of lymphocytes undergo blastic transformation into large pyroninophilic cells which then divide repeatedly (Gowans, 1962),

(c) lymphocytes from tolerant donors when injected into recipients which are susceptible to a GVH reaction neither transform into blasts nor do they initiate a GVH reaction (McCullagh and Gowans, 1967).

It was also suggested that division of the large pyroninophilic cells generated a new population of small lymphocytes (Gowans *et al.*, 1962).

These experiments exploited the systemic GVH reaction which follows the i.v. injection of lymphocytes from an inbred rat into an F_1 hybrid between the donor strain and a second strain. Lymphocytes from the parental strain react against the transplantation antigens which the F_1 hybrid has inherited from the other parental strain. The F_1 hybrid accepts the donor cells because his tissues express the identical antigens so that he is naturally tolerant of them. However host cell proliferation in GVH reactions does start after several days (Davies and Doak, 1960; Fox, 1962). The stimulus to this late host response remains a mystery.

In the past few years, since GVH reactions were comprehensively reviewed (Elkins, 1971), several groups have returned to the parental *v.* F_1 hybrid system in both rats and mice. The use of whole-body irradiation of the host before injection of the donor cells has been useful in largely eliminating unwanted host lymphocytes. This recent work has filled in several gaps in knowledge and has been paralleled to a remarkable extent by experiments on the proliferation of lymphocytes *in vitro* in response to transplantation antigens as measured in one-way mixed lymphocyte culture (Bach, Chapter 5).

Which cell-type initiates GVH reactions?

An inoculum of parental strain cells consisting entirely of lymphocytes from the thoracic duct population produced a lethal GVH reaction when injected i.v. into an F_1 hybrid recipient. In subsequent experiments the cell responsible for initiating the response was narrowed down to the small lymphocyte since large lymphocytes were eliminated before injection by incubation of the cells *in vitro* for 24 hours (Gowans, 1962).

The identity of the initiator cell can now be defined even more precisely. Three lines of evidence indicate that thymus-derived T lymphocytes are uniquely capable of initiating GVH reactions. These are—

(a) T lymphocytes alone are fully effective,
(b) B lymphocytes alone are ineffective, and
(c) the GVH activity of a mixed population of B and T lymphocytes is a function of the number of T lymphocytes present; there is no synergy between B and T lymphocytes in contrast with that found in a number of antibody responses.

Some of the details of this evidence are as follows:

(a) Thymus-cell suspensions have consistently been found to have low but detectable GVH activity (Miller and Osoba, 1967). Most or all of this activity is attributable to the cortisone-resistant lymphocytes in the medulla which were as active in causing splenomegaly in F_1 hybrid mice as were spleen cells (Blomgren and Andersson, 1969; Cohen *et al.*, 1970). Cortisone-resistant thymus-cells have many of the properties of thymus-derived cells in the spleen and lymph-nodes but it is not certain that they are fully representative of mature T cells. A more satisfactory piece of evidence consisted of removing B cells from a rat thoracic duct population by passing it through a glass bead column. The non-adherent cells, which were almost entirely T cells by several criteria, had at least as great GVH activity as the starting population (Hunt, 1973).

(b) Early evidence that B lymphocytes cannot initiate GVH reactions was the failure of lymphocytes from neonatally thymectomized mice to cause splenomegaly in F_1 hybrids (Miller *et al.*, 1967). The same assay was used more recently by Cantor (1972) who found that treatment of spleen or lymph-node cells with anti-theta serum completely inhibited their GVH activity. In other experiments thoracic duct lymphocytes were obtained from rats which had been thymectomized, irradiated and restored with small doses of bone-marrow cells. The GVH activity of these lymphocytes was usually undetectable by the sensitive popliteal lymph-node assay and where small reactions were found the activity was depressed by a factor of at least 20. These very slight reactions were probably due to a small minority ($<3\%$) of residual T cells (Rolstad and Ford, 1973).

(c) Synergy between thymus cells and bone marrow cells has not been found when mixtures of parental cells were injected into non-irradiated F_1 hybrid mice (Hilgard, 1970; Bennett, 1972). The latter found that thymus cells alone were more effective in producing death than the same number of thymus cells combined with marrow cells. Hilgard found that thymus cells and bone-marrow cells acted synergistically only with respect to splenomegaly and only in *irradiated* F_1 hybrid recipients. In this case F_1 hybrid bone-marrow cells were as effective in increasing the spleen weight as were parental bone-marrow cells and therefore the rôle of bone-marrow cells may simply be to supply precursors for the host response, which is not directly induced by antigen. In the case of the reaction in the rat popliteal lymph-node no synergy was found when varying excesses of B lymphocytes were injected together with a constant dose of normal thoracic duct lymphocytes (about two-thirds T cells) (Rolstad and Ford, 1973).

However there is good evidence of synergy between different sub-populations of T cells in producing splenomegaly and death in F_1 hybrid mice (Cantor and Asofsky, 1970, 1972). Mixtures of thymocytes and either blood lymphocytes or lymph-node cells produce responses which are greater than the sum of each population alone. Both subpopulations require to be responsive to the alloantigen against which the reaction is directed. It has been proposed that one subpopulation (T_2) is derived from the other (T_1) largely as a consequence of antigenic stimulation. The degree of synergy is less dramatic than between T and B lymphocytes in certain antibody responses and the mechanism of this interesting effect remains to be fully clarified (Cantor, 1972b).

In the course of a GVH reaction alloantibody directed against the recipient is produced (Cerottini *et al.*, 1971) just as after skin allografting alloantibody directed against donor tissue is manufactured by the host. These alloantibody-forming cells presumably arise by activation of B lymphocytes as in other antibody responses (Miller and Mitchell, 1969) but it is probable that the precursor B cells which respond to alloantigens are far fewer than the responsive T cells and so make a negligible contribution to the proliferative response as assessed by an enlarged spleen or lymph node.

The proportion of T lymphocytes responsive to each strong transplantation antigen

Snell (1953) distinguished strong and weak transplantation antigens on the simple basis of differences in skin graft rejection times and whether or not certain tumors were transferable between different strains of mice. Subsequently GVH and MLC studies have suggested that antigenic strength is not a continuously variable quantity but rather that transplantation antigens can be divided into two distinct groups. The division may be according to whether or not the antigens elicit detectable stimulation in MLC or according to the number of lymphocytes required to give a standard GVH response against the antigen. Table 2.1 shows that about 100 times as many rat lymphocytes are required to produce a popliteal lymph-node reaction of 10 mg in a weak (Ag–B identical) compared to a strong strain combination. Between different strong strain combinations there is only a three-fold range of variation in GVH activity. Recent work has suggested the unexpected possibility that most of this variation is in the responder strain—that is each strain sees the range of Ag–B antigens as about equally strong but there is a 2–3 fold variation in the responsiveness of different strains (Dorsch and Roser, 1973a). This is compatible with the data of Table 2.1.

Table 2.1 *Number of parental strain thoracic duct lymphocytes required to produce lymph-node enlargement to* 10.0 *mg in* F_1 *hybrid recipients*

	Donor strain	*Ag-B type*	*Recipient strain*	*Ag-B antigen*	*Number of TDLs* $\times 10^6$
Ag-B different	AS	1	(AS × BN)F_1	3	0.4
	AS	1	(AS × AS2)F_1	not 1	0.3
	F	1	(F × BN)F_1	3	0.4
	AS2	not 1	(AS2 × AS)F_1	1	0.5
	AO	2	(AO × DA)F_1	4	0.25
	AO	2	(AO × HO)F_1	5	0.25
	BN	3	(BN × F)F_1	1	0.4
	DA	4	(DA × AO)F_1	2	0.6
	HO	5	(HO × DA)F_1	4	0.4
Ag-B identical	AS	1	(AS × F)F_1	1	30
	F	1	(F × AS)F_1	1	20
	AU	5	(AU × HO)F_1	5	50
	(AS × BN)F_2*	1/3	(AS × BN)F_1	1/3	50

* = heterozygous at Ag-B locus
F = Fisher
AU = August

An early hint that an exceptionally high proportion of lymphocytes respond to each strong transplantation antigen came from GVH experiments in rats in which labelled lymphocytes were injected i.v. into newborn allogeneic recipients. After 24 hours 30% of the labeled lymphocytes seen in the recipients' spleens had undergone blastic transformation (Porter and Cooper, 1962). Unfortunately this remarkable figure was difficult to relate to the proportion of *injected* cells transforming since the spleen may have selected out the reacting cells from a larger population than was actually present within it 24 hours after injection. In the chicken, Nisbet *et al.* (1969) used a limiting dilution assay in which allogeneic spleen cells were injected into chicken embryos. Progressively smaller doses of cells were injected until donor cell proliferation in the spleen was no longer detectable. Statistical analysis of the frequency of responses at low donor cell numbers (50–500) showed that at least 1–2% of cells were reactive and several reasons were given for believing that this might be an underestimate.

Recently we have used three different methods to estimate the proportion of parental strain T lymphocytes which recognize and respond to transplantation antigen in irradiated F_1 recipients (Ford and Atkins, 1972). One method involved detecting by scintillation counting labeled lymphocytes which had ceased to recirculate as a consequence of antigenic recognition. This produced a figure of 12% ±2% in both AO→(DA × AO)F_1 and AO→(HO × AO)F_1 combinations. Two autoradiographic methods consisted of counting (1) the proportion of labeled donor cells which transformed into large, pyroninophilic cells in the recipient spleen 24 hours after the i.v. injection of lymphocytes labeled *in vitro* with ^{3}H-uridine and (2) the proportion of donor lymphocytes in the thymus-dependent area of the recipient's spleen which had taken up ^{3}H-thymidine infused into the recipient for 24 hours after cell injection. In both experiments cell division was prevented by colcemid and the small 'background' of transformation after syngeneic transfer was subtracted. It was observed that 16% to 19% of donor lymphocytes present in the recipient's spleen had responded by blast transformation or by entering DNA synthesis. When correction was made for the finding that about 50% of the injected cells had visited the spleen immediately after leaving the blood but at 24 hours only 20% were present in the spleen the number of responding lymphocytes was estimated to be at least 7% of the starting population of T cells.

The conclusion that 7–12% of cells respond to an Ag-B antigen in GVH is reconcilable with the careful estimate of 1–3% responding in MLC (Wilson *et al.*, 1968) if allowance is made for the use of peripheral blood lymphocytes in MLC, of which some are B lymphocytes, variation in antigenic strength between different Ag-B incompatible strains and finally that some potentially responsive cells may succumb *in vitro* before they have a chance to become activated by antigen.

The anomalous aspects of T cell responses to strong transplantation antigens can be explained by a frequency of responders in a non-immune population in the region of 1 in 10 to 1 in 10^2 in contrast to 1 in 10^5 to 1 in 10^6 for non-transplantation antigens (e.g. Armstrong and Diener, 1968). The origin of the high proportion of responders is an unsolved problem but the possibility that immunization by cross-reacting environmental antigens may be responsible has been discounted by the finding that germ-free rats have levels of activity in both MLC and GVH assays which are at least as high as in normals (McDonald and Zimmerman, 1971; Nielsen, 1972).

Different T cells respond to different transplantation antigens

The evidence that different antibody-forming cell precursors (B lymphocytes) respond to different antigens is satisfactory; B lymphocytes are somehow committed to respond to one particular antigen before that antigen is ever encountered. However, the conclusion that such a high proportion of T cells respond to some antigens calls for a critical examination of the evidence that T cells are strictly precommitted, each to a single antigen. The extreme possibility is that each competent T cell can recognize and respond to the whole range of strong transplantation antigens. This idea would put alloimmune responses in a basically different category from other immune responses as has been proposed by Lafferty *et al.* (1973).

Four independent groups have produced evidence that different lymphocytes respond to different transplantation antigens as is the case in other immune responses. Two of these methods required the elimination of cells which have reacted in MLC. In a secondary culture the remaining (non-responding) cells produced a response to a different antigen but not to the same antigen as was present in the first culture (Zoschke and Bach, 1971; Salmon *et al.*, 1971). The other two groups exploited irradiated allogeneic rats or semiallogeneic (F_1 hybrid) rats as antigen-bearing columns to 'absorb out' the reactive cells. Lymphocytes were injected i.v. and the non-reactive majority of cells were recovered from the lymph. Loss of reactivity from this population was shown to be specific by GVH assay (Ford and Atkins, 1971) or by restoring the capacity of an irradiated recipient to reject first-set skin grafts in the normal time (Dorsch and Roser, 1973a). Both of these groups argued against other possible mechanisms of loss of specific responsiveness.

None of these four experiments excluded the possibility that each lymphocyte may be able to recognize a small number of strong transplantation antigens. For example if 10% of lymphocytes are responsive to antigen A and 10% to antigen B then the two subpopulations may overlap so that 1% can react to both antigens. Evidence that subpopulations of lymphocytes which recognize different antigens do in fact overlap comes from experiments of Howard and Wilson (1973). They selected lymphocytes responding to a strong transplantation antigen in two stages. Firstly one-way MLCs were maintained for 6 days by which time the non-responding cells had died. The surviving cells were transferred to syngeneic rats which had been deprived of their own T cells. When T lymphocytes of donor origin were subsequently recovered from the thoracic duct of these recipients, their GVH activity was increased by a factor of 8. The most interesting point was that their GVH activity against a different transplantation antigen was approximately the same as that of non-immune lymphocytes. Therefore substantial enrichment of cells reactive against one antigen did not automatically deplete the population of cells reacting against a second antigen.

This is not compatible with completely separate subpopulations if it is accepted that at least 5% of cells were initially reactive.

The probable overlapping of these subpopulations can be explained in two ways. Either each lymphocyte has recognition structures for more than one antigen or alternatively strong transplantation antigens are compounded of 10–100 different determinants and only a small minority of lymphocytes are capable of reacting to each determinant in the antigenic complex. The sharing of determinants by several antigen complexes would result in a unipotential cell reacting to different complexes which happen to include the same determinant. The latter explanation is more orthodox and therefore less interesting if it should turn out to be correct.

Cell proliferation in GVH reactions

Most small lymphocytes in the blood and lymph are in a dormant stage of their cell cycle. Their life-span, i.e. the time from one mitosis to either the next mitosis or cell death, has been measured in terms of months or years, depending on species (Robinson *et al.*, 1965; Buckton *et al.*, 1967). However, when T lymphocytes are injected into an F_1 hybrid recipient, they re-enter the active phases of the cell cycle. Several hours after transformation into large, pyroninophilic cells DNA synthesis begins as has been shown by administration of ^{3}H-thymidine to F_1 hybrid recipients of parental strain lymphocytes (Sprent and Miller, 1972a). Soon after the S phase, antigenically stimulated small lymphocytes enter mitosis as was well shown when rat lymphocytes were injected i.v. into lethally-irradiated mice. The burst of mitosis which started after 24 hours in the recipients' spleens was found by chromosome analysis to be almost entirely due to dividing donor cells (Gowans, 1962).

Both the transformation into DNA synthesizing cells and mitoses are more prominent in the thymus-dependent areas of the spleen than in the thymus-dependent areas of lymph nodes. This is doubtless because most cells injected i.v. localize initially in the spleen and due to the faster rate of migration through the splenic pulp, some are later redistributed to lymph nodes which lymphocytes take on average three times as long to pass through (Ford and Simmonds, 1972).

Activated T lymphocytes continue to proliferate within the spleen through several cycles (Ford *et al.*, 1966; Sprent and Miller, 1972b). By 2–4 days after injection the daughter cells suddenly regain the migratory capacity of the initiator cells and are released into the blood. This has been shown by injecting the lymphocytes into an irradiated F_1 hybrid recipient whose thoracic duct had been cannulated. For the first 36 hours after injection only the non-responsive donor cells recirculate into the lymph with the normal tempo of syngeneic cells (Figure 2.1). A dramatic change is seen by 48 hours in the rat (Ford and Atkins, 1971) and 84 hours in the mouse (Sprent and

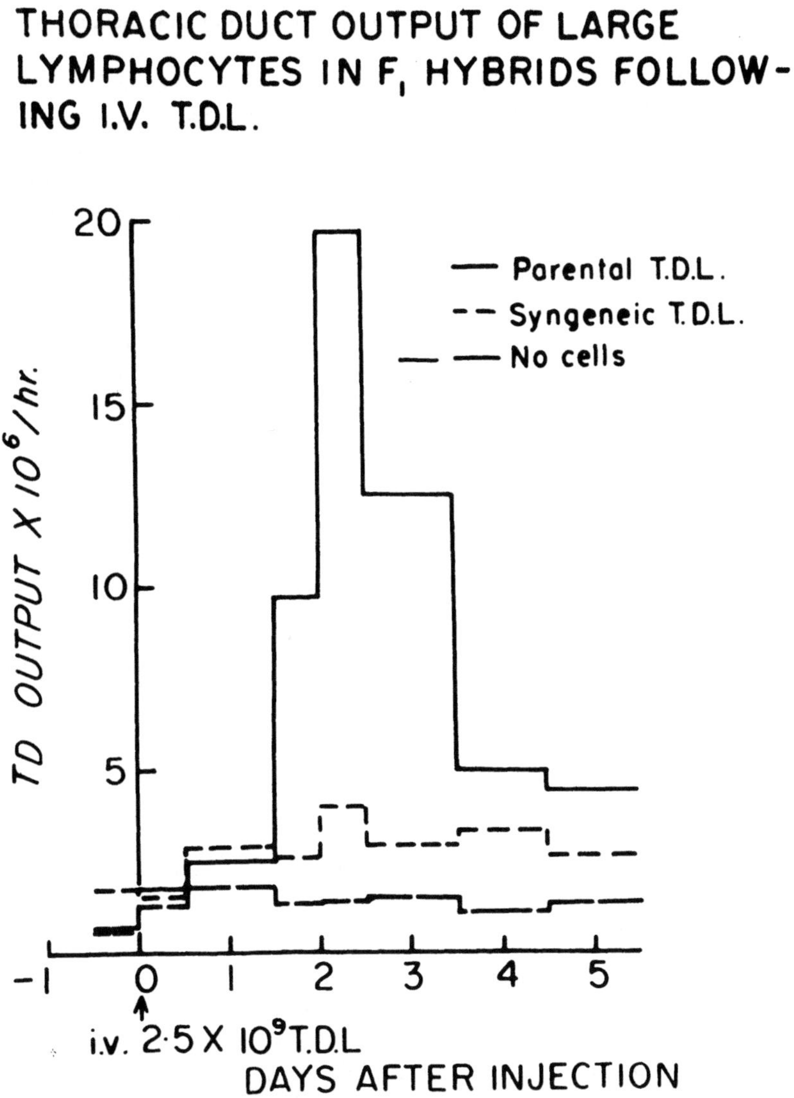

Figure 2.1 *2.5×10^9 thoracic duct lymphocytes from a parental strain (AO) rat donors were injected into an (AO $\times$ HO)F_1 hybrid recipient which had been given 400 rads of whole-body γ-irradiation 3 days previously. The output of large lymphocytes from the thoracic duct of the recipient (unbroken line) showed a massive increase beginning at 36 hours which consisted almost entirely of donor cells. The output of small lymphocytes of donor origin followed a similar pattern (Ford and Atkins, 1971). The immunological properties of these activated T lymphocytes are discussed in the text especially in relation to Sprent and Miller's data on mice (1972a, 1972b, 1972c)*

Miller, 1972b). In both species there is an outpouring of donor type cells (of which about half are large lymphocytes) into the thoracic duct of the F_1 recipient. In the mouse experiments it was found that these donor lymphocytes, large and small, had been produced by cell division after injection into the recipient; they were virtually all labelled when the recipient was injected with ^{3}H-thymidine at 8-hourly intervals (Sprent and Miller, 1972b). Moreover these newly produced cells retained the properties of thymus-derived lymphocytes in that they were susceptible to anti-theta serum and they recirculated from blood to lymph when returned to a syngeneic mouse. This thorough evidence confirmed earlier results in the rat which supported the sequence of small lymphocyte → large pyroninophilic cell → small lymphocytes (Figure 2.2) (Ford *et al.*, 1966).

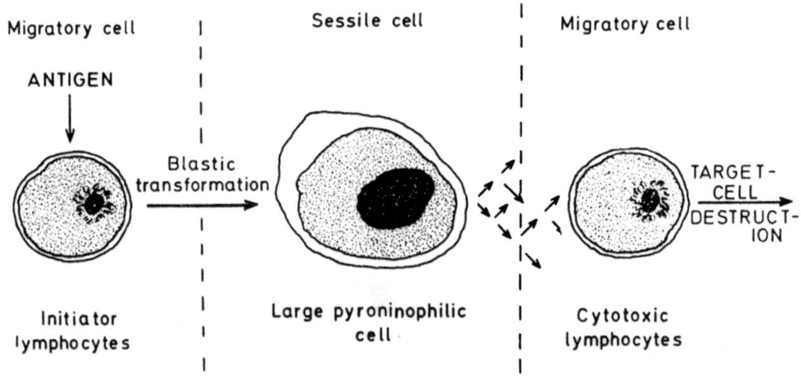

Figure 2.2 *Scheme of the antigen-induced transformation of small lymphocytes into large pyroninophilic cells which divide repeatedly to produce a new population of small lymphocytes*

The conclusion that activation of T cells does not result in plasma cell production is in line with the evidence that the rôle of T lymphocytes in co-operative antibody responses is not that of an antibody-forming cell precursor; the latter belong to the B lymphocyte population (Miller and Mitchell, 1969). This was anticipated from the electron microscopic appearance of transformed T cells since the lack of endoplasmic reticulum and abundance of polyribosomes did not suggest a development towards plasma cells (Burwell, 1962; Gowans and McGregor, 1965). The ultrastructure of transformed T cells has been described in detail by Greaves and Janossy (1972). It is very similar, whether the transforming agent is an antigen or a mitogen like phytohemagglutinin.

The production of cytotoxic lymphocytes (CL) in GVH reactions

The progeny of proliferating T cells in systemic GVH reactions includes lymphocytes which are specifically cytotoxic for target cells bearing the antigens which originally activated the virgin T cells. This crucial point has recently been established by Sprent and Miller (1972c) who studied the lymphocytes which were released in large numbers into the thoracic duct lymph of a heavily irradiated F_1 hybrid recipient between 4 and 5 days after the injection of parental strain thymocytes or thoracic duct lymphocytes. They showed that almost all of the cells were of donor origin and that they had powerful cytotoxic activity against DBA/2 mastocytoma cells provided that the F_1 hybrid recipient expressed the H-2^d antigenic complex (as does the DBA/2 strain). Moreover when CBA lymphocytes activated in (CBA × C57BL)F_1 hybrids were returned to neonatally thymectomized CBA mice they brought about prompt rejection of C57BL grafts (H-2^b) but BALB/C grafts (H-2^d) continued to survive indefinitely.

The production of cytotoxic lymphocytes in the course of a GVH reaction has also been documented by Cerottini *et al.* (1971), who recovered donor cells from the spleens of F_1 hybrid recipient mice. They found specific target cell killing *in vitro* which was

(a) inhibited by anti-theta serum
(b) unaffected by anti Fab or anti μ-chain sera and
(c) complement independent.

In all these respects target cell lysis by alloantibody forming cells was different.

In view of this evidence it can be assumed that the new production of T lymphocytes in response to transplantation antigens is a necessary step in GVH disease and that these specifically sensitized lymphocytes do not act by secreting antibody. Several questions regarding the pathogenesis of GVH disease remain unanswered, especially the distribution and fate of cytotoxic lymphocytes in an intact F_1 hybrid from which the cells are not drained by a thoracic duct fistula.

The production of initiator lymphocytes (IL) in GVH reactions

The spleen weight assay in the mouse (Simonsen, 1962a) and the popliteal lymph node assay in the rat (Ford *et al.*, 1970) are popular methods of assaying GVH activity. The basic point that these are measures of lymphoid cell proliferation and not host cell damage has often been overlooked. Mixed lymphocyte culture is also a measure of cell proliferation. The question has been raised in different forms of whether the antigen sensitive cell which initiates proliferation in GVH and MLC is the same cell or whether it is a different cell from that which is specifically cytotoxic in assays of target cell destruction. In the present context the former has been called an initiator lymphocyte following Howard (1973) and the latter a cytotoxic lymphocyte. Operative terms are used because great confusion has been caused by three ambiguous terms—effector cell, memory cell and target cell. The last is used here to mean a cell which is liable to attack by cytotoxic lymphocytes.

When a mouse (Simonsen, 1962b), chicken (Warner and Szenberg, 1964) or rat (Ford and Simonsen, 1971) has been immunized against a strong transplantation antigen, e.g. by skin grafting, there is little or no change in the GVH activity of its lymphocytes against that antigen, suggesting that the number of initiator lymphocytes has not increased. By contrast, immunization appears to be a prerequisite for the production of cytotoxic lymphocytes since cytotoxic activity is not detectable by sensitive assays when a non-immune lymphoid population is given the opportunity to attack suitable target cells for up to 24 hours. (Admittedly non-immune lymphocytes may be cytotoxic if they are artificially attached to target cells by phytohemagglutinin (Perlmann and Holm, 1969) but this is probably not relevant to the argument).

The evidence that immunization by an allograft produces cytotoxic lymphocytes (CL) with little or no expansion of initiator lymphocytes (IL) does not prove that these are always distinct populations. It remains possible that in an immune population some cells can both kill target cells and proliferate in response to antigen. The powerfully cytotoxic population produced by activation of parental strain lymphocytes in an F_1 hybrid recipient has reduced GVH activity in secondary recipients in the mouse (Sprent and Miller, 1972c) and in the rat (Ford and Atkins, 1971) which favors separate IL and CL populations. However, when these cells are set up in one-way MLC with the same antigens against which they were activated, a high proportion of them respond initially by entering DNA synthesis but the response is not sustained; many of the cells do not continue to mitosis (Cheers *et al.*, 1973). A similarly rapid and transient response is also found when blood lymphocytes from rats immunized with a skin allograft are tested in MLC (Wilson and Nowell, 1971).

In conclusion it seems likely that although CLs are derived from ILs they are functionally separate populations. This raises further questions as follows:

1. Are the specific suppressor cells which can markedly inhibit a GVH reaction (Elkins, 1972) in fact CLs which inhibit the induction of ILs in a similar way to the feedback inhibition by antibody on the induction of antibody responses?

2. Is the cell proliferation induced by transplantation antigen entirely directed to the production of CLs or do only a minority of the ILs differentiate into appropriate CLs? The latter alternative is favored by the exquisite specificity of CLs when they apparently discriminate between patterns of overlapping antigenic specificities (Brondz, 1971) suggesting that a wide diversity of CLs must exist and therefore the

frequency of precursors of each type of CL must be very low according to clonal selection principles. If this reasoning is sound then most of the 1–10% of ILs which respond to each strong antigen are not precursors of the cells which are cytotoxic for target cells bearing that antigen.

Summary

The initiation of many antibody responses requires a complicated interaction between the precursor B lymphocytes, T lymphocytes and macrophages but GVH reactions are apparently simpler in that they are initiated by T lymphocytes without the aid of other cells. Activated T lymphocytes transform into large pyroninophilic cells which proliferate to produce a new population of lymphocytes. This newly generated population is very limited in its capacity to divide when re-exposed to the antigen responsible for its production but it does include cytotoxic lymphocytes which can kill the appropriate target cells *in vitro*.

ALLOGRAFT REJECTION

The initiation of the lymphocytic response to allografts

An orthotopic allograft of skin gives rise to a proliferative reaction in the regional lymph node which later extends to the spleen (Billingham *et al.*, 1954). Allografts in other sites are followed by a similar reaction in the draining lymph nodes, in the spleen, or in both (e.g. Porter *et al.*, 1964; Pedersen and Morris, 1970) but such grafts have been studied much less than have skin grafts.

The response in lymphoid tissue follows the activation of immunologically competent host cells by the transplantation antigens of the graft. This section is concerned with the identity of the host cell which initiates the reaction and the site at which it interacts with antigen. It will not deal with the important question of which structures in the graft are responsible for the immunogenic stimulus and in particular the contribution made by passenger leukocytes (Guttmann *et al.*, 1969).

The meeting place of antigen and antigen sensitive cells may be the draining lymph node which antigenic material from the graft reaches via the afferent lymphatics. Alternatively, lymphocytes may migrate from the blood into the graft, become activated 'peripherally' and then pass via the lymphatics to the regional node where they settle down and they proliferate. The long delay in the rejection of skin allografts on an alymphatic skin pedicle is consistent with either mechanism but the observation that these grafts are eventually rejected suggests that peripheral activation *can* occur (Tilney and Gowans, 1971).

Whether 'peripheral' or 'central' activation of lymphocytes is the more important depends, as might be expected, on which tissue has been grafted and its situation. This is most clearly shown by experiments in which the lymphatic coming directly from an allograft has been cannulated. In the case of a skin graft on a sheep there was little or no increase in the number of lymphocytes passing up the afferent lymphatic from the graft site but a spectacular increase in the flow of lymphocytes and a lymphoblastic response were seen in the efferent lymph issuing from the draining node (Hall, 1967). By contrast collection of lymph from a kidney allograft (lymph which had not passed through a lymph node) showed an enormous increase in the flow of cells, many of which were blast cells (Pedersen and Morris, 1970). This evidence that lymphocytes are activated within kidney grafts confirms earlier work which showed that the kidney grafts could sensitize a recipient without an intact lymphatic drainage (Hume and Egdahl, 1955; Strober and Gowans, 1965).

Some of the evidence that allograft rejection is initiated by lymphocytes can be summarized as follows:

1. In animals which have been rendered tolerant by neonatal inoculation of F_1 hybrid marrow cells long standing allografts are rejected soon after the injection of purified lymphocytes from normal syngeneic donors (Gowans *et al.*, 1963);

2. A near lethal dose of whole-body irradiation delays first-set allograft rejection (Micklem and Loutit, 1966; Dorsch and Roser, 1973b) but if the irradiated recipient is replenished with lymphocytes from a normal syngeneic donor the first-set rejection time is restored to normal (Dorsch and Roser, 1973b);

3. Lymphocytes from tolerant rats fail to restore the capacity of a heavily irradiated recipient to reject a specific skin allograft in the normal time. However the rejection of allografts expressing different antigens is restored to normal in these circumstances (Dorsch and Roser, 1973b).

These experiments show that lymphocytes play a necessary rôle in graft rejection which depends on them being specifically reactive to the antigens of the graft. This is most economically explained by supposing that their specific rôle is that of antigen recognition. Experiments which implicate the T lymphocyte in particular are—

4. Rodents deficient in T lymphocytes, for example neonatally thymectomized mice (Miller, 1962) and rats (Arnason *et al.*, 1962), are very slow to reject skin allografts. Particularly spectacular prolongation of allograft survival has been noted in athymic (*nu/nu*) mice (Wortis, 1971).

5. Removal of the bursa of Fabricius from chickens at the time of hatching is followed by a defective capacity for antibody production which has been attributed to a lack of antibody-forming cell precursors. The development of the thymus and the rejection of allografts are unaffected (Cooper *et al.*, 1969).

6. In thymectomized mice carrying a thymus graft which had chromosomally marked cells the proliferative response to a skin allograft was largely due to division of the thymus-derived cells (Davies *et al.*, 1966).

Despite all this positive evidence there are several situations in which profound lymphocytopenia is associated with little or no change in the first-set rejection time of allografts. Examples are chronic thoracic duct drainage (McGregor and Gowans, 1964), lymphocytopenia induced by continuous β-irradiation of the spleen and lymph nodes (Roser and Ford, 1972) and early intra-uterine thymectomy of lambs followed by ALS treatment (Silverstein and Prendergast, 1973). In all these cases it is only grafts expressing strong antigens which are rejected in the normal time and so a ready explanation lies in the exceptionally high proportion (say 1–10%) of lymphocytes which can react to each strong antigenic complex. If this were reduced by say 99% it is conceivable that there are still more lymphocytes reactive to these antigens than there are reactive to weak antigens in the normal animal. The idea that there is a large surplus of cells reactive to strong antigens has received support from Dorsch and Roser's recent work (1973c) on the effect of whole body X-irradiation of rats before skin allografting. Whereas 750 rads substantially prolonged graft survival, 600 rads was ineffective, although the great majority of lymphocytes were destroyed by the latter dose. Transfer of only 10^7 lymphocytes from a normal rat to a recipient which had been given 750 rads restored the first-set rejection time to normal. The recirculating lymphocyte pool of normal adult rats contains about 200×10^7 small lymphocytes (Gowans and Knight, 1964) and about 20×10^7 are usually required to give a maximum effect in restoring other immune responses to irradiated recipients. In conclusion, evidence which suggested that small lymphocytes are not necessary for graft rejection can now be interpreted as showing that very few lymphocytes are necessary for rejecting certain types of allograft.

The sites and tempo of the proliferative response

Landsteiner and Chase found that a heightened reaction to certain skin sensitizing agents (1942) and delayed hypersensitivity to tuberculin (Chase, 1945) could be elicited from previously untreated guinea-pigs by giving them lymphoid cells from actively immunized guinea-pigs but transfer of serum from similar donors was ineffective. Allograft rejection was put in the same category by Mitchison (1954) who studied an allogeneic sarcoma the rejection of which was accelerated by active immunization. He observed that accelerated tumor rejection occurred in a mouse which had not been actively immunized if it had received lymph node fragments from an animal which had been inoculated with the tumor. He went on to make three supplementary observations which have been repeatedly confirmed in principle—

1. The lymph nodes draining the site of the immunizing graft increase in weight over several days to reach 2–3 times their normal size.

2. The draining lymph nodes are more effective in transferring immunity than are other lymph nodes.

3. Both the increased weight of the regional node and its ability to confer adoptive immunity are transient; 20 days after transplantation the lymph node has returned to normal in both respects (Mitchison, 1955). Also in 1954 Billingham, Brent and Medawar described experiments of the same basic design in which accelerated, second-set rejection of a skin allograft was found as a consequence of injecting lymph node cells from a mouse which had rejected a similar graft.

The histological changes in lymph nodes draining skin allografts in rabbits were described in detail by Scothorne and McGregor (1955) and André *et al.* (1962). A striking change was the appearance, 2–5 days after grafting of large, pyroninophilic cells in the lymph node cortex. This cell-type has a large, pale vesicular nucleus with a prominent nucleolus. The cytoplasm is deeply basophilic and pyroninophilic. Both the perinuclear membrane and cytoplasmic boundary are distinct. The ultrastructure of these cells was described by Burwell (1962) and André-Schwartz (1964); lack of endoplasmic reticulum and an abundance of polyribosomes in the cytoplasm are the outstanding features. Thus this cell is morphologically identical to the large, pyroninophilic cell into which small lymphocytes transform early in GVH reactions. There is still no agreement on the most suitable name for a morphologically transformed T lymphocyte. Immunoblast (Dameshek, 1963), large lymphoid cell (Scothorne and McGregor, 1955) and large, pyroninophilic cell are all equally appropriate for activated B lymphocytes which are distinguishable by the presence of endoplasmic reticulum (Greaves and Janossy, 1972) as well as functionally.

Other changes which have been noted in the regional lymph-nodes are a slight increase in the number of plasma-cells in the medulla and a late increase in the number of germinal centres (Micklem and Loutit, 1966). These increases in thymus-independent cells (like the concentration of alloantibody in the serum) generally reach a maximum after rejection of the graft in contrast to the earlier blast cell reaction in the thymus-dependent paracortex and there is no evidence that they are necessary events for graft rejection.

Direct evidence that large, pyroninophilic cells are a frequently dividing population was obtained by Prendergast (1964) who injected ^{3}H-thymidine into the base of rabbit skin allografts tissue daily from day 2 until day 7 after grafting. Of the large lymphoid cells scored in imprints 93% were labeled by this regime and in tissue sections most of the large, pyroninophilic cells in the lymph node cortex were labeled. The fate of large pyroninophilic cells in a lymph node reacting to the contact sensitizing agent, oxazolone was analyzed by Oort and Turk (1965). The morphology of this reaction is the same as that which follows allografting. Injections of ^{3}H-thymidine at intervals after the application of oxazolone provided convincing evidence of the production of small lymphocytes by the division of large pyroninophilic cells as occurs in GVH reactions.

Recently radioactive DNA precursors have been used to study the tempo of the lymph node proliferative response. In mice given a single pulse of ^{125}I-IUDR at daily intervals after grafting two well-defined peaks of uptake into the nodes draining an allograft were seen. Eleven days after grafting the uptake reached 5 times that of the autografted control; an earlier and lower peak occurred 3 days after grafting (Lance and Cooper, 1972). In allografted rats which had been given single pulses of ^{3}H-thymidine a monophasic response was found with a maximum at days 6–8 at a level of 6–7 times the ^{3}H-thymidine uptake of the contralateral node (Figure 2.3). The uptake per mg of node was increased by a factor of 3 which showed that cell division within the nodes had been stimulated; the increase in weight was not only due to to retention of cells from the blood (Tilney and Ford, 1973).

Further evidence for the increased production of small lymphocytes within lymph nodes draining grafts was obtained by cannulation of the efferent lymphatic of the sheep popliteal lymph node. As is the case with lymph nodes responding to non-transplantation antigens an impressive rise in the efflux of lymphocytes from the node was recorded. The flow of small lymphocytes was substantially increased and there was an even greater increase in the number of large, basophilic cells which reached 40% of the lymph-borne cells compared to 5–10% from a resting node. Of these large cells 60% incorporated ^{3}H-thymidine after exposure for 1 hour *in vitro* indicating a short generation time. One surprising aspect of this work was the lateness of the response to grafting which did not begin until 8 days and peaked at 15 days after the graft had been applied (Hall, 1967).

The proliferative response of lymphoid tissue to skin allografts has usually been found to extend to the spleen (Figure 2.2) (Scothorne and McGregor, 1955; Blamey and Evans, 1971), and a small increase in the rate of cell division in non-draining lymph-nodes has sometimes been detected (Micklem and Loutit, 1966). The response in the spleen is later than in the draining lymph-nodes and may be due to seeding of the blast cells released from the draining nodes which lodge there and continue to proliferate for a limited time. However, some of the lymphocytic response of the spleen may be a consequence of transplantation antigen reaching it via the blood or alternatively lymphocytes which have been activated in the blood in contact with the vascular endothelium of the graft may settle and proliferate in the spleen. Neither removal of the regional lymph nodes (Billingham *et al.*, 1954) nor splenectomy

(Krohn and Zuckerman, 1954) has an appreciable effect on graft rejection probably because of the wide dispersal of the lymphocytic reaction.

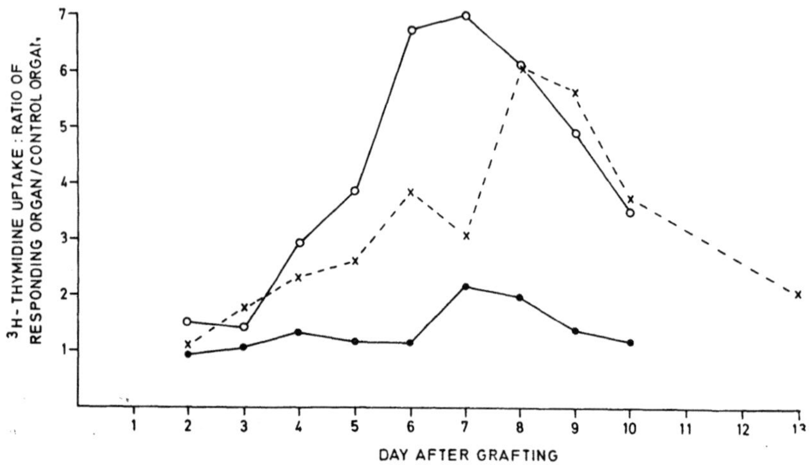

Figure 2.3 *Proliferative responses to a skin allograft in the draining lymph-nodes (axillary and brachial), contralateral lymph-nodes and spleen of rats. Each received 1 μCi/g of body weight of ^{3}H-thymidine 4 hours before sacrifice.*

——O—— *–Ag–B incompatible allograft, ratio of radioactivity in draining nodes/contralateral nodes (no response was apparent in the contralateral nodes).*

– – –X– – – *–Ag–B identical allograft, ratio of radioactivity in draining nodes/contralateral nodes.*

——●—— *–Ag–B incompatible allograft, ratio of splenic uptake/uptake by recipient of a syngeneic graft.*

The uptake in the draining lymph-node increased by a factor of 6–7 and in the weak strain combination, peaked two days later than in the strong. The splenic uptake was double that of the control on days 7 and 8 after grafting. Each point is the mean of two recipients (data of Tilney and Ford)

The expected changes have been observed in lymphocytes in the blood following grafting. By 4–5 days after allografting, the proportion of lymphocytes in rat blood which took up ^{3}H-thymidine *in vitro* was greatly increased (Siciu-Foca *et al.*, 1972) and the use of this principle as a test for kidney graft rejection in man is under critical assessment (e.g. Hayry *et al.*, 1972).

The lymphoid cell response to weak and strong transplantation antigens

In rats weak skin allografts, i.e. from an Ag–B identical donor, evoked a proliferative response in the regional lymph node which was only slightly less and only two days later than was the response to strong allografts, i.e. Ag–B incompatible (Figure 2.3; unpublished data of Tilney and Ford). This was despite the hundred-fold difference in the number of lymphocytes required to produce a standard GVH response. Similarly the injection of F_1 hybrid lymph-node cells into the footpad of a parental strain recipient ($F_1 \rightarrow P$) provoked an allograft reaction in the popliteal lymph-node which was slightly less in weak than in strong strain combinations but the difference was again much less marked than with parental to F_1 transfer (Dorsch and Roser, 1973a). The rather slight differences in the proliferative responses between weak and strong combinations is reflected in the marginal difference between first-set survival times of skin allografts which is only a day or two longer in Ag-B incompatible than in Ag-B identical strain combinations (Roser and Ford, 1972). It is only if the recipient is depleted of lymphocytes by thoracic duct drainage (McGregor and Gowans, 1964) or by continuous local irradiation of the spleen (Roser and Ford, 1972) that a large difference in rejection times between weak and strong combinations becomes apparent matching the sharp contrast in GVH activity and MLC activity which are both enormously greater in strong combinations. The number of germinal centres provoked in mouse lymph nodes by weak (H-2 identical) or strong allografts is the same (Mariani *et al.*, 1972) which is consistent with other evidence that thymus-independent cells do not appreciate the distinction between strong and weak alloantigens.

Second-set rejection and the production of cytotoxic lymphocytes

Several methods have been used to study the process of sensitization which originally meant development of the capacity to reject grafts with the accelerated response characteristic of the second of two grafts from the same donor. Recently sensitizaton has been extended to mean any specifically altered reactivity of the host lymphocytes. The time course of sensitization can be studied most simply by varying the time between the first and second grafts. By this method it was found that the capacity to give a second-set response in rodents begins before rejection of the first graft and persists for at least 200 days (Billingham *et al.*, 1954; Lehrfield *et al.*, 1954; Steinmuller and Weiner, 1963). This method only provides a semi-quantitative estimate of the level of sensitization and is not informative about events at the cellular level which can be studied either in adoptive transfer systems or by cytotoxic assays.

Adoptive transfer experiments are clearly relevant to graft rejection in an intact recipient since what is actually scored is rejection of a similar graft on a secondary recipient. This secondary recipient may have been manipulated, for example by inducing tolerance or by depletion of T cells, so that its own primary response has been delayed or abolished. Alternatively the secondary recipient may be fully capable of mounting its own primary response in which case adoptive transfer from a sensitized donor may only accelerate graft rejection by 2–3 days if an H-2 different or an Ag-B different strain combination is used. Cells from a lymph node draining the site of a skin allograft were found to be particularly effective in the adoptive transfer of allograft sensitivity. The spleen has usually proved to be a good second best (Mitchison, 1955; Billingham *et al.*, 1963). Lymphocytes in the blood and thoracic duct population also transfer sensitivity as do peritoneal exudate cells and cells from non-draining lymph nodes. The maximum effectiveness of draining lymph node cells is reached at about 11 days after application of a skin allograft. This is followed by a steady waning of effectiveness but adoptive transfer can be achieved by large doses of cells as long as one year after grafting mice (Billingham *et al.*, 1963).

The assay of specific cytotoxic activity against antigenic target cells is a more rapid and less laborious method of measuring at the cell population level the altered reactivity which follows allografting (Bach, Chapter 5). The cytotoxic activity of immune cells is confined to target cells which express antigens present on the immunizing graft or inoculum (Wilson, 1963; Mauel *et al.*, 1970; Brondz, 1972). The relevance of this measurement to graft rejection in an intact animal is widely assumed when it is described as an '*in vitro* model of graft rejection'. There is no evidence against this although the relevance of cytotoxicity tests is not so obvious *a priori* as are adoptive transfer experiments. Cytotoxic cells can be removed *in vitro* from an immune population by incubation in contact with a target cell monolayer of fibroblasts (Goldstein *et al.*, 1971; Lonai *et al.*, 1973). The easily detached majority of cells are very deficient in cytotoxic activity and also have reduced GVH activity (Lonai *et al.*, 1973) so apparently both initiator and cytotoxic lymphocytes are specifically adherent.

In response to an allograft of skin cytotoxic activity is first detectable in the draining lymph nodes after 3–5 days. It usually reaches a peak at 7–8 days after grafting (Canty and Wunderlich, 1971; Peter and Feldman, 1972). As with other methods of assessing the lymph-node response, such as ^{3}H-thymidine uptake (Lance and Cooper, 1972) and numbers of alloantibody forming cells (Micklem *et al.*, 1970), a biphasic response has sometimes been observed (Canty and Wunderlich, 1971). In these cases it is possible that the secondary peak is a consequence of the increased liberation of antigen from the graft as it begins to break down. In the spleen cytotoxic activity is at a maximum one or two days after the peak in the draining lymph nodes. Cytotoxic cells have also been found in the blood lymphocyte population and in non-draining lymph nodes. The short duration of the cytotoxic response to skin grafts is rather consistent—they cannot be found after 14–21 days (Canty and Wunderlich, 1971; Peter and Feldman, 1972).

After a kidney allograft in the rat cytotoxic activity reached a maximum in the spleen 5 days later. The cytotoxic activity of lymph node cells was much less (Biesecker, 1973). The injection of DBA/2 mastocytoma cells i.p. into allogeneic recipients was also followed by a sharp peak of cytotoxic activity in the spleen after 10–11 days. The usual sudden decline was succeeded by a prolonged plateau and substantial cytotoxic activity was still detectable after 70 days (Brunner *et al.*, 1970).

The question of whether accelerated second-set rejection is due to the persistence of cytotoxic lymphocytes from the first graft or whether an anamnestic reaction occurs with the greatly increased numbers of cells entering division which is characteristic of secondary antibody responses, has been debated for many years. In a response to a second graft the lymph node reaction is only slightly greater in terms of weight gain and is more transient (Burwell, 1962; André *et al.*, 1962) which fits in well with the ephemeral response produced by lymphocytes generated in the course of a GVH reaction when they re-encounter alloantigen in MLC (Cheers *et al.*, 1973). Similarly, the reappearance of cytotoxic cells after a second immunization with allogeneic spleen cells is barely distinguishable from the response to primary immunization (Biesecker, 1973). This suggests that accelerated rejection is *not* due to a faster proliferative response involving more initiator lymphocytes at least when the graft expresses strong transplantation antigens. On the other hand when only weak transplantation antigens are involved accelerated rejection may well be partly or wholly attributable to an increased number of initiator lymphocytes as has been suggested by the greatly increased GVH activity following allogeneic immunization (Simonsen, 1970).

The difficulty in ascribing accelerated rejection to the persistence of cytotoxic cells is that they have often been found to disappear in a much shorter time (2–3 weeks) than the disappearance of second-set responsiveness in an intact recipient (up to 1 year). The explanation may simply be that most cytotoxic assays are insensitive; when the highly susceptible mastocytoma cells were used as target cells a detectable level of cytotoxic activity was found to persist in the spleen for two months at least (Brunner *et al.*, 1970).

Do cytotoxic lymphocytes enter grafts?

Before grafts are rejected they become infiltrated with mononuclear cells including lymphocytes and macrophages (Wiener *et al.*, 1964; Jacobisiak, 1971). Most of these mononuclears are produced by recent division of their precursors since about 90% of them were labeled by frequent injections of ^{3}H-thymidine which were started after skin grafting (Gowans *et al.*, 1962). They are therefore not a random sample of the mononuclear cells in the blood of which only a minority are labeled by such a regime. Recently mononuclear cells have been recovered from skin grafts by enzymatic digestion (Jacobisiak, 1971) and cytotoxic assay of these cells may settle this question. However, several groups have investigated whether the lymphocytes generated in response to a skin allograft (including cytotoxic lymphocytes and probably others) can be found in the graft following their release into the blood. Three series of experiments have been reported in which lymphocytes produced in response to a skin graft were selectively labeled (Najarian and Feldman, 1962; Prendergast, 1964; Hall, 1967). There was a general agreement that (a) only a small minority of the lymphocytes in a graft had been produced in response to grafting (clearly not contradictory to the statement that they had been produced after grafting) and (b) the selectively labeled lymphocytes entered specific grafts and unrelated third party grafts with equal facility since as far as the autoradiographic method of scoring could resolve there was no preferential accumulation of sensitized lymphocytes in specific skin allografts. However, this is an insensitive method for detecting minor differences in cell localization.

Recent studies on mice (Lance and Cooper, 1972) and on rats (Tilney and Ford, 1973) have measured the concentration of labeled lymphocytes in skin allografts by radioactive counting of the whole graft. In both studies, labeled lymphocytes produced in response to a particular type of graft were transferred to syngeneic recipients which had previously received specific and third-party grafts. There was agreement that the concentration of labeled cells was higher in the specific than in the third party grafts although the degree of preference was variable. These results do not necessarily indicate that lymphocytes are attracted into grafts bearing the antigen against which they are reactive; it is perhaps more likely that a random selection of the lymphocyte specificities in the blood enter grafts but the minority which respond to the antigen are retained there while the remainder pass on into the lymphatics. In antigen bearing lymphoid tissue a selective retention of lymphocytes is known to occur (Rowley *et al.*, 1972) and there is a steady traffic of lymphocytes through normal skin from which reactive cells could be selected (Smith *et al.*, 1970).

That the entry of sensitized lymphocytes into grafts is essential for rejection still lacks rigorous proof although it became a reasonable assumption when Algire *et al.*

(1954), showed that allografts protected from host cells in diffusion chambers survived indefinitely even in sensitized recipients. The evidence that there is some preferential localization of sensitized lymphocytes in specific allografts makes it an even more likely assumption but it should not be forgotten that the majority of mononuclear cells in a skin graft are probably not immunologically active against the graft antigens. Many of them have been recently derived from dividing precursors in the bone marrow and probably belong to the monocyte/macrophage series (Giroud *et al.*, 1970).

Do cytotoxic lymphocytes act alone?

Since cytotoxic lymphocytes are in a minority among the cells which infiltrate a graft the ratio of attacker cells to the target cells which are subsequently destroyed is probably very low—perhaps several orders less than 1:1. On the other hand *in vitro* models of target cell damage often require ratios of 100:1 to 1000:1 in order to kill the majority of target cells. This has raised the question of whether other cells are recruited by specifically reactive lymphocytes to aid the destructive process or whether the rôle played by macrophages in particular is simply to deal with cell debris produced by the destructive action of lymphocytes acting alone. This question cannot be answered at present partly because of the difficulty of producing in an animal a complete lack of monocytes and macrophages throughout the period normally required for graft rejection.

The phagocytic activity of macrophages is increased in an immune mouse following the exposure of its sensitized lymphocytes to the antigen against which it had been immunized (Mackaness and Blanden, 1967). This mechanism is of protective value against certain bacterial infections but the 'angry' macrophages are indiscriminately active against a number of bacterial species. If graft rejection requires the local recruitment of macrophages (or other cells) then it seems unlikely that such helpers would be indiscriminate in their action. This is because of experiments in which grafts have consisted of a mixture of cells of which one component was antigenic and the other was not. For example when non-immunogenic tumor cells were included in a great excess of strongly immunogenic cells rejection of the latter did not impair growth of the former (Klein and Klein, 1956). Also, when a graft from an allophenic mouse consisted of an intimate mixture of cells of which one component was syngeneic with the recipient, the syngeneic cells were largely unaffected by the lethal attack on the adjacent allogeneic cells (Mintz and Silvers, 1970).

Recently some experiments have indicated that macrophages may be recruited by sensitized lymphocytes in such a way that they do acquire the capacity to recognize antigenic cells. Cytotoxic activity *in vitro* against two mouse lymphomas was found to be implemented by macrophages which have been 'armed' by some recognition molecule as a consequence of the exposure of immune lymphoid cells to antigen (Grant *et al.*, 1972; Den Otter *et al.*, 1972). It was suggested that the recognition substance was liberated by T lymphocytes and that it might not be a conventional antibody since it was not neutralized by anti-mouse Ig. (Grant *et al.*, 1972) but neither of these propositions is yet certain. One attraction of this model is that it is so similar to the mechanism of initiating thymus-dependent antibody responses which is thought to follow the binding of antigen to a receptor on the surface of an immune T lymphocyte, the release of the receptor and the antigen as a complex and the adsorption of this complex on the surface of macrophages. The presentation of antigen in this way to B lymphocytes may be uniquely effective in activating them (Feldmann, 1972). Of course it is the implementation of cell-mediated immunity which is under discussion and Feldmann's model is concerned with the initiation of antibody responses but there seems no reason why the same mechanism should not be exploited at different stages in the two classes of immune response.

It would be easy to jump to the conclusion that such a mechanism operates in graft rejection as originally proposed by Granger and Weiser (1966) but it is still possible that cytotoxic lymphocytes may act much more efficiently *in vivo* than they do *in vitro* and thus do without the aid of other cells. A rather unattractive idea is that lymphocytes directed against antigens other than those expressed by the graft may be recruited to exert a non-specific cytotoxic action. Although a mitogenic factor for lymphoid cells is released by the interaction of sensitized lymphocytes and antigen (Vischer, 1972) it is not known to have any significance *in vivo*.

Conclusions

The cellular events in allograft rejection, graft-versus-host reactions and prolonged mixed lymphocyte cultures (Bach, Chapter 5) resemble each other in that (1) the reactions are initiated by the activation of T lymphocytes by transplantation antigens which by several criteria fall in two rather distinct categories—'strong' and 'weak', (2) activated T lymphocytes transform into larger cells which undergo a limited number of cell divisions, (3) after a lag period of 2–4 days specific cytotoxic lymphocytes are produced. The peak of cytotoxic activity follows the peak of cell proliferation by a few days. These seem good reasons for assuming that the three systems are reflections of the same basic phenomenon in different environments and consequently that GVH reactions and MLC are legitimate methods for the study of certain aspects of graft rejection.

References

Algire, G. H., Weaver, J. M. and Prehn, R. T. (1954). *J. nat. Cancer Inst.*, **15,** 493

André, J. A., Schwartz, R. S., Mitus, W. J. and Dameshek, W. (1962). *Blood,* **19,** 313

André-Schwartz, J. (1964). *Blood,* **24,** 113

Armstrong, W. D. and Diener, E. (1968). *J. exp. Med.*, **129,** 371

Arnason, B. G., Jankovic, B. D., Waksman, B. K. and Wennersten, C. (1962). *J. exp. Med.*, **116,** 177

Bennett, M. (1972). *Cell. Immunol.*, **3,** 531

Biesecker, J. L. (1973). *Transplantation,* **15,** 298

Billingham, R. E., Brent, L. and Medawar, P. B. (1954). *Proc. roy. Soc. B.*, **143,** 58

Billingham, R. E., Silvers, W. K. and Wilson, D. B. (1963). *J. exp. Med.*, **118,** 397

Blamey, R. W. and Evans, D. M. (1971). *Brit. J. Cancer,* **25,** 527

Blomgren, H. and Andersson, B. (1969). *Exp. Cell Res.*, **57,** 185

Brondz, B. D. (1972). *Transplant. Res.*, **10,** 112

Brunner, K. T., Mauel, J., Rudolf, H. and Chapius, B. (1970). *Immunology,* **18,** 501

Buckton, K. E., Court-Brown, W. M. and Smith, P. G. (1967). *Nature,* **214,** 470

Burwell, R. G. (1962). *Ann. N.Y. Acad. Sci.*, **99,** 821

Cantor, H. (1972a). *Cell. Immunol.*, **3,** 461

Cantor, H. (1972b). *Progr. Biophys. molec. Biol.*, **25,** 73

Cantor, H. and Asofsky, R. (1970). *J. exp. Med.*, **131,** 235

Cantor, H. and Asofsky R. (1972). *J. exp. Med.*, **135,** 764

Canty, T. G. and Wunderlich, J. R. (1971). *Transplantation,* **11,** 111

Cerottini, J.-C., Nordin, A. A. and Brunner, K. T. (1971). *J. exp. Med.*, **134,** 553

Chase, M. W. (1945). *Proc. Soc. exp. Biol. Med.*, **59,** 134

Cheers, C., Sprent, J. and Miller, J. F. A. P. (1973). *Cell. Immunol.* (In press)

Cohen, J. J., Fishbach, M. and Claman, H. N. (1970). *J. Immunol.*, **105,** 1146

Cooper, M. D., Cain, W. A., Van Alten, P. J. and Good, R. A. (1969). *Int. Arch. Allergy,* **35,** 242

Dameshek, W. (1963). *Blood,* **21,** 243

Davies, A. J. S. and Doak, S. M. A. (1960). *Nature,* **187,** 610

Davies, A. J. S., Leuchars, E., Wallis, V. and Koller, P. C. (1966). *Transplantation,* **4,** 438

Den Otter, W., Evans, R. and Alexander, P. (1972). *Transplantation,* **14,** 220

Dorsch, S. and Roser, B. J. (1973a). *Aust. J. exp. Biol. med. Sci.* (In press)

Dorsch, S. and Roser, B. J. (1973b). *Aust. J. exp. Biol. med. Sci.* (In press)

Dorsch, S. and Roser, B. J. (1973c). *Aust. J. exp. Biol. med. Sci.* (In press)

Elkins, W. L. (1971). *Progr. Allergy,* **15,** 70

Elkins, W. L. (1972). *Cell. Immunol.*, **4,** 192

Feldmann, M. (1972). *J. exp. Med.*, **136,** 737
Ford, W. L. and Atkins, R. C. (1971). *Nature New Biol.*, **234,** 178
Ford, W. L. and Atkins, R. C. (1972). *Microenvironmental Aspects of Immunity*, p. 255 New York: Plenum Press
Ford, W. L., Burr, W. and Simonsen, M. (1970). *Transplantation*, **10,** 258
Ford, W. L., Gowans, J. L. and McCullagh, P. J. (1966). In *Ciba Foundation Symposium on the Thymus*, p. 58 London: J. A. Churchill
Ford, W. L. and Simmonds, S. J. (1972). *Cell Tiss. Kinet.*, **5,** 175
Ford, W. L. and Simonsen, M. (1971). *J. Exp. Med.*, **133,** 938
Fox, M. (1962). *Immunology*, **5,** 489
Giroud, J. P., Spector, W. G. and Willoughby, D. A. (1970). *Immunology*, **19,** 857
Goldstein, P., Svedmyr, E. A. J. and Wigzell, H. (1971). *J. Exp. Med.*, **134,** 1385
Gowans, J. L. (1962). *Ann. N.Y. Acad. Sci.*, **99,** 432
Gowans, J. L. and Knight, E. J. (1964). *Proc. Roy. Soc. B.*, **159,** 257
Gowans, J. L. and McGregor, D. D. (1965). *Progr. Allergy*, **9,** 1
Gowans, J. L., McGregor, D. D. and Cowen, D. M. (1963). *Ciba Foundation Study Group*, **16,** 20
Gowans, J. L., McGregor, D. D., Cowen, D. M. and Ford, C. E. (1962). *Nature*, **196,** 651
Guttmann, R. D., Lindquist, R. R. and Ockner, S. A. (1969). *Transplantation*, **8,** 837
Granger, G. A. and Weiser, R. S. (1966). *Science*, **151,** 97
Grant, C. K., Currie, G. A. and Alexander, P. (1972). *J. exp. Med.*, **135,** 150
Greaves, M. and Janossy, G. (1972). *Transplant. Rev.*, **11,** 87
Hall, J. G. (1967). *J. exp. Med.*, **125,** 737
Hayry, P., Lalla, M. and Pasternak, A. (1972). *Ann. clin. Res.*, **4,** 100
Hilgard, H. R. (1970). *J. exp. Med.*, **132,** 317
Howard, J. C. (1973). *Transplant. Proc.* (In press)
Howard, J. C. and Wilson, D. B. (1973). *Science.* (In press)
Hume, D. M. and Egdahl, R. H. (1955). *Surgery*, **38,** 194
Hunt, S. V. (1973). *Immunology*, **24,** 699
Jakobisiak, M. (1971). *Transplantation*, **12,** 364
Klein, G. and Klein, E. (1956). *Nature*, **178,** 1389
Krohn, P. L. and Zuckerman, A. (1954). *Brit. J. exp. Path.*, **35,** 223
Lafferty, K. J., Walker, K. Z., Scollay, R. G. and Killby, V. A. A. (1972). *Transplant. Rev.*, **12,** 198
Lance, E. M. and Cooper, S. (1972). *Cell. Immunol.*, **5,** 66
Landsteiner, K. and Chase, M. W. (1942). *Proc. Soc. exp. Biol.*, **49,** 688
Lehrfield, J. W., Taylor, A. C. and Converse, J. M. (1954). *Proc. Soc. exp. Biol.*, **86,** 848

Lonai, P., Eliraz, A., Wekerle, H. and Feldman, M. (1973). *Transplantation*, **15**, 368
Mackaness, G. B. and Blanden, R. V. (1967). *Progr. Allergy*, **11**, 89
Mariani, T., Damhof, J. and Good, R. A. (1972). In *Microenvironmental Aspects of Immunity*, p. 597 New York: Plenum Press
Mauel, J., Rudolf, H., Chapius, B. and Brunner, K. T. (1970). *Immunology*, **18**, 517
McCullagh, P. J. and Gowans, J. L. (1967). In *The Lymphocyte in Immunology and Haemopoiesis*, p. 234 London: E. Arnold
McDonald, J. C. and Zimmerman, G. (1971). *Proc. Soc. exp. Biol. Med.*, **136**, 987
McGregor, D. D. and Gowans, J. L. (1964). *Lancet*, **i**, 629
Micklem, H. S. and Loutit, J. F. (1966). In *Tissue Grafting and Radiation*. New York: Academic Press
Micklem, H. S., Asfi, C., Staines, N. A. and Anderson, N. (1970). *Nature*, **227**, 947
Miller, J. F. A. P. (1962). *Proc. roy. Soc. B.*, **156**, 415
Miller, J. F. A. P. and Mitchell, G. P. (1969). *Transplant. Rev.*, **1**, 3
Miller, J. F. A. P., Mitchell, G. P. and Weiss, N. S. (1967). *Nature*, **214**, 992
Miller, J. F. A. P. and Osoba, D. (1967). *Physiol. Rev.*, **47**, 437
Mintz, B. and Silvers, W. K. (1970). *Transplantation*, **9**, 497
Mitchison, N. A. (1954). *Proc. roy. Soc. B.*, **142**, 72
Mitchison, N. A. (1955). *J. exp. Med.*, **102**, 157
Najarian, J. S. and Feldman, J. D. (1962). *J. exp. Med.*, **115**, 1083
Neilsen, H. E. (1972). *J. exp. Med.*, **136**, 417
Nisbet, N. W., Simonsen, M., and Zaleski, M. (1969). *J. exp. Med.*, **129**, 459
Oort, J. and Turk, J. L. (1965). *Brit. J. exp. Path.*, **46**, 147
Pedersen, N. C. and Morris, B. (1970). *J. exp. Med.*, **131**, 936
Perlmann, P. and Holm, G. (1969). *Advanc. Immunol.*, **11**, 117
Peter, H.-H. and Feldman, J. D. (1972). *J. exp. Med.*, **135**, 1301
Porter, K. A. and Cooper, E. H. (1962). *J. exp. Med.*, **115**, 997
Porter, K. A., Peart, W. S., Kenyon, J. R., Joseph, N. H., Hoehn, R. J. and Calne, R. Y. (1964). *Ann. N.Y. Acad. Sci.*, **120**, 472
Prendergast, R. A. (1964). *J. exp. Med.*, **119**, 337
Robinson, S. H., Brecher, G., Lourie, S. I. and Maley, J. E. (1965). *Blood*, **26**, 281
Rolstad, B. and Ford, W. L. (1973). MS submitted for publication
Roser, B. J. and Ford, W. L. (1972). *Aust. J. exp. Biol. med. Sci.*, **50**, 185
Rowley, D. A., Gowans, J. L., Atkins, R. C., Ford, W. L. and Smith, M. E. (1972). *J. exp. Med.*, **136**, 499
Salmon, S. E., Krakauer, R. S. and Whitmore, W. F. (1971). *Science*, **172**, 490
Scothorne, R. J. and McGregor, I. A. (1955). *J. Anat.*, **89**, 283
Siciu-Foca, N., Buda, J. A. and Thiem, T. (1972). *Transplantation*, **14**, 711

Silverstein, A. M. and Prendergast, R. A. (1973). In *Microenvironmental Aspects of Immunity*, p. 383 New York: Plenum Press

Simonsen, M. (1962a). *Progr. Allergy*, **6,** 349

Simonsen, M. (1962b). *Ciba Foundation Symposium on Transplantation*, p. 185 London: Churchill

Simonsen, M. (1970). *Transplant. Rev.*, **3,** 22

Smith, J. B., McIntosh, G. H. and Morris, B. (1970). *J. Anat.*, **107,** 87

Snell, G. D. (1953). *J. nat. Cancer Inst.*, **14,** 691

Sprent, J. and Miller, J. F. A. P. (1972a). *Cell. Immunol.*, **3,** 361

Sprent, J. and Miller, J. F. A. P. (1972b). *Cell. Immunol.*, **3,** 385

Sprent, J. and Miller, J. F. A. P. (1972c). *Cell. Immunol.*, **3,** 213

Steinmuller, D. and Weiner, L. J. (1963). *Transplantation*, **1,** 97

Strober, S. and Gowans, J. L. (1965). *J. exp. Med.*, **122,** 347

Tilney, N. L. and Ford, W. L. (1973). *Transplantation* (In press)

Tilney, N. L. and Gowans, J. L. (1971). *J. exp. Med.*, **133,** 951

Vischer, T. L. (1972). *J. Immunol.*, **109,** 401

Warner, N. L. and Szenberg, A. (1964). *Aust. J. exp. Biol. med. Sci.*, **42,** 100

Wiener, J., Spiro, D. and Russell, P. S. (1964). *Amer. J. Path.*, **44,** 319

Wilson, D. B. (1963). *J. cell. comp. Physiol.*, **62,** 273

Wilson, D. B. and Billingham, R. E. (1967). *Advanc. Immunol.*, **7,** 189

Wilson, D. B. and Nowell, P. C. (1971). *J. exp. Med.*, **133,** 142

Wilson, D. B., Blyth, J. L. and Nowell, P. C. (1968). *J. exp. Med.*, **128,** 1157

Wortis, H. H. (1971). *Clin. exp. Immunol.*, **8,** 305

Zoschke, D. C. and Bach, F. H. (1971). *Science*, **172,** 1350

3
Chemistry of HL-A Antigen: Separation, Assay and Biological Properties

D. A. L. Davies

INTRODUCTION

It is almost normal practice to greet a newly described biological phenomenon by naming a substance by which one hopes it is mediated. Even if the phenomenon has been correctly described a simple mediator may not account for it; if incompletely or incorrectly described, search for a simple mediator is at best a hazard. Mediation may be by an array of components, e.g. like a chain of enzymes. Complexity mounts as we delve deeper into biological phenomena and their inter-relationships; there are the multiple components of complement, of coding, of capping, of clotting.

One might ask, what happened to transplantation antigens? What went wrong? When Billingham *et al.* (1956, 1958) showed that transplantation immunity could be attributed to something less than living cells, the door seemed to be open to the identification and characterization of a substance to mediate the effects, and it was given the name 'transplantation antigen'. True, it would differ among different individuals but with the concept of specific tolerance for self, the idea of a tolerogen emerged. We still do not have a transplant tolerogen, although 'specific graft prolongation' is a reality and a variety of model systems show the concept to be still valid.

The first problem which arose in chemical studies was the association of histocompatibility antigens, which were then taken to be the same as transplantation antigens, with cell membranes. The era of characterization of soluble proteins had not provided any methods for dissociating membrane complexes and methods were not and are not available for studying insoluble preparations. There followed difficulties in assay, especially *in vivo* and the *in vitro* methods may even now be misleading us.

Then the complexity of the polymorphism of the major loci and the multiplicity of loci became apparent from genetic work.

The dissociation of the matrices in which cells lie corresponds to the work on microbial cells of components lying outside the plasma membrane: peripheral 'antigens' of various kinds and cell wall to protect from osmotic stress, from which our cells are not at risk. Only erythrocyte membranes had been studied, a most aberrant kind of cell which provides a model for no other. Even now red cell membrane components are far from being sorted out to everyone's satisfaction. Conceptually the lymphocyte membrane is greatly clarified but the sheer complexity of its exposed components is bewildering. Membrane models constructed by the physico-chemists do not concern us greatly here because we are concerned with minutiae, not with 'surface protein', we are concerned about the expression of the products of more than forty genes, for example, on mouse lymphocyte membranes. There is every reason to suppose that man has as many as the mouse, probably the same number as reasons for supposing full homology of components become compelling. The role of all this paraphernalia is mostly obscure, but a connection with control of differentiation and homeostasis seems probable (Bennett *et al.*, 1972). There are enough histocompatibility loci to have two per chromosome and the presence in mice of one on the X chromosome (Bailey, 1963) and one on the Y chromosome (Goldberg *et al.*, 1971; Heslop, 1973) suggests it is at least unlikely that any has none.

In any event in the context of transplantation and especially of tolerance we may have been led astray by the skin graft model, valuable though it is. From the practical point of view, skin allografts are much more difficult to maintain than the organs now transplanted in the clinic. HL-A matched siblings reject each other's skin grafts in 20–30 days (Amos *et al.*, 1969); one would like to interpret this in the light of mouse skin allograft results where the outcome is greatly influenced by a large number of non-H-2 histocompatibility loci. This may be due at least in part to the necessity for a skin graft to become vascularized while a kidney graft has its blood supply provided. Indeed a newborn mouse heart allograft inserted subcutaneously in the ear behaves much like a skin graft while a rat heart sewn in abdominally is influenced almost exclusively by the major locus (Ag-B). ABO antigens are strong transplantation antigens for human skin (Dausset and Rapaport, 1966) and although ABO matching is usual for human kidney transplants some early attempts with ABO incompatibility were successful. The fact remains that ability to transplant allogeneic skin would be of greater practical clinical value than kidneys and hearts on account of the high incidence of accidental burns. Nevertheless what follows is an account of the major histocompatibility locus (MHL) products because non-HL-A incompatibilities can be covered adequately by mild non-specific immunosuppression in clinical transplantation of purposefully vascularized organs.

As it is my intention to pool the data obtained from studies of several animal species, it is necessary to assess the justification for accepting the genetic homology of the MHL in those species. Why do we feel confident in arguing from mouse H-2 to rat Ag-B to human HL-A as was done in the previous paragraph? The evidence comes from a variety of sources because there are many characteristics associated with the mouse H-2 locus which can be sought in other species. HL-A resembles mouse H-2 in being the dominant genetic system involved with histocompatibility in the species, having similar complexity and the same kind of arrangement in (at least) two sub-loci ('segregant series') referred to as 'K' end and 'D' end in the mouse, and as 'Four' series and 'LA' series in man. In both, incompatibilities permit graft versus host reactions without preimmunization, mixed lymphocyte reactions and other cell interactions measurable *in vitro**. The gene products, in so far as they can be detected by serological methods, have the same cellular location and tissue distribution and are glycoproteins which can be extracted by the same methods from mouse or human sources (Davies *et al.*, 1968). Associated with both systems are immune responsiveness genes (Ir genes) (McDevitt *et al.*, 1972) although some are linked to other minor loci. The presence of H-2 on mouse red cells and absence of HL-A from human red cells is considered to be a trivial difference; H-2 is very poorly represented on mouse red cells, many specificities being undetectable, and evidence has been given for HL-A specificities on human erythroblasts (Harris and Zervas, 1969). The most convincing evidence for genetic homology, if more were needed is of very recent date; there is another complex genetic locus in the mouse, T locus (Gluecksohn-Waelsch and Erickson, 1970) responsible for development of the mouse embryo on its long axis, and this, like H-2, is in the IXth linkage group. The new finding (Amos, personal communication) that spina bifida is linked to HL-A in man indicates that a homologous chromosomal region exists, greater in extent than the H-2/HL-A regions themselves. There must be some very basic reason for this stability over such a long evolutionary period. Without listing further H-2/HL-A similarities, it may be said that the only obvious differences reside in the range of specificities of the gene products, but even these overlap (Ivašková *et al.*, 1972). For other animal species studied one or usually more of the principal features of a MHL are clear, especially so for the rat (Ag-B locus) and sub-human primates (Balner *et al.*, 1971; Barnes and Hawker, 1972; Downing *et al.*, 1972; Dersjant *et al.*, 1973). So there is PL-A (Viza *et al.*, 1970) or SL-A (Vaiman *et al.*, 1972) in the pig, DL-A in the dog (Westbroek *et al.*, 1972),

*In the mouse there is at least one non-H-2 locus ('M') where incompatibility gives an MLC reaction (Festenstein *et al.*, 1972).

RL-A in the rabbit (Tissot and Cohen, 1972) etc. For the guinea pig the histocompatibility locus distinguishing line 2 and 13 inbred strains (unnamed) has not been properly defined as an MHL. In the chicken the B blood group locus (Gleason and Fanguy, 1964) is a histocompatibility locus, probably the major one but one would not with present knowledge regard this as a homologue in comparison of gene products (Malchow *et al.*, 1972).

Non-H-2 loci have been extensively studied in mice (Graff, 1970) but so far have received little attention in other species. They are most in evidence as mediators of skin graft rejection where they are frequently 'weak' and rarely stronger than a single H-2 specificity difference. Multiple non-H-2 incompatibilities may give as rapid rejection of skin grafts as an H-2 difference; graft versus host reactions are generally only found following preimmunization of the donor (Davies, 1963) and cell–cell interactions *in vitro* are not usually detectable. These antigens should not be forgotten while correlation between tissue typing and the fate of kidney grafts is rather poor. A badly neglected area of study is that of tissue-specific alloantigens (non-MHL); there are some data for the mouse, e.g. there are skin specific (*Sk*-1, Scheid *et al.*, 1972), lymphocyte specific (*Ly-A* and others, Boyse *et al.*, 1968a; Boyse *et al.*, 1971), thymocyte specific (TL, Boyse *et al.*, 1968c) alloantigens and some of rather limited distribution such as theta (Reif and Allen, 1964). A hint of the existence of heart-specific alloantigenicity exists for the mouse (Judd and Trentin, 1972). Human kidney tissue should be examined with a similar possibility in mind.

The difficulties of direct *in vivo* assay are considerable. Both immunogenicity and tolerogenicity are not directly related to amount of antigen injected, the dose response curve is too flat. Of the variety of *in vitro* assays, complement mediated cytotoxicity inhibition is much the most used. It was more than an article of faith that this reaction truly detected a product of the H locus but later discussion does now call in question whether the H locus as seen this way or something closely genetically linked to it (not seen this way) is the true immunogen involved in transplant rejection, as will be discussed later (Yunis and Amos, 1971; Boyse *et al.*, 1970).

Other reviews relevant to the topic of this chapter are as follows: transplantation antigens (Davies, 1968; Nathenson, 1970) H-2 genetic model (Klein and Shreffler, 1971), cell surface glycoproteins (Hughes, 1973).

Separation

The injection of a critical small number of leukocytes into mice about two weeks before skin grafting under antithymocyte globulin (ATG) can lead to donor specific prolongation in mice (Kilshaw *et al.*, 1973) and similar treatment of rats leads to heart transplant prolongation without any other treatment and is presumed to be active enhancement (MacDonald *et al.*, 1972). Nevertheless hopes rest mainly on extracted material to induce tolerance although it is not self-evident that the high and low dose tolerance models apply in cellular immune situations. The other purposes of purification reside especially in the interpretation of functions of the MHL genetic region since in the presence of impurities only limited deductions can be made about the properties of the gene products.

Sources

Animals

The mouse has been, and still is the main source of information about MHL; human studies come second in line. The other animal species in use have their own advantages for particular studies; rats in enhancement, pigs in liver transplantation studies, dogs in reacting more like man for kidney transplants, sub-human primates where it is necessary to model closely on human clinical situations. Rabbits, guinea pigs, sheep, chickens etc. have their uses but have contributed little novel chemical information.

Tissues

Lymphoid tissue is the principal source of material for extraction because of the relatively high content of active material and ease of access (e.g. spleens). In the mouse it is possible to increase the yield up to 10-fold by using suitable lymphomas that give 1 g (wet wt.) spleens, or strain specific ascites tumors may be used. Since human leukemic lymphocytes can be obtained in useful numbers from patients or grown in culture, it should be mentioned that, e.g. mouse F_1 lymphomas can be subjected to immunoselection in parental lines so that they lose some of their H-2 antigens (Bjaring and Klein, 1968). It seems that this is a true loss and not akin to the situations in so-called non-specific ascites tumors where removal of neuraminic acid may affect transplantability over H-2 incompatibilities (Sanford and Codington, 1971). However, one such selected tumor did, *on extraction*, produce material having a specificity considered to have been lost by immunoselection (our unpublished observations). Otherwise tumor cells, or at least leukemic cells, are an adequate source although there are both antigenic gains and losses on record. HL-A losses from cells in lymphoma patients have been reported (Seigler *et al.*, 1971) and evidence given for the absence of H-2 antigens from Ehrlich ascites tumor of mice (Chen and Watkins, 1970), however extraction of Ehrlich cells gives H-2 antigen which can be purified in the usual way (our unpublished observations). In the last few years it has been shown that for a variety of different tumors, the cell surface tumor-specific antigen can be extracted, solubilized and purified by the methods described below for transplantation antigens (Baldwin and Glaves, 1972) and thus becomes a potential contaminant. This is of little consequence, however, because a variety of other histocompatibility antigens behave likewise and at least one (Tl, thymus-leukemia antigen) can be separated from H-2 antigen by ion exchange chromatography (Davies *et al.*, 1969). In any case white cells from any source are a heterogeneous collection of cell types and subtypes probably all having characteristic cell-type antigens (studied to some extent in mice) and even for man granulocyte-specific antigens are known (Lalezari *et al.*, 1970) and homologues of the mouse series are certain to exist corresponding to, e.g. Ly antigens, Pc plasma cell antigen, theta etc.

Liver has been used as source most often after spleen and other lymphoid tissue. Crude extracts have somewhat different properties from those of spleen, described later, and soluble preparations tend to have a component of lower molecular weight (Davies, 1970). In the context of the unexpected behavior of pig liver transplants (Chapter 12) it may be important that whereas whole spleens may be stored for up to a week at 4 °C with only a small loss of units of activity (cytotoxicity inhibition) by the sixth and seventh days, livers may be similarly stored but show a progressive increase in total units up to 15-fold (our unpublished observations). The replacement time for H-2 and HL-A removed from lymphocyte membranes by papain is about 6 h (see below); the turnover time is probably about the same. Liver may therefore have a more rapid turnover. This is not a finding of great use in practice because the yield of protein that can be solubilized after such storage is increased more than 15-fold, so that the specific activity (i.e. units/mg protein) is lower for crude extracts which constitute the starting point for purification.

Of the many other tissues which have been extracted none is specially convenient. Placenta is a poor source. Of general interest is the demonstration of HL-A on human sperm, where a haploid expression has been suggested (Fellous and Dausset, 1970); this requires confirmation however, as very careful serological analysis of mouse sperm has not revealed haploid expression of H-2 (Goldberg *et al.*, 1970; Vojtískova and Pokorná, 1971), and the presence of HL-A activity in seminal plasma complicates the issue (Singal *et al.*, 1971). HL-A is present in trophoblast (Loke *et al.*, 1971). Brain, thought for many years to lack H-2 antigens because no specificity could be shown by absorption methods, does have H-2 antigen as seen by its ability to sensitize for hastened skin graft rejection between H-2 congenic mice (Barnes, 1964).

It has been reported that cultures of human and mouse skin can lose their HL-A/H-2 alloantigenicity allowing allotransplantation without rejection (Summerlin *et al.*, 1972). This important observation awaits confirmation in the light of conflicting information for rabbit skin (Friedman and Valenti, 1966).

No convenient source of soluble antigen has been found comparable to ovarian cyst fluids for ABO mucopolysaccharides, which has resulted in this being the only isoantigenic system where detailed structural studies and biosynthetic pathways have been elucidated. There is 'soluble' HL-A material in human serum (Van Rood *et al.*, 1970) but this is most likely debris on its way to the 'disposal machine'. On fractionation some truly soluble material appears but this is to be expected. HL-A7 specific activity is found associated with the β-lipoprotein fraction of human serum (Charlton and Zmijewski, 1970).

Cells

Tissue culture cell lines are becoming a popular source. Mouse 'L' cell fibroblasts were shown to be good $H\text{-}2^k$ cells after 20 years in culture (Davies and Hutchison, 1961; Gangal *et al.*, 1966). Other mouse tumor lines have been studied recently and no typing anomalies found (Klein *et al.*, 1970). Now that cultured human lymphoblasts are available for study it is rather suspicious that certain anomalies have appeared. Some sublines from one donor yield more or less antigen than the original; others when examined serologically show either increased or decreased reactivities with HL-A typing sera or appear to have more than the 4 antigens (if heterozygous at both subloci) than the HL-A genetic model permits (McDonald *et al.*, 1970; Sasportes *et al*, 1971; Belpomme *et al.*, 1969; Dick *et al.*, 1972). Either the model is inadequate or the HL-A typing sera have non HL-A reactivities. Broadly speaking, however, the cell lines are a welcome addition to available sources of antigen (Reisfeld *et al.*, 1970) because more thousands of mouse spleens can be produced for any phenotype under study but while one human spleen is unique, it does not provide enough starting material to prepare pure material for analysis.

At the cell level, lymphocytes and tumor cells have been most studied. H-2 and HL-A antigens are almost exclusively cell-surface located but do occur on nuclear membranes (Albert and Davies, 1973). In culture their expression varies with the cell cycle (Cikes, 1970; Pasternak *et al.*, 1971). The low yields of material on extraction and logistic problems of starting material for purification are explained by estimates of the number of molecules per cell. For a single HL-A specificity in a heterozygous individual 7000 has been calculated (Sanderson and Welsh, 1973). For rats a figure of 37 500 sites was found using serum distinguishing two Ag-B different lines (i.e. for 4 antigens), (Batchelor *et al.*, 1973); if an HL-A model for Ag-B is accepted then for a single specificity in a homozygous rat there are 19 000 molecules per cell. These two studies were carried out under quite different conditions yet give figures of the same order, which is rather convincing. If we give a figure of 4×10^4 daltons for the HL-A molecule then the total HL-A content of an average sized human spleen is about half a milligram. Whereas a good yield of crude extract can be obtained in terms of recovery of units of activity, the yields of purified soluble antigen are rarely better than a few percent.

Purification

Crude extracts

The separation from cells of MHL activity, measured *in vitro* or *in vivo*, is rather easy on account of its location in the plasma membrane fraction. In recent years a variety of methods has become available for purifying plasma membranes from various cell types, the only restriction upon these being the necessity for providing conditions in which the antigens are stable. This forbids the use of most detergents, organic solvents, heat and pH outside the physiological range. In practice the preparation of pure membrane fractions is unnecessary or undesirable for three reasons; the antigen content is so low that removal of small amounts of non-plasma membrane material is a waste of time; secondly antigen is easily lost during the preparation, only a proportion of the antigen content can actually be solubilized and this loss reduces that fraction; thirdly simple washing of cell suspensions in the absence of Ca^{2+} releases virtually all of the activity, which can be recovered from the cell washings by high speed centrifuging (Davies, 1966). Hypotonic conditions are usually used and the degree of hypotonicity has to be found for the cell type used, e.g. lymphoma cells can best be eluted in 0.3% NaCl whereas 0.8% NaCl is adequate for lymphoid cells (Davies *et al.*, 1967). Similar membrane derived activity can be recovered from ascitic fluid in the case of mouse-grown tumor cells or culture fluids in which human lymphoid cell lines have been grown.

These crude preparations cannot be fractionated in the sense of separating different gene products from one another, in spite of having been shown to carry all of a variety of alloantigens sought (in the mouse, H-2, TL, Ly-A, B and C, theta, H-Y, etc.; in the human, HL-A, ABO, Rh, MN, 5^b etc.; our unpublished observations). The reason is connected with the poorly understood way in which membranes retain their structural integrity. Removal of lipid or solution in, e.g. deoxycholate leads to some fragmentation (Allan and Crumpton, 1971) but limited information came from early studies of detergent solubilization where Triton X100 was the most useful (Kandutsch and Stimpfling, 1963). There are, of course, any number of methods for dissolving membranes but we are concerned only with those whose conditions allow recovery of the very labile molecules having MHL specificity. Crude membrane material has been used extensively as a source of activity in biological experiments as described later but the presence of non-MHL immunogenicity confuses many interpretations of the results. The material is glyco-lipoprotein whose overall chemical composition has been described in the context of membrane structural studies.

Soluble extracts

A certain fraction of the MHL activity as measured by *in vitro* assays and some *in vivo* methods is released spontaneously in soluble form from the preparations just referred to. 'Spontaneous' requires some explanation, however, and proves to be really enzymic. Thus if membrane preparations are stored at 4 °C even for a few days, soluble material with H-2, or HL-A etc. activity remains in the supernatant after high speed centrifuging, having a molecular weight variously estimated at between 35 000 and 55 000. This has been described as autolytically solubilized antigen and the yields may be increased by incubation at 37 °C (Nathenson and Davies, 1966a). All the methods referred to here were first used with mouse products but have been employed with equal success in HL-A studies. Soluble antigen (H-2 and HL-A) released by sonic disintegration is no doubt of the same origin but the conditions provided for very low yields. Another style in the use of autolytic enzymes, either 'cathepsins' or membrane bound proteases (but cathepsins have not been studied in this context) is the use of 3 M KCl at 4 °C for 16 h. This method and sonic disintegration have been reviewed by Reisfeld and Kahan (1971). It was to be hoped that the latter method was non-enzymic in nature but removal of the soluble fraction at the start (source of enzyme) or inclusion of inhibitors of proteolysis abolish the solubilization (Mann, 1972). This was a disappointing outcome because proteolysis, however controlled, is not a desirable starting point for material to be purified for analytical studies as heterogeneity is likely to be introduced right at the start. Heterogeneity has indeed been found in the most highly purified preparations made so far though the reason for it may not be the initial enzymic step. Indeed there are some reasons for thinking that initial proteolysis, either autolytic or by the addition of proteases affects not the antigen itself but the membrane material in its vicinity. These reasons are that specificities common to different genotypes may be released in different amounts relative to other specificities from mice of different genotype (e.g. H-2.5 from H-2^k, H-2^b or H-2^n mice; this effect has not been studied for HL-A specificities), furthermore, indistinguishable products are released by a variety of enzymes (autolysis used in different ways, papain, ficin or bromelin; our unpublished observations).

So to obtain molecules having a restricted array of gene products we are still confined to enzymic methods and the addition of known pure enzyme is generally preferred to autolysis although it is not easy to have the former without the latter because some proteolytic activity appears to be bound into membranes and cannot be washed out beforehand. Ficin and papain have been most used (Nathenson and Davies, 1966b; Shimada and Nathenson, 1969; Nathenson *et al.*, 1970) and it is clear that prolonged incubation with these enzymes is destructive; different specificities (of H-2 and of HL-A) are probably released at different rates and are certainly destroyed at different rates. The rather good yield of autolytically derived antigen obtainable by prolonged incubation at 4 °C in 3 M KCl (Reisfeld and Kahan, 1971) is probably due to restricted destruction, where protease tends to hydrolyse only those peptide bonds to which it has the greatest affinity, when acting under conditions far from the optimum.

Solubilization with deoxycholate has recently been studied again (Hayman and Crumpton, 1972) and gives some variety of soluble molecular products that can be fractionated. The degree of complexity of molecules which might carry alloantigenic activity is not yet clear. Indeed this is not fully clarified for H-2 and HL-A in the sense that for the better studied H-2 material it has not been shown that all non-H-2 alloantigens have been removed. Some progress has been made in that direction, however, because it can be seen (McPherson *et al.*, 1971) that a whole family of glycoproteins is present in crude enzymically solubilized preparations, possibly 20 or more, but only a few of these carry recognized MHL specificities. Some others do carry non-MHL specificities and can be separated, e.g. TL (thymus–leukemia antigen) from H-2, already referred to, and H-6 from H-2 (Lilly and Nathenson, 1968). It remains a possibility that other glycoproteins carry MHL gene products that have no serological marker yet recognized, if such exist. In addition to what antigens can be separated from each other on subsequent fractionation, at least many remain in the insoluble fraction after proteolysis or are destroyed in the incubation (for the mouse, e.g. Ly-A, B, C and theta). The close similarity in the properties of lymphocytes from different species with respect to those activities mediated directly or indirectly by their plasma membrane components, leads one to believe at this time that homologues exist for all the components involved although the degree of multiple allelism outside MHL has hardly been studied; it would seem permissible to imagine an alloantigen in one species not to be an alloantigen in another species but the material would still be present to perform its physiological role and exist as an impurity in the context of purifying any other molecule. Biosynthetic methods for assembling molecules composed of products of several unlinked genes have been clarified for immunoglobulins, but at this time there is no clear evidence that H-2 or HL-A purified products are complexes of gene products.

Fractionation

These methods will not be dealt with in detail because necessarily lengthy instructions will be found in papers referred to. Whereas the variety of conditions making use of molecular size and charge obtainable with polyacrylamide gel electrophoresis and isotachophoresis could lead in theory to single or 'oligo'-stage isolation methods, this cannot be achieved because the yield is too small from the amounts of material for which these methods can cater. For this reason methods have not changed greatly since the time when soluble H-2 and HL-A antigens first became available (Nathenson and Davies, 1966b; Davies, 1967; Shimada and Nathenson, 1969). Ammonium sulfate precipitation of antigen may be used to reduce volumes for more convenient handling. Gel infiltration is used to separate impurities of higher and lower molecular size. DEAE ion exchange chromatography has been a principal standby and CM ion exchange has also been used to remove impurities because the required product is not adsorbed. Polyacrylamide gel electrophoresis (PAGE) is essential and isotachophoresis, where ampholines are interpolated, has additional resolving power (Hess and Davies, 1973). Methods in general have been dealt with elsewhere (Davies, 1973).

Fractionation on DEAE ion exchange columns leads to some separation of different H-2 (Davies, 1969) or HL-A (Colombani *et al.*, 1970) specificities. It is therefore not sufficient to monitor a column serologically with a single mono- or oligo-specific antiserum if the product is required to fully represent the phenotype of the starting material. This is equally true on PAGE fractionation where MHL specificities will also separate from one another (H-2, Hess and Davies, 1973; HL-A, O'Neill and Davies, 1971). In addition gel filtration may resolve some specificities on account of there being Class I and Class II molecules of different sizes (Yamane and Nathenson, 1970).

Class I and II molecules are not substantially different in size but there are much larger and much smaller specific molecules that deserve mention. A large but soluble molecular complex has been described (for H-2, Hämmerling *et al.*, 1971; Davies *et al.*, 1971b; for HL-A, Davies *et al.*, 1971a) that was solubilized by use of sodium dodecylsulfate and starch stearate. The complex carrying H-2 also has specificities for other gene products and is hence of little use for studying the MHL product analytically. This is probably similar to products described earlier, solubilized with Triton X100 and snake venom. Small molecules with H-2 specificity have been prepared, having molecular weights of the order of 10 000 (Edidin, 1967; Davies, 1970; Kerman *et al.*, 1972) but these have not been studied in the context of H-2 structure in spite of their obvious importance in this regard. This seems to be due to difficulties over obtaining sufficient material for study. In addition, the MHL product carries common specificities recognizable with xenoantisera (Staines *et al.*, 1973) and a fragment has been described which is 'non-specific' and may indicate that this part of the molecule can be detached from that bearing the allo-epitopes (Miyakawa *et al.*, 1973).

Chemical properties

The only kind of product extensively studied is that released by gentle proteolysis, either autolytic or assisted. A direct comparison of H-2 and HL-A thus prepared was made by Mann and Nathenson (1969) and few differences were found between their properties other than those due to immunological specificity. They were described as 'strikingly similar', the amino acid compositions showed relatedness of a non-coincidental kind, there were some differences in carbohydrate composition. The substances are glycoproteins having about 9% of carbohydrate made of 4–5% neutral sugar (galactose, mannose and fucose), 3–4% *N*-acetyl-glucosamine (0.5% for HL-A) and about 1% sialic acid. Galactosamine is conspicuously absent though found in many of the other glycoproteins present in the crude unfractionated products of membrane proteolysis. Whereas *N*-glycollyl-neuraminic acid has not been found from any human source (but commonly found elsewhere, e.g. pig mucopolysaccharides), polymers containing *N*-glycollyl- but not those having only *N*-acetyl-neuraminic acid are non-specific inhibitors of H-2 cytotoxic antisera acting upon mouse lymphocytes (our unpublished observations). The possibility that the carbohydrate moiety contributes to specificity has always seemed unlikely although the question has been difficult to formally exclude. No differences have been found between glycopeptides from starting material of different H-2 genotype (pronase digestion products), nor between lymphocyte and tumor derived products of the same H-2 genotype (Muramatsu and Nathenson, 1970). Neuraminic acid can be removed without loss of activity and most of the remaining sugars also; the situation has been summarized in a review by Nathenson and Muramatsu (1971). Nevertheless a carbohydrate involvement has been suggested for some HL-A specificities (Sanderson *et al.*, 1971). There is a likelihood that sugars are involved with the reaction of xenoantisera with the specific products but otherwise the matter is not likely to be finally settled until the epitopes are absolutely identified and the reasons for the extreme temperature and pH lability accounted for. It should be noted that both for temperature and pH, lability is independently variable and depends on the specificity tested for. Hence it is a property closely associated with the molecular structures involved in reaction with antibody and not denaturation of a more general kind (our unpublished observations).

Studies of the protein moieties have shown differences in peptide fingerprinting that make likely candidates for specificity differences (Yamane *et al.*, 1972). For such studies the purity of the products being compared are the features to be focussed upon as no claim has yet been made by anyone for a product even approaching homogeneity of amino-acid end group. This raises the question of how many molecules carry the recognizable epitopes of a particular H-2 or HL-A phenotype. It is clear from membrane surface topography studies that 'K' and 'D' end specificities are remote from each other (Boyse *et al.*, 1968b). This point is not settled for the two sub-loci (Four and LA series) of HL-A but other features of topography mouse and man have in common (Legrand and Dausset, 1971; Neauport-Sautes *et al.*, 1972). Thus it is evident that different sub-locus determinants are on different molecules and this is seen in molecular studies. For a heterozygous mouse four separable gene products have been demonstrated, two for D-end specificities and two for K-end specificities (Cullen *et al.*, 1972). This study also showed that a heterozygous individual does not make a hybrid molecule. How many specificities are carried then on a single molecule? A range of H-2 specificity separations have been described (Davies, 1969) some of which, in the light of more recent work and clarification of antibody specificities, are of doubtful validity. However at least three substantial separations are clear, on the other hand groups of specificities can be shown by antibody binding experiments to be located on the same molecule (Davies, 1970; Cullen and Nathenson, 1971).

The most purified preparations are polydisperse as indicated by the diffuse spread of the polyacrylamide gel band although immunologically reactive for HL-A or H-2 markers. Possible reasons for this have recently been suggested (Hess and Davies, 1973). Amino acid compositions have been given (Mann *et al.*, 1969) which show HL-A and H-2 to be very similar.

BIOLOGICAL STUDIES

Assays

The earliest attempts to follow purification of transplantation antigens made use of tumor enhancement (Kandutsch, 1960) but the difficulties and especially the lack of precision of *in vivo* methods led to the use of serological techniques of various kinds. Complement mediated cytolysis inhibition quantitated by ^{51}Cr release (Sanderson, 1965; Wigzell, 1965) became the favored method but much discussion centered on whether this measured the gene product which mediated *in vivo* activities. This question has now been raised again because in the following decade increasing complexity revealed in the MHL genetic region seemed to allow a distinction between serologically definable regions and an 'MLR' (mixed lymphocyte reaction) region, possibly coinciding with an 'Ir' (immune-responsiveness) region. For this and other reasons a search is being made for Ir gene products whose relationship to K and D (Four and LA) genes remains obscure. Also it cannot be denied that while inhibitory activity in serological assays increases progressively on purification, there is no such increase in the capacity of the products to mediate *in vivo* activity although they will hasten rejection of skin grafts when appropriately administered (Harris *et al.*, 1971; Graff and Nathenson, 1971). There are several possible reasons which might account for this poor biological activity; the true mediator may be separating as an 'impurity' in the course of serological monitoring; the activity may suffer by loss of these impurities by removal of adjuvanticity, or loss of carrier effects if the molecules carry only one determinant of each kind. The last is suggested by some limitation in reaction with antibody such that precipitation cannot be induced.

The range of assays which have been tried, many with limited success, will not be listed again here (see Davies, 1968). Most used are cytotoxic inhibition, immune fluorescence, and radioimmune assay (Miyakawa *et al.*, 1971). A version of cytotoxicity assay which seems to permit monitoring of MHL material from any animal species, in the absence of any immunogenetic data, makes use of xenogeneic anti-spleen or anti-thymus serum whose cytotoxicity is mainly directed against a common specificity located on the same molecule (Staines *et al.*, 1973). Since ALS cytotoxicity does not correlate with its immunosuppressive action, then the immunosuppressive antibody is not one reacting with the MHL product which emerges from cytotoxic monitored procedures. In this context the antibody, in 'enhancing' alloantisera, may have similar features and in both cases be directed at e.g. Ir gene products rather than K/D, Four/LA products for which we have serological markers.

Direct *in vivo* assays following either hastened graft rejection or tolerance induction have proved too difficult to use for following antigen purification and while heated discussion continues on what *in vitro* model truly reflects these activities and graft versus host reactions in addition, the 'right' *in vitro* test system cannot be decided upon.

Biological properties

The characteristic biological property of the isolated substances is their exquisite specificity which truly reflects that exhibited by the tissue of origin and shows that major damage has not been wrought in the course of isolation. This is not to say that the literature does not contain misleading descriptions of products for which adequate specificity controls were not carried out. Evidence that the soluble molecules studied are not quite 'complete' comes from a discrepancy in molecular weights, the NP40 solubilized material being about 6000 daltons larger than the product of papain digestion (Schwartz and Nathenson, 1971b; Nathenson *et al.*, 1972). This might be a component responsible for integrating the specific part of the molecule into the membrane structure. Removal of antigen by papain directly from living cell surfaces is not lethal and regeneration takes place in 4–6 hours (H-2, Schwartz and Nathenson, 1971a; HL-A, Turner *et al.*, 1972).

It should be mentioned in passing that there is a cross reaction between a component of group A streptococci and transplantation antigens of many species including man and this overrides allo-differences. There is no interpretation for this in molecular terms nor any precedent for such a situation. The reactivity has been variously attributed to protein or carbohydrates; it is certainly not due to the type specific polysaccharide of type 1 strains (to which this reactivity is confined) (our unpublished observations). On the whole it seems most likely to involve the 'M' protein of the bacterial cell (Hirata and Terasaki, 1970).

Immunogenicity of crude (insoluble) membrane preparations is much more easily demonstrated by *in vivo* effects than that of the truly soluble molecules. In this context and in the light of differences between the transplantability of liver and kidney in man, it has long been known that whereas spleen derived crude extracts are strongly sensitizing, similar material from liver is not. Moreover in treatment with both preparations even by independent routes into the same animal, the sensitizing activity of the spleen product is abrogated (Mandel *et al.*, 1965; Manson and Palm, 1966). This effect has become almost anecdotal on account of lack of recent study and interpretation.

Soluble antigens are rather poor inducers of cytotoxic antibodies. This is not a serious matter in mouse studies because of the good selection of congenic strains available, over which purified materials offer no special advantages. It is unfortunate for human studies since immunization of volunteers with lymphoid cells for eliciting tissue-typing alloantisera presents certain problems. In this situation soluble purified HL-A antigen would have advantages in safety and in eliminating non-HL-A antibodies which help to confuse HL-A serology.

Of a more pressing practical nature are studies of induction of specific immunological unresponsiveness. The tolerance models using purified protein and carbohydrate antigens, and which have provided a set of rules, are in fact measures of reduced antibody production. It is becoming less clear that such rules apply in situations mediated, or at least dominated by a cellular immunity. A study bearing exactly on this point (Law *et al.*, 1972) showed that purified H-2 antigen could be used to induce specific unresponsiveness as measured by cytotoxic alloantibody production, but did not affect the fate of skin grafts in the same animals. A different view could be derived from the new interpretation of the major histocompatibility gene complexes suggested by Amos and Yunis (1971). This view would be, as referred to earlier, that the serological markers have led us astray and a closely linked gene product is the immunogen (tolerogen) required.

Be this as it may, soluble antigens, not so very highly purified, have been shown to mediate specific transplant prolongation. Whether this is tolerance old style (elimination of recognizing clones), tolerance new style (serum blocking factors), enhancement (antibody mediated) or a complexes affair is not clear. The situations are all multiparametric; a graft may release antigen to complex with injected or elicited antibody (passive or active enhancement) and graft derived antigen may raise antibodies to complex with injected soluble antigen. Thus the alternative view to the different gene product idea seems to be that all signposts point to complexes. While the following references are consistent with the latter, they are not inconsistent with the former. Rat renal allografts can be prolonged by administration of antigen and antibody (Stuart *et al.*, 1970) or skin grafts by antigen helped with ALS (Sumerska *et al.*, 1971). Mouse skin graft survival can be prolonged by antigen alone (but not substantially) (Rosenberg *et al.*, 1971), or with antigen helped by cyclophosphamide (Halle-Pannenko *et al.*, 1971a). Very impressive mouse skin graft prolongation can be arranged by use of antigen (not solubilized) given two weeks before grafting, helped with ALS and *Pertussis* vaccine (Brent *et al.*, 1973).

Several papers record unsuccessful attempts to achieve 'low dose tolerance' with H-2 soluble antigens but they have tested insufficient variables to justify any conclusions. That low dose tolerance cannot be obtained with the products now available could be concluded from an experiment where groups of mice were maintained with a circulating purified H-2 preparation of molarities 10^{-8} to 10^{-13} by daily injections for two months without affecting subsequent skin graft survival in two different H-2 incompatibilities (our unpublished observations).

The frequent finding that skin grafts are not favourably affected by a situation arranged to prolong the survival of kidney, liver or heart from the same donor could be due to skin-specific alloantigenicity which is known to exist in mice (Scheid *et al.*, 1972).

Among other *in vivo* activities obtained with soluble preparations are active and passive tumor enhancement in mice (Law *et al.*, 1971), inhibition of graft versus host reaction in mice (Halle-Pannenko *et al.*, 1971b) etc. MLC reaction can be stimulated with HL-A antigens (Viza *et al.*, 1968). A set of conclusions can hardly be drawn from so cursory a coverage of this subject. Help would most likely come from some realistic interpretation of the normal physiological role of the MHL gene products as membrane components and their polymorphism, if the role is not just to carry that polymorphism. It might be hoped that the polymorphism extending to a new specificity for every mouse deme may be partly artifactual by limitations of serology to high affinity antibody. It is some relief that cross reactions between H antigens of different species is on record.

It remains only for me to tender my apologies to the authors of the many thousands of papers to which it has not been possible to refer in the allotted space.

References

Albert, W. H. W. and Davies, D. A. L. (1973). H-2 antigens on nuclear membranes. *Immunology*, **24**, 1

Allan, D. and Crumpton, M. J. (1971). Solubilization of pig lymphocyte plasma membrane and fractionation of some of the components. *Biochem. J.*, **123,** 967

Amos, D. B., Seigler, H. F., Southworth, J. G. and Ward, F. E. (1969). Skin graft rejection between subjects genotyped for HL-A. *Transplant. Proc.*, **1,** 342

Amos, D. B. and Yunis, E. J. (1971). A new interpretation of the major histocompatibility gene complexes of man and mouse. *Cell. Immunol.*, **2,** 517

Bailey, D. W. (1963). Histoincompatibility associated with the X chromosome in mice. *Transplantation*, **1,** 70

Baldwin, R. W. and Glaves, D. (1972). Solubilization of tumor-specific antigen from plasma membrane of an aminoazo-dye-induced rat hepatoma. *Clin. Exp. Immunol.*, **11,** 51

Balner, H., Gabb, B. W., Dersjant, H., Van Vreeswijk, W. and Van Rood, J. J. (1971). Major histocompatibility locus of rhesus monkeys (RhL-A). *Nature New Biol.*, **230,** 177

Barnes, A. D. (1964). A quantitative comparison study of immunizing ability of different tissues. *Ann. N.Y. Acad. Sci.*, **120,** 237

Barnes, A. D. and Hawker, R. J. (1972). Leukocyte antigens in baboons: a preliminary to tissue typing for organ grafting. *Transplant. Proc.*, **4,** 37

Batchelor, J. R., Shumak, K. H. and Watts, H. G. (1973). ^{125}I-labeled rat transplantation alloantibody. *Transplantation*, **15,** 80

Belpomme, D., Le Borgne de Kaouel, C., Ajuria, E., Jasmin, C. and Dore, J. F. (1969). Increase in antigenicity of permanent tissue culture lines ICI 101, ICI 104 and ICI 202 established from human leukemic blood. *Nature (London)*, **222,** 890

Bennett, D., Boyse, E. A. and Old, L. J. (1972). Cell surface immunogenetics in the study of morphogenesis. In *Cell Interactions*, Third Lepetit Colloquium, p. 247 (L. G. Silvestri, editor). Amsterdam: North Holland)

Billingham, R. E., Brent, L. and Medawar, P. B. (1956). The antigenic stimulus in transplantation immunity. *Nature (London)*, **178,** 514

Billingham, R. E., Brent, L. and Medawar, P. B. (1958). Extraction of antigens causing transplantation immunity. *Transplant. Bull.*, **5,** 377

Bjaring, B. and Klein, G. (1968). Antigenic characterization of heterozygous mouse lymphomas after immunoselection *in vivo*. *J. Nat. Cancer Inst.*, **41,** 1411

Boyse, E. A., Miyazawa, M., Aoki, T. and Old, L. J. (1968a). Ly-A and Ly-B: two systems of lymphocyte isoantigens in the mouse. *Proc. Roy. Soc. (London) B*, **170,** 175

Boyse, E. A., Old, L. J. and Stockert, E. (1968b). An approach to the mapping of antigens on the cell surface. *Proc. Nat. Acad. Sci. USA.*, **60,** 886

Boyse, E. A., Stockert, E. and Old, L. J. (1968c). Properties of four antigens specified by the *Tla* locus. Similarities and differences. In *International Convocation on Immunology*, p. 353 (N. R. Rose and F. Milgrom, editors). Basel: S. Karger

Boyse, E. A., Flaherty, L., Stockert, E. and Old, L. J. (1970). Histoincompatibility attributable to genes near H-2 that are not revealed by hemagglutination or cytotoxicity tests. *Transplantation*, **13,** 431

Boyse, E. A., Itakura, K., Stockert, E., Iritani, C. A. and Miura, M. (1971). Ly-C: a third locus specifying alloantigens expressed only on thymocytes and lymphocytes. *Transplantation*, **11,** 351

Brent, L., Hansen, J. A., Kilshaw, P. J. and Thomas, A. V. (1973). Specific unresponsiveness to skin allografts in mice. I. Properties of tissue extracts and their synergistic effect with antilymphocyte serum. *Transplantation*, **15,** 160

Charlton, R. K. and Zmijewski, C. M. (1970). Soluble HL-A7 antigen: localization in the β-lipoprotein fraction of human serum. *Science*, **170,** 636

Chen, L. and Watkins, J. F. (1970). Evidence against the presence of H-2 histocompatibility antigens in Ehrlich ascites tumour cells. *Nature (London)*, **225,** 734

Cikes, M. (1970). Relationship between growth rate, cell volume, cell cycle kinetics, and antigenic properties of cultured murine lymphoma cells. *J. Nat. Cancer Inst.*, **45,** 979

Colombani, J., Colombani, M., Viza, D. C., Degani, Bernard, O., Dausset, J. and Davies, D. A. L. (1970). Separation of HL-A transplantation antigen specificities. *Transplantation*, **9,** 228

Cullen, S. E. and Nathenson, S. G. (1971). Distribution of H-2 alloantigenic specificities on radiolabelled papain-solubilized antigen fragments. *J. Immunol.*, **107,** 563

Cullen, S. E., Schwartz, B. D., Nathenson, S. G. and Cherry, M. (1972). The molecular basis of codominant expression of the histocompatibility-2 genetic region. *Proc. Nat. Acad. Sci. USA.*, **69,** 1394

Dausset, J. D. and Rapaport, F. T. (1966). The role of blood group antigens in human histocompatibility. *Ann. N.Y. Acad. Sci.*, **129,** 408

Davies, D. A. L. (1963). The presence of non-H-2 histocompatibility specificities in preparations of mouse H-2 antigens. *Transplantation*, **1,** 562

Davies, D. A. L. (1966). Mouse histocompatibility isoantigens derived from normal and from tumor cells. *Immunology*, **11,** 115

Davies, D. A. L. (1967). Soluble H-2 isoantigens. *Transplantation*, **5,** 31

Davies, D. A. L. (1968). Transplantation Antigens. Chapter 38 in *Human Transplantation* (F. T. Rapaport and J. Dausset, editors). New York: Grune and Stratton

Davies, D. A. L. (1969). The molecular individuality of different mouse H-2 histocompatibility specificities determined by single genotypes. *Transplantation*, **8,** 51

Davies, D. A. L. (1970). Transplantation antigens: some features of mouse H-2 molecules and their relevance to HL-A in man. In *Blood and Tissue Antigens*, p. 101 (D. Aminoff, editor). New York: Academic Press

Davies, D. A. L. (1973). Preparation of antigens from tissues and fluids. Chapter 11 in *Handbook of Experimental Immunology*, 2nd Ed. (D. M. Weir, editor). Oxford: Blackwell Scientific Publications

Davies, D. A. L. and Hutchison, A. M. (1961). The serological determination of histocompatibility activity. *Brit. J. Exp. Pathol.*, **42**, 587

Davies, D. A. L., Alkins, B. J., Boyse, E. A., Old, L. J. and Stockert, E. (1969). Soluble TL and H-2 antigens prepared from a TL positive leukaemia of a TL negative mouse strain. *Immunology*, **16**, 669

Davies, D. A. L., Boyse, E. A., Old, L. J. and Stockert, E. (1967). Mouse isoantigens: separation of soluble TL (thymus-leukaemia) antigen from soluble H-2 histocompatibility antigen by column chromatography. *J. Exp. Med.*, **125**, 549

Davies, D. A. L., Manstone, A. J., Viza, S. C., Colombani, J. and Dausset, J. (1968). Human transplantation antigens: the HL-A (Hu-1) system and its homology with the mouse H-2 system. *Transplantation*, **6**, 571

Davies, D. A. L., Colombani, J., Viza, D. C. and Hämmerling, U. (1971a). Extraction of HL-A transplantation antigen in high molecular weight soluble form. *Clin. Exp. Immunol.*, **8**, 801

Davies, D. A. L., Hämmerling, U. and Alkins, B. J. (1971b). Transplantation antigens in a high molecular form. II. Non H-2 mouse antigens and membrane structure. *Immunochemistry*, **8**, 17

Dersjant, H., Van Vreeswijk, W. and Balner, H. (1973). Relation between chimpanzee leukocyte antigens and HL-A. In *Immunobiological Standardization* Symposia series No. 18, p. 61 (R. H. Regamey and J. V. Spärck, editors). Basel: S. Karger

Dick, H. M., Steel, C. M. and Crichton, W. B. (1972). HL-A typing of cultured peripheral lymphoblastoid cells. *Tissue Antigens*, **2**, 85

Downing, H. J., Brain, P., Hammond, M. G., Vos, G. H. and Webb, G. R. (1972). Leukocyte antigens of baboons. *Transplant. Proc.*, **4**, 33

Edidin, M. (1967). Preparation of single soluble antigens of the mouse histocompatibility-2 complex. *Proc. Nat. Acad. Sci. USA.*, **57**, 1226

Fellous, M. and Dausset, J. (1970). Probable haploid expression of HL-A antigens on human spermatozoon. *Nature (London)*, **225**, 191

Festenstein, H., Abbafi, K., Sachs, J. A. and Oliver, R. T. D. (1972). Serologically undetectable immune responses in transplantation. *Transplant. Proc.*, **4**, 219

Friedman, E. A. and Valenti, C. (1966). Persistence of individual specific transplantation antigens in long term cultures of rabbit skin. *Transplantation*, **4**, 747

Gangal, S. G., Merchant, D. J. and Shreffler, D. C. (1966). Characterization of the H-2 antigens of L-M mouse cells grown in culture. *J. Nat. Cancer Inst.*, **36,** 1151

Gleason, R. E. and Fanguy, R. C. (1964). The relationship of blood groups to skin graft survival in chickens. *Transplantation*, **2,** 509

Gluecksohn-Waelsch, S. and Erickson, R. P. (1970). The T-locus of the mouse: implications for mechanisms of development. *Curr. Top. Dev. Biol.*, **5,** 281

Goldberg, E. H., Aoki, T., Boyse, E. A. and Bennett, D. (1970). Detection of H-2 antigens on mouse spermatozoa by the cytotoxicity test. *Nature (London)*, **228,** 570

Goldberg, E. H., Boyse, E. A., Bennett, D., Scheid, M. and Carswell, E. A. (1971). Serological demonstration of H-Y (Male) antigen on mouse sperm. *Nature (London)*, **232,** 478

Graff, R. J. (1970). Polymorphism of histocompatibility genes in the mouse. *Transplant. Proc.*, **2,** 15

Graff, R. J. and Nathenson, S. G. (1971). Immunogenic properties of papain-solubilized alloantigen. *Transplant. Proc.*, **3,** 249

Halle-Pannenko, O., Martyré, M. C. and Jolles, P. (1971a). Conditioning of allogeneic mice with crude and purified H-2 extracts, alone and combined with cyclophosphamide, for skin graft prolongation. *Transplant. Proc.*, **3,** 257

Halle-Pannenko, O., Martyré, M. C. and Mathé, G. (1971b). Prevention of graft-versus-host reaction by donor pretreatment with soluble H-2 antigen. *Transplantation*, **11,** 414

Hämmerling, U., Davies, D. A. L. and Manstone, A. J. (1971). Transplantation antigens in a high molecular weight form. I. Mouse H-2 antigens. *Immunochemistry*, **8,** 7

Harris, R. and Zervas, Z. D. (1969). Reticulocyte HL-A antigens. *Nature (London)*, **221,** 1062

Harris, T. N., Harris, S. and Ogburn, C. A. (1971). Solubilization of H-2 histocompatibility antigens of the mouse by Triton X100 and Butanol. *Transplantation*, **12,** 448; Harris, T. N., Harris, S., Ogburn, C. A., Bocchieri, M. H. and Farber, M. B. (1971). Accelerated rejection of allogeneic skin grafts in the mouse after injections of histocompatibility antigens solubilized by Triton, Butanol, and Papain. *Transplantation*, **12,** 459

Hayman, M. J. and Crumpton, M. J. (1972). Isolation of glycoproteins from pig lymphocyte plasma membrane using *Lens culinaris* phytohemagglutinin. *Biochem Biophys. Res. Commun.*, **47,** 923

Hess, M. and Davies, D. A. L. (1973). Structure of histocompatibility antigens. On the reduction and alkylation of mouse histocompatibility antigens. *Eur. J. Biochem.* (In press)

Heslop, B. F. (1973). The male antigen in the rat. *Transplantation*, **15**, 31

Hirata, A. A. and Terasaki, P. I. (1970). Cross-reactions between streptococcal M proteins and human transplantation antigens. *Science*, **168**, 1095

Hughes, R. C. (1973). Glycoproteins as components of cellular membranes. In *Progress in Biophysics and Molecular Biology*, p. 191 (J. A. V. Butler and L. Noble, editors). Oxford: Pergamon Press

Ivǎsková, E., Dausset, J. and Iványi, P. (1972). Cytotoxic reactions of anti-H-2 sera with human lymphocytes. *Folia Biol. (Prague)*, **18**, 194

Judd, K. P. and Trentin, J. J. (1972). Tolerance induction to murine cardiac allografts with anti-thymocyte globulin (ATG) and cell fiee antigens. *Transplantation Abstracts of the Fourth International Congress of the Transplantation Society*, p. 154 (S. L. Kountz, editor). New York: Grune and Stratton

Kandutsch, A. A. (1960). Intracellular distribution and extraction of tumour homograft-enhancing antigens. *Cancer Res.*, **20**, 264

Kandutsch, A. A. and Stimpfling, J. H. (1963). Partial purification of tissue isoantigens from a mouse sarcoma. *Transplantation*, **1**, 201

Kerman, R. H., Harris, T. N. and Harris, S. (1972). Preparation of dialyzable histocompatibility antigen from Balb/c mice. *Proc. Nat. Acad. Sci. USA.*, **69**, 223

Kilshaw, P. J., Brent, L. and Thomas, A. V. (1973). *Transplantation* (In press)

Klein, D., Merchant, D. J., Klein, J. and Shreffler, D. C. (1970). Persistence of H-2 and some non-H-2 antigens on long-term-cultured mouse cell lines. *J. Nat. Cancer Inst.*, **44**, 1149

Klein, J. and Shreffler, D. C. (1971). The H-2 model for the major histocompatibility systems. *Transplant. Rev.*, **6**, 3

Lalezari, P., Thalenfeld, B. and Weinstein, W. J. (1970). The third neutrophil antigen. In *Histocompatibility Testing*, p. 319 (P. I. Terasaki, editor). Copenhagen: Munksgaard

Law, L. W., Appella, E., Strober, S., Wright, P. W. and Fischetti, T. (1972). Induction of immunological tolerance to soluble histocompatibility-2 antigens of mice. *Proc. Nat. Acad. Sci. USA.*, **69**, 1858

Legrand, L. and Dausset, J. (1971). Cell surface interaction between HL-A antigen determinants. *Nature New Biol.*, **234**, 271

Lilly, F. and Nathenson, S. G. (1968). Solubilization of the H-6A isoantigen of the mouse. In *Advance in Transplantation*, p. 279 (J. Dausset, J. Hamburger, and G. Mathé, editors). Copenhagen: Munksgaard

Loke, Y. W., Joysey, V. C. and Borland, R. (1971). HL-A antigens on human trophoblast cells. *Nature (London)*, **232**, 403

MacDonald, A. S., Davies, D. A. L., and Calne, R. Y. (1972). Factors governing antigen and antibody enhancement of the rat heart allografts. *Transplantation Abstracts of the Fourth International Congress of the Transplantation Society*, p. 180 (S. L. Kountz, editor). New York: Grune and Stratton

McDonald, J. C., Jacobbi, L. and Williams, R. W. (1970). HL-A antigen studies with leukocyte cell lines. *Transplantation*, **10,** 499

McDevitt, H. O., Deak, B. D., Shreffler, D. C., Klein, J., Stimpfling, J. H. and Snell, G. D. (1972). Genetic control of the immune response: mapping of the IR-1 locus. *J. Exp. Med.*, **135,** 1259

McPherson, J. C., Clamp, J. R. and Manstone, A. J. (1971). Carbohydrate analysis of membrane derived glycoproteins carrying some cell surface expressed antigens. *Immunochemistry*, **8,** 225

Malchow, D., Droege, W. and Strominger, J. L. (1972). Solubilization and partial purification of lymphocyte specific antigens in the chicken. *Eur. J. Immunol.*, **2,** 30

Mandel, M. A., Monaco, A. P. and Russell, P. S. (1965). Destruction of splenic transplantation antigens by a factor present in liver. *J. Immunol.*, **95,** 673

Mann, D. L. (1972). The effect of enzyme inhibitor on the solubilization of HL-A antigens with 3M KCl. *Transplantation*, **14,** 398

Mann, D. L. and Nathenson, S. G. (1969). Comparison of soluble human and mouse transplantation antigens. *Biochemistry*, **64,** 1380

Mann, D. L., Rogentine, G. N., Fahey, J. L. and Nathenson, S. G. (1969). Human lymphocyte membrane (HL-A) alloantigens: isolation, purification and properties. *J. Immunol.*, **103,** 282

Manson, L. A. and Palm, J. (1966). Mouse transplantation antigens: blocking by liver and kidney microsomal lipoproteins of homograft immunity induced by H-2 transplantation antigens. *IXth Internat. Congress of Microbiology, Moscow*. Abstracts, p. 642

Miyakawa, Y., Tanigaki, N., Yagi, Y. and Pressman, D. (1971). Human transplantation antigens: isolation and radioimmunoassay. *Proc. Soc. Exp. Biol. Med.*, **136,** 899

Miyakawa, Y., Tanigaki, N., Yagi, Y. and Pressman, D. (1973). Common antigenic structures of HL-A antigens. I. Antigenic determinants recognizable by rabbits on papain-solubilized HL-A molecular fragments. *Immunology*, **24,** 67

Muramatsu, T. and Nathenson, S. G. (1970). Studies on the carbohydrate portion of membrane-located mouse H-2 alloantigens. *Biochemistry*, **9,** 4875

Nathenson, S. G. (1970). Biochemical properties of histocompatibility antigens. *Ann. Rev. Genet.*, **4,** 69

Nathenson, S. G. and Davies, D. A. L. (1966a). Solubilization and partial purification of mouse histocompatibility antigens from a membranous lipoprotein fraction. *Proc. Nat. Acad. Sci. USA.*, **56,** 476

Nathenson, S. G. and Davies, D. A. L. (1966b). Transplantation antigens: studies of the mouse model system, solubilization and partial purification of H-2 isoantigens. *Ann. N.Y. Acad. Sci.*, **129,** 6

Nathenson, S. G. and Muramatsu, T. (1971). Properties of the carbohydrate portion of mouse H-2 alloantigen glycoproteins. In *Glycoproteins of blood cells and plasma*, p. 245 (G. A. Jamieson, editor). Philadelphia: J. B. Lippincott Co.

Nathenson, S. G., Schwartz, B. D. and Cullen, S. E. (1972). Immunochemical properties and genetic relationships of H-2 histocompatibility alloantigens. In *Membrane and Viruses in Immunopathology*, p. 117 (S. C. Day and R. A. Good, editors). New York: Academic Press

Nathenson, S. G., Shimada, A., Yamane, K., Muramatsu, T., Cullen, S. E., Mann, D. L., Fahey, J. L. and Graff, R. (1970). Biochemical properties of papain-solubilized murine and human histocompatibility alloantigens. *Fed. Proc.*, **29,** 2026

Neauport-Sautes, C., Silvestre, D., Niccolai, M. G., Kourilsky, F. M. and Levy, J. P. (1972). Ultrastructural localization of human HL-A membrane antigens by use of hybrid antibodies. *Immunology*, **22,** 833

O'Neill, G. J. and Davies, D. A. L. (1971). Behaviour of mouse H-2 specificities on polyacrylamide gel electrophoresis and polyacrylamide gel electrofocussing. *Biochim. Biophys. Acta*, **243,** 337

Pasternak, C. A., Warmsley, A. M. H. and Thomas, D. B. (1971). Structural alterations in the surface membrane during the cell cycle. *J. Cell Biol.*, **50,** 562

Reif, A. E. and Allen, J. M. V. (1964). The AKR thymic antigen and its distribution in leukaemias and nervous tissues. *J. Exp. Med.*, **120,** 413

Reisfeld, R. A. and Kahan, B. D. (1971). Extraction and purification of soluble histocompatibility antigens. *Transplant. Rev.*, **6,** 81

Reisfeld, R. A., Pellegrino, M., Papermaster, B. W. and Kahan, B. D. (1970). HL-A antigens from a continuous lymphoid cell line derived from a normal donor *J. Immunol.*, **104,** 560

Rosenberg, E. B., Mann, D. L., Hill, J. J. and Fahey, J. L. (1971). Prolonged skin allograft survival in mice pretreated with soluble transplantation antigens. *Transplantation*, **12,** 402

Sanderson, A. R. (1965). Cytotoxic reactions of mouse isoantisera: the scope of an assay using radiolabelled target cells. *Transplantation*, **3,** 557

Sanderson, A. R., Cresswell, P. and Welsh, K. I. (1971). Involvement of carbohydrate in the immunochemical determinant area of HL-A substances. *Nature New Biol.*, **230,** 8

Sanderson, A. R. and Welsh, K. (1973). Quantitation of transplantation (HL-A) antigen sites on peripheral human lymphocytes. *Biochem. Soc. Trans.* (In press)

Sanford, B. H. and Codington, J. F. (1971). Further studies on the effect of neuraminidase on tumour cell transplantability. *Tissue Antigens*, **1,** 153

Sasportes, M., Dehay, C. and Fellous, M. (1971). Variations of the expression of HL-A antigens on human diploid fibroblasts *in vitro*. *Nature (London)*, **233,** 332

Scheid, M., Boyse, E. A., Carswell, E. A. and Old, L. J. (1972). Serologically demonstrable alloantigens of mouse epidermal cells. *J. Exp. Med.*, **135,** 938

Schwartz, B. D. and Nathenson, S. G. (1971a). Isolation of H-2 alloantigens solubilized by the detergent NP-40. *J. Immunol.*, **107,** 1363

Schwartz, B. D. and Nathenson, S. G. (1971b). Regeneration of transplantation antigens on mouse cells. *Transplant. Proc.*, **3,** 180

Seigler, H. F., Kremer, W. B., Metzgar, R. S., Ward, F. E., Haung, A. T. and Amos, D. B. (1971). HL-A antigenic loss in malignant transformation. *J. Nat. Cancer Inst.*, **46,** 577

Shimada, A. and Nathenson, S. G. (1969). Murine histocompatibility-2 (H-2) alloantigens. Purification and some chemical properties of soluble products from $H\text{-}2^b$ and $H\text{-}2^d$ genotypes released by papain digestion of membrane fractions. *Biochemistry*, **8,** 4048

Singal, D. P., Berry, R. and Naipaul, N. (1971). HL-A inhibiting activity in human seminal plasma. *Nature New Biol.*, **233,** 61

Staines, N. A., O'Neill, G. J., Guy, K. and Davies, D. A. L. (1973). Xenoantisera against lymphoid cells: specificity and use in monitoring purification of mouse and human histocompatibility antigens. *Tissue Antigens*, **3,** 1

Stuart, F. P., Fitch, F. W. and Rowley, D. A. (1970). Specific suppression of renal allograft rejection by treatment with antigen and antibody. *Transplant. Proc.*, **2,** 483

Sumerska, T., Betel, I. and Balner, H. (1971). Skin graft prolongation in rats using ALS and soluble histocompatibility antigens. *Radiobiological Institute TNO, Annual Report*, p. 101 (151 Lange Kleiweg, Rijswijk, Holland)

Summerlin, W. T., Faanes, R. B. and Good, R. A. (1972). Homologous transplantation of cultured skin. *Transplantation Abstracts of the Fourth International Congress of the Transplantation Society*, p. 280 (S. L. Kountz, editor). New York: Grune & Stratton

Tissot, R. G. and Cohen, C. (1972). Histocompatibility in the rabbit: identification of the major locus. *Tissue Antigens*, **2,** 267

Turner, M. J., Strominger, J. L. and Sanderson, A. R. (1972). Enzymic removal and re-expression of a histocompatibility antigen, HL-A 2, at the surface of human peripheral lymphocytes. *Proc. Nat. Acad. Sci. USA.*, **69,** 200

Vaiman, M., Garnier, H., Kunlin, A., Hay, J. M., Parc, R., Bacour, F., Fagniez, P. H.,

Villiers, P. A., Lecointre, J., Bara, M. F. and Nizza, P. (1972). The SL-A histocompatibility system in the *Sus scrofa* species. *Transplantation*, **14**, 541

Van Rood, J. J., Van Leeuwen, A. and Van Santen, M. C. T. (1970). Anti HL-A2 inhibitor in normal human serum. *Nature* (*London*), **226**, 366

Viza, D. C., Degani, O., Dausset, J. and Davies, D. A. L. (1968). Lymphocyte stimulation by soluble human HL-A transplantation antigens. *Nature* (*London*), **219**, 704

Viza, D., Sugar, J. R. and Binns, R. M. (1970). Lymphocyte stimulation in pigs: evidence for the existence of a single major histocompatibility locus, PL-A. *Nature* (*London*), **227**, 949

Vojtíšková, M. and Pokorná, Z. (1971). Developmental expression of H-2 antigens in the spermatogenic cell series: possible bearing on haploid gene action. *Folia Biol.* (*Prague*), **18**, 1

Westbroek, D. L., Silberbusch, J., Vriesendorp, H. M., Van Urk, H., Roemeling, H. W., Schönherr-Scholtes, Y. and de Vries, M. J. (1972). The influence of DL-A histocompatibility on the function and pathohistological changes in unmodified canine renal allografts. *Transplantation*, **14**, 582

Wigzell, H. (1965). Quantitative titration, kinetic behaviour and inhibition of cytotoxic mouse isoantisera. *Immunology*, **9**, 287

Yamane, K. and Nathenson, S. G. (1970). Murine histocompatibility-2 (H-2) alloantigens: purification and some chemical properties of a second class of fragments (Class II) solubilized by papain from cell membranes of H-2^b and H-2^d mice. *Biochemistry*, **9**, 1336

Yamane, K., Shimada, A. and Nathenson, S. G. (1972). Peptide comparison of two histocompatibility-2 (H-2b and H-2d) alloantigens. *Biochemistry*, **11**, 2398

Yunis, E. J. and Amos, D. B. (1971). Three closely linked genetic systems relevant to transplantation. *Proc. Nat. Acad. Sci. USA.*, **68**, 3031

4

Tissue Typing in Human Kidney Transplantation

P. I. Terasaki, G. Opelz, and A. Ting

Transplantation antigens have been found on the cell surface of virtually all tissues of an animal. Differences in these antigens between members of the same species may be a reflection of small chemical changes in these antigens. Surgical transfer of an organ from one individual to another will in most instances be followed by an immunological reaction against these small differences.

One of the most remarkable findings of the past 30 years has been that the major transplantation antigens for many animal species are determined by a single locus on a pair of homologous chromosomes. In mice this locus has been designated the H-2, in rats the Ag-B, in chickens the B, in dogs the D-LA, and in humans the HL-A ('H' stands for human, 'L' for leukocyte, and 'A' for the first locus to be described). The antigens determined by the main locus are, fortunately, detectable serologically, with antibodies produced after immunization by pregnancy, blood transfusion, or organ transplantation from an allogeneic animal. With the production of a wide battery of reagent antisera in immunized hosts, it has been possible to define the different tissue 'types' (transplantation antigens) of a species.

In humans, 27 antigens have been relatively well established. Of these, 11 have been given official designations by the World Health Organization: HL-A1 to HL-A13. The other 16 specificities, which are not as well defined, have provisional 'workshop' designations prefixed with a 'W' (Table 4.1). These antigens can be divided into two series of mutually exclusive alleles as shown in Table 4.1. It is assumed, however, that other series of antigens may exist, and presumably more antigens remain to be demonstrated in the two established series, since the gene frequencies of the detected alleles for each series do not total one in any race studied thus far. The frequency of the 27 antigens in the random population of three races is given in Table 4.1. Marked variations in the frequencies of certain antigens between the races can be noted. For example, HL-A1, HL-A8, and W14 are common in Caucasians, rare in Negroes, and absent in Orientals.

Table 4.1 *HL-A Antigens and their Phenotype Frequencies*

First Segregant Series				*Second Segregant Series*			
	Caucasian	*Negro*	*Oriental*		*Caucasian*	*Negro*	*Oriental*
HL-A1	28	14	0	HL-A5	11	6	43
HL-A2	50	26	48	HL-A7	24	24	10
HL-A3	26	22	3	HL-A8	21	8	0
HL-A9	20	26	60	HL-A12	29	26	12
W23	4	19	0	HL-A13	4	1	2
W24	16	7	60	W5	18	27	20
HL-A10	12	13	27	W10	12	4	34
W25	5	2	2	W14	8	4	0
W26	7	11	25	W15	10	3	13
HL-A11	11	2	10	W16	9	6	12
W28	9	22	4	W17	9	21	2
W29	9	7	0	W18	8	9	0
W30	9	28	14	W21	6	6	2
W32	7	3	0	W22	5	13	10
				W27	6	4	0

The serology of HL-A is undergoing constant change, for although the antigens given in Table 4.1 are generally accepted as specific entities, recent studies have shown that a number of these antigens can be subdivided into factors (Thorsby *et al.*, 1971; Dausset, 1971). For example, HL-A5 has been split into A5-AJ and A5-non-AJ, W22 into AJ, non-AJ, W21 into ET* and SL-ET, and HL-A12 into Te87 and Te88 (Ting *et al.*, to be published). Furthermore, certain well-defined antigens can be classed together into 'cross-reacting groups' (Dausset, 1971), the antigens within each of which are thought to be structurally more similar than antigens between groups. Despite the complexity of the HL-A antigens, however, the well-defined antigens listed in Table 4.1 may represent the immunodominant HL-A specificities and those pertinent to clinical transplantation.

The tissue type of an individual is determined by two HL-A genes on two chromosomes (haplotypes), one paternal and the other maternal in origin (Table 4.2). Since only one paternal and one maternal chromosome are involved, four different genotypes (two haplotypes) are possible in the children; so one quarter of the siblings would be expected to have the same genotype and, therefore, tissue type. Between either parent and a child there is always one haplotype in common; the other will be different except on the rare occasion when the other parent has the same haplotype and the child inherits it.

Table 4.2 *Inheritance of HL-A antigens: The specificities determined on each chromosome (haplotype) are inherited as 'packets', so that only four types of children result from any mating.* The numbers are HL-A designations and a, b refers to the paternal and c, d to the maternal chromosomes

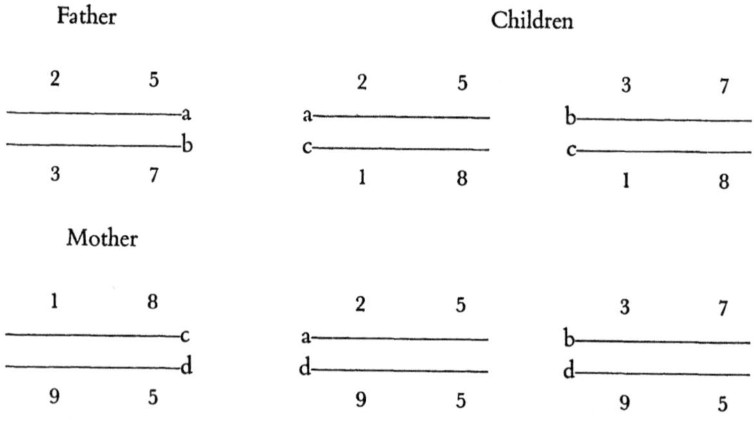

METHODOLOGY

The major concern in the early period of research in histocompatibility was to determine what kinds of tests might best detect these antigens.

The leukoagglutination test, in which leukocytes are agglutinated by antisera, much as red cells are typed, was the most logical first step. Despite numerous problems with reproducibility in this test (particularly since the granulocytes tend to agglutinate non-specifically), Dausset (1958) was able to distinguish an antigen which he called 'Mac', and van Rood (1963) was able to establish allelic specificities 4a and 4b. The subsequent rapid development of the field was promoted by van Rood's introduction of computer technology in sorting out specificities.

Detection of the antigens on lymphocytes by the use of cytotoxicity was introduced by Terasaki *et al.* (1964) and by Walford *et al.* (1964). This method was subsequently made practical for large-scale testing by introduction of microtechniques (Terasaki and McClelland, 1964). Basically, the test consists of reacting lymphocytes with antibody and complement; if the reaction is positive, the lymphocytes are killed, as indicated by the uptake of dye introduced at the end of the test. Since 1967 this test has, with minor modifications, been the most commonly employed and standardized conditions (the 'NIH' conditions) have been agreed upon. This process consists of reacting 0.001 ml of reagent antisera with 1000–2000 lymphocytes and incubating for 0.5 hour at room temperature (22–25 °C), then adding 0.005 ml of rabbit complement and incubating for another hour, then staining and fixing the reaction. Eosin dye or trypan blue (which would be taken up by dead cells but excluded by living cells) has commonly been used.

The antibodies used to type the cells are most commonly found in sera obtained from multiparous women or persons who have been accidentally or deliberately immunized with leukocytes from other humans. During pregnancy, mothers become immunized to the foreign antigens present in the fetus which were inherited from the father. Much of the immunization occurs during labor, when bleeding across the placenta results in fetal blood entering the maternal circulation. To what extent immunization proceeds continuously during pregnancy is not known, although there is some evidence that production can occur during the first pregnancy (Overweg and Engelfriet, 1969). Because most women are immunized by two specificities of a haplotype (or sometimes, in two consecutive pregnancies, from two specificities of each of the two haplotypes of the father), most antisera are multispecific. The same problem occurs even when immunizing volunteer donors. It has therefore been difficult to identify sera which have a single antibody producing strong, clear-cut reactions. Identifying and obtaining sufficient quantities of such high-quality typing reagents has been and continues to be a difficult but important task for the field of HL-A typing.

Clarification of the genetic inheritance and serologic identification of the antigens has surpassed all expectation. Over the past five years laboratories have demonstrated that serologic tests can reliably detect antigens present on lymphocytes and platelets with almost the same level of accuracy as the red cell antigens can be detected—at least with respect to several antigens. Five years ago, no one would have suspected that such a high level of knowledge could have been reached in such a short time.

ROLE OF TISSUE TYPING IN KIDNEY TRANSPLANTS

A high level of perfection can be achieved in kidney transplants between siblings determined by tissue typing to be HL-A identical. With only minimal doses of immunosuppressive drugs, such transplants provide a level of function indistinguishable from that of a normal kidney. But despite the success of transplants between these 'perfectly matched' donors and recipients, the role of histocompatibility testing in selecting donors is currently being questioned for a variety of reasons.

GENETIC BASIS FOR HISTOCOMPATIBILITY TESTING

Proof of the genetic basis for histocompatibility is provided by the finding that kidney transplants from monozygotic twins do exceptionally well without immunosuppression and that kidney transplants taken from other genetically related individuals function better than those from unrelated donors (Tenth Report of the Human Transplant Registry, 1972). Thus, the chances of successful transplants are considerably better if we resort to matching according to 'blood' relationships. This fact was established in man largely as a result of the pioneering kidney transplantation studies of Hamburger *et al.* (1962) and Starzl (1964). Since that time, many compilations of survival rates in kidney transplants have absolutely confirmed the marked difference in results depending on the genetic relationship of the donor to the recipient. The Human Renal Transplant Registry has now compiled 10 reports, and the single most outstanding finding throughout has been the marked difference shown when cadaver donor transplants are compared to related donor transplants. This means that the genetic compatibility between the donor and recipient can be demonstrated to have more effect upon transplant success than any other single factor (such as differences in immunosuppressive therapy, differences in experience between transplant centers, differences among surgeons, etc.).

It is well recognized that some patients are more immunocompetent than others and also that given drugs may be more effective in some patients than others. But in spite of these variables, the fact that a clear difference can be found only by dividing patients on the basis of whether they have received a transplant from a related or an unrelated donor suggests that the difference in results between these two groups is directly attributable to histocompatibility matching.

In fact, if unrelated donor transplants could be done with the same success as those from related donor transplants, a major step toward complete acceptance of kidney transplants as a therapeutic measure would have been accomplished. The success rate from related donor transplants is more than 70 per cent at one year. Removal of kidneys from healthy donors cannot, however, be thought to be a satisfactory practice in the future. It is generally recognized that cadaver donors must be the principal source of organs for transplantation. Currently, more than three quarters of the transplants being done in the United States and more than 90 per cent of those being done in Europe are from such cadaver donors. Transplants of other organs, such as hearts and livers, which cannot be taken from living donors will of course require cadaver donors.

HL-A ANTIGENS AS THE TRANSPLANTATION ANTIGENS IN MAN

The strongest proof that HL-A antigens are the main transplantation antigens in man comes from the results of kidney transplantation from HL-A identical sibling donors. In an extensive analysis of transplants done since January 1, 1969, for the 215 transplants between HL-A identical siblings, the survival rate was 90 per cent at one year (Opelz *et al.*, 1973). In approximately 100 other transplants from HL-A identical siblings which have been reported (Stickel *et al.*, 1970; Amos *et al.*, 1971; Kissmeyer-Nielsen and Thorsby, 1970; Patel and Myrberg, 1970; Dausset and Hors, 1971; Hors *et al.*, 1971; Worham *et al.*, 1971), essentially perfect kidney function was obtained. It is highly unlikely that this large number of transplants could have resulted in such excellent results by chance alone. Laboratory evidence that longer skin graft survival can be obtained in HL-A identical siblings (Dausset *et al.*, 1965; van Rood *et al.*, 1966, Ceppellini *et al.*, 1966) and that they do not stimulate each other by the mixed leukocyte culture test (Bach and Voynow, 1966) indicates strongly that transplants between HL-A identical siblings are a special group of transplants. Since these results were obtained by many transplant centers and different typing laboratories, variations in the management of patients and in the serologic grading schemes do not influence this single strongest evidence that HL-A antigens are the principal transplantation antigens in man. It should be noted that there is evidence that the ABO red cell antigens are also strong antigens in transplantation, based principally on skin transplantation experiments (Ceppellini *et al.*, 1966; Dausset *et al.*, 1970).

If other histocompatibility loci not closely linked to HL-A were of importance to kidney transplantation, it would be expected that some of the HL-A identical siblings would have been incompatible at these loci. The fact that the transplants functioned well in spite of these incompatibilities indicates that for practical purposes, with the current development of immunosuppression and kidney transplantation, the other loci can be ignored. Certainly, products of other histocompatibility loci can have a marked effect without immunosuppression and with other organs. This is most evident in skin transplants which are rejected in approximately 21 days in untreated HL-A identical siblings. Thus, many loci probably control transplantation in man as they do in mice; but as in mice, one strong histocompatibility locus stands out as the principal one. It is becoming evident that in humans, as in mice, the strongest locus stimulates the formation of antibodies; and quite conveniently for our purposes, these antibodies can then be used to type for the antigens of the strongest histocompatibility locus. Our work has been initiated under this assumption (Terasaki *et al.*, 1965), and the work of the past 5 years has not yielded results contradictory to this assumption.

CORRELATION OF HL-A TYPING WITH CLINICAL OUTCOME

HL-A Chromosome (allele)

Evidence that the HL-A chromosome governs the most important antigens of transplantation is incontrovertible from the findings with HL-A identical siblings. This complex is responsible for three distinct risk categories among siblings: 90 per cent survival at one year for 215 with two HL-A identical chromosomes, 67 per cent for 126 patients with one HL-A identical chromosome, and 59 per cent for 30 with no HL-A identical chromosomes (Opelz *et al.*, 1973). Subdivision of sibling donors into these three distinct risk groups is not possible by any means other than HL-A typing. Mixed leukocyte culture (MLC) tests cannot readily separate one- and two-HL-A haplotype-different siblings, and no transplant survival rates based on MLC reactivity have been published for non-identical siblings.

All cadaver transplants can be classified as two-HL-A chromosome different—in contrast to parental donors, who are one-chromosome different. On the basis of HL-A chromosome difference alone, then the three main risk groups of HL-A identical, HL-A one-haplotype different, and HL-A two-haplotype different can be distinguished. In simplified terms, no HL-A chromosome difference (HL-A identical siblings) yields 90 per cent one-year success, one-chromosome difference gives 70 per cent, and two-chromosome difference (two-haplotype different sibling and cadaver transplants) yields 55 per cent survival.

These conclusions are essentially those arrived at by Simonsen (1965) and suggest that a single locus is involved as the major histocompatibility locus. The realization that only one genetic locus is of importance is of critical significance clinically for sibling donors, since it provides a means by which two-allele different donors can be eliminated in favor of comparable cadaver donors.

Nevertheless, for selection between mother and father or between different possible combinations of cadaver donor and recipient, no real advantage is gained by the identification of the HL-A chromosome itself. One allele of difference for either parent would exist by definition; and 99 per cent of the time, two alleles of difference can be assumed to exist in any random cadaver combination. Means by which differences can be distinguished within the groups of one- and two-chromosome different donors are therefore necessary.

This brings us to the attempts to look more closely at the HL-A chromosomes, at the individual specificities which comprise the two locii of HL-A (Table 4.2). Three ways in which the specificities have been used are: (1) totalling numbers of specificities; (2) distinguishing between strength of each specificity; and (3) considering cross-reaction between donor and recipient specificities.

Number of incompatible HL-A specificities

One logical way in which choices can be made between two parents who are each one-haplotype different from the recipient is to count up the *number* of specificities that are incompatible. A parent who is HL-A1, 8, 2, 12 may be a better donor for a recipient who is 1, 8, 2, 7 (one-antigen mismatch: 12) than the other parent who is 3, 5, 2, 7 (two-antigen mismatch: 3 and 5). A shorthand notation to describe the difference was introduced by us to describe the above matches as a C match (one-antigen incompatible) and D match (two-antigens incompatible). An A match indicates identity, a B match indicates compatibility (e.g. 1, 8, 2 donor for a 1, 8, 3, 7 recipient) and E match stands for three or four antigens incompatible.

This type of enumeration of mismatched antigens assumes that each antigenic specificity is about equal in strength and that two mismatches would be worse than one, and three worse than two. As a first approximation, such an assumption would appear to be reasonable. From the results of rather extensive studies over 4 years of parental and cadaver donor transplants, we have come to the conclusion that this ranking of incompatibilities on the basis of the number of mismatches is inadequate for clinical purposes (Terasaki and Mickey, 1971; Mickey *et al.*, 1971).

Our work was based on the approximately 70 per cent of transplant patients who were shown not to have cytotoxic antibodies prior to transplantation. Among such patients, no correlation of kidney transplant outcome with the number of incompatibilities was found in subsequent studies by others (van Hooff *et al.*, 1972; van Rood, 1971). Van Rood notes that the number of HL-A incompatibilities is important in presensitized recipients (and, we can infer, *not* important to the majority of the patients who are not presensitized) (Van Rood *et al.*, 1973). Moreover, it has recently been claimed that the second locus antigens are important (the first locus antigens must therefore *not* be important) (Oliver *et al.*, 1972; van Hooff *et al.*, 1972). However, in our series, no difference was noted for first and second locus antigens in 1740 cadaver donor transplants (Opelz *et al.*, 1973).

There has been a tendency in all the published series (including our own) toward the generalization that the fewer antigens mismatched, the better the chances. However, the point to be made is that simple counting of the number of incompatibilities *alone* will not be a sufficiently sensitive practicable guide to donor selection.

Number of compatible HL-A specificities

The method of counting the number of compatible HL-A specificities is similar to counting mismatched antigens, but it has the advantage that a higher grade is given if the typing is more complete by being based on four identified antigens per person. A match for three antigens with one group undetermined in the donor would thus be regarded as a one-antigen mismatch on the assumption that the fourth has not been identified by current serologic reagents. Simply to state that one antigen is mismatched does not tell us whether there is a possibility that a second one is not also mismatched. As an example, a match between a donor 1, 2, 8 and recipient 1, 8 is a two-antigen match and a one-antigen mismatch. To say that one antigen is mismatched is to ignore the possibility that actually another antigen might also be mismatched. The donor could be a 1, 8, 2, X, so that both 2 and X may be mismatched.

This type of argument is the basis for the Net Histocompatibility Ratio (NHR) calculations proposed by Dausset and Rapaport (1970), which compute the possibility that the 'blank' in the chromosome is occupied by a yet undetected antigen. But this focus of attention on incomplete typing and the recognition of missing alleles has not actually led to a significant improvement in the correlation of typing to transplant outcome, as several studies of NHR have shown (Halgrimson *et al.*, 1971; Terasaki and Mickey, 1971; Morris, 1971).

Dausset and Hors have recently improved the NHR measure by taking into account the possibility of homozygocity. This corrects for the chance that the donor or recipient are homozygous and therefore have less than four antigens. For example, the 1, 8, 2 donor could have been genotypically 1, 8/2, 8 rather than 1, 8/2, X as postulated earlier. The match would thus be a true one-antigen mismatch to a 1, 8 recipient. Unfortunately, because of the low frequency of most antigens aside from HL-A2, the correction did not alter the poor correlation noted in our series (Opelz *et al.*, 1973), though it seems to have produced a significant correlation in the French series (Dausset and Hors, 1972).

Conversion of matches to the 'worst possible match' by counting all blanks as mismatches, has been done by Kissmeyer-Nielsen who thereby noted some association in the Scandinavian transplants (Kissmeyer-Nielsen *et al.*, 1972).

The rationale behind all these corrections is that if the direct counting of the number of mismatches is not correlated to outcome, then perhaps taking into account the missing antigens will correct the situation. The problem is, however, that the missing antigens add to the mismatches, making each transplant appear to be a worse match. But this does nothing to help determine the clinical significance of mismatches. Most of the non-correlation is contributed by mismatched transplants which work well, not by matched grafts which fail. It has been our view that even with the known antigens there are too many mismatches which succeed. The way to explain these clinical successes is to determine why the known mismatches are *practicable*. A thorough discussion providing evidence for the belief that technical errors in tissue typing are not responsible has been given (Terasaki and Mickey, 1971).

Quality of mismatch (antigenic strength)

There is no reason not to suppose that a given antigen might be more antigenic than another. Extrapolating from the human red cells and mouse H-2, it is actually rather surprising that there has not been more evidence of gradations in antigenic strength. There has been some indication that HL-A2 is a strong antigen (Dausset, 1969); but if it were, one might expect a greater effect from mismatching for this antigen. It is clear that no single HL-A antigen is so strong that a mismatch would uniformly result in failure of a kidney transplant.The strongest antigen has about a 55 per cent failure rate, which is not essentially different from any other antigen (Opelz *et al.*, 1973). Thus, there are, to date, no specific antigens which we can say should be avoided in mismatching—as for example RhD must be in blood transfusions. If all the antigens are of equal importance, then it seems reasonable that the number of mismatches should be counted up as described in the previous section. A partial compromise solution is offered by Oliver *et al.* (1972) and van Hooff *et al.* (1972), who suggest that half of the HL-A antigens are not significant (first locus), whereas the antigens of the second locus are significantly associated with the outcome. These findings await confirmation in other series, since such an effect is not seen in our data (Opelz *et al.*, 1973).

The concept of relative antigenic strength must also be clarified. When an antigen is said to be a strong antigen, do we mean only that the immunological response to the antigen is strong? Moreover, when the response is strong (for example, to RhD) what is generally meant is that more people respond to RhD than to RhC. If the clonal selection theory of antibody response is accepted, then one might say that lymphocytes having receptors for D are present in many Rh-negative persons, and lymphocytes having receptors for C are much rarer, occurring in only a few per cent of the Rh-negative persons. The selective absence of lymphocytes with certain receptors and the corresponding inability to respond to certain mismatches could explain the non-immunogenicity of some antigens.

The possibility that a given antigen could be incompatible with a certain antigen but not with another, has been given (Terasaki and Mickey, 1971). A haplotype may also be acceptable or non-acceptable to a certain other haplotype. This concept could then explain why certain incompatible transplants fail whereas others do not. Empirical knowledge of the risks involved for each type of mismatch will require an extensive data base. With the aid of computers the possibility of developing programs which draw on prior experience is not entirely out of the question.

Cross-reactivity of donor and recipient antigens

One might assume that if certain antigens cross-react (i.e. are chemically similar to each other), then no reaction might occur when they are mismatched. Studies of kidney transplants have to date shown a slight improvement in the association when this factor is considered (Dausset and Hors, 1971; Kissmeyer-Nielsen *et al.*, 1971). The problem is that from the cross-reactive groups known, insufficient numbers of mismatches were 'correctable' by cross-reactivity. It can be noted that cross-reactivity does correct the results of mismatching in the needed direction by changing a combination which is mismatched into a matched one. However, a re-analysis taking into account a larger pattern of cross-reactivity as recently established (Mittal and Terasaki, 1972) did not yield markedly superior associations (Mickey *et al.*, 1972).

Some relationship of cross-reactivity to immunogenicity seems reasonable, since antibody formation in pregnant women appears to be related to cross-reactivity (Staub Nielsen and Svejgaard, 1972; Mickey *et al.*, 1972). It may be of importance that all studies have noted a shift in the right direction, though not of statistical significance, when cross-reactivity was taken into account. The conclusion therefore is that cross-reactivity is helpful, but by itself does not solve all the problems in associating the HL-A typing results with transplant outcome.

RECIPIENT RESPONSIVENESS

(*i*) *Preimmunization.* In distinct contrast to the above search for association, we noted a marked association of preimmunization with poor outcome (Terasaki *et al.*, 1971), and this effect has now been well confirmed (Patel and Briggs, 1971; Opelz and Terasaki, 1972a; van Rood *et al.*, 1973). This state of preimmunization is detected by the presence of lymphocytotoxic antibodies. The possibility that cellular immunity could also be utilized has been tested on a small scale (Tanaka *et al.*, 1971; Garovoy *et al.*, 1973) but has not been utilized clinically. Among cadaver transplant recipients without cytotoxic antibodies, the one-year survival rate was 55 per cent as compared to 36 per cent in patients with antibodies. Some refinements have been provided by data showing that if the antibodies are directed at the mismatched antigen(s), the survival rate is decreased to 20 per cent (Opelz *et al.*, 1973). If the antibody cross-reacts with the mismatch or is entirely unrelated to the mismatch, it is not as deleterious. This means that presensitization is specific to certain antigens and not a generalized state of reactivity.

On the other hand, those who respond to certain antigens may also be prone to respond to others, giving the appearance that the preimmunized state already identifies patients who are non-specific immunologic 'responders'. Patients with cytotoxins and negative crossmatches with the donor have been noted to reject transplants at higher rates than patients without cytotoxins (Opelz and Terasaki, 1972a). One explanation for this effect is that preimmunization for the donor's antigens had existed, but that the crossmatch test had not been sensitive enough. And retesting of sera from patients with early graft failure by more sensitive tests had indeed yielded a significant increase in the number of sera with antibodies (Ting *et al.*, 1973). Another common source of error lies in the great fluctuation of antibodies in the serum of patients (Terasaki and Mickey, 1971; Caseley *et al.*, 1971; Opelz and Terasaki, 1972a), which may have resulted in the use of sera for crossmatching at a time when antibodies had disappeared. A common example of the use of inappropriate serum samples (Dossetor and Olson, 1972) is the missing of latent sensitization acquired by women during pregnancy because the serum is not obtained until many years later, when a transplant is required. Antigenic specificities against which such patients could be potentially sensitized could be avoided by typing the husbands.

From the foregoing, it appears that presensitization is specific for certain antigens; and if the common pitfalls are avoided, preimmunized patients could have the same chances of transplant success as those who are not preimmunized. In summary, preimmunized patients must be matched carefully by (1) testing for humoral cytotoxins following all transfusions, (2) crossmatching using the most positive serum, (3) crossmatching with a sensitive test, and (4) avoiding HL-A specificities in the donor which are present in (a) the recipients' serum antibodies, (b) a prior transplant donor, and (c) the husband if the patient has been pregnant.

(*ii*) *Non-responsiveness.* Identification of patients who were immunologically non-responsive to HL-A provides the key explanation for the incompatible transplants which continue to function. Patients who were repeatedly challenged by blood transfusions but who did not make cytotoxins were found to accept transplants from incompatible donors with a one-year transplant survival rate of 85 per cent (Opelz *et al.*, 1972a). Those patients without a response to transfusions were unreactive against incompatible transplants. In subsequent studies (Opelz *et al.*, 1973), cytotoxicity negative patients who had never been challenged by transfusions were found to have even a lower rate of transplant survival (29%) than those with 1–10 (48%) or with 10 or more transfusions (80%). Quite surprisingly, transfusions increase the survival rate rather than decreasing it as was previously thought. Thus, while transfusions can have the effect of immunizing patients, they can also make them less responsive (enhanced). Active enhancement effect rather than simple genetic unresponsiveness must be postulated since prior transfusions appear to *improve* the results of transplantation rather than simply serving to select out the non-responders.

To say that certain patients are unresponsive implies that those patients may not react against *any* donor. Though some patients may have such anergy, there is evidence that it is more likely that unresponsiveness, like responsiveness, is more specific. Perhaps the best evidence is that from the second transplant experience. If 50 per cent of the population were non-responders and 50 per cent were responders, the 50 per cent random cadaver donor success rate, the 50 per cent immunization rate of patients on hemodialysis, and the 50 per cent rate at which pregnant women make antibodies against their fetuses would be explainable. If those who reject a transplant are the responders, one might expect that a second graft into these same selected responders would result uniformly in transplant failure. Yet this does not occur. As we (Terasaki and Mickey, 1971; Opelz and Terasaki, 1972b) and others (Hume *et al.*, 1966; Barnes *et al.*, 1968; Morris *et al.*, 1968) have shown, random second cadaver donor grafts survive at the same rate as first grafts. These findings are more compatible with the notion that selective non-responsiveness exists and that the chance of receiving an 'acceptable' donor is the same the first time as the second.

A somewhat paradoxical situation arises in second grafts, in that more patients who receive them have preformed cytotoxins than do those receiving first grafts, yet the survival rates overall are the same for first and second grafts. If the second grafts are split into those with and without antibodies, then, as noted earlier (Terasaki and Mickey, 1971), a higher failure rate is found for those with antibodies (Opelz and Terasaki, 1972b). The conclusion seems unavoidable: to compensate for the higher failure rates among presensitized patients, there must be some patients who are actually helped by rejecting a transplant. Enhancement could be induced by the rejection of a graft just as it is by transfusion (Opelz *et al.*, 1972b). A similar situation was noted among females who have twice the frequency of cytotoxins as males and yet do not have a correspondingly poor outcome in transplantation (Beliel *et al.*, 1972). The only reasonable explanation thus far has been that some opposing factor such as enhancement works in favor of transplants into females.

If unresponsiveness and responsiveness are specific, some patients must be specifically unresponsive to certain antigens *and* responsive to others. Thus, following multiple transfusions from random donors, patients sometimes respond by producing antibodies of limited numbers of specificities. This may mean that these patients are specifically responsive only to those specificities and not to the others. Conceivably, transfusions can be utilized to ascertain the specific responsiveness profile of recipients before kidney transplantation. Transfusion failures (production of cytotoxins) can then be used to select certain antigens to be avoided and certain others to be utilized for kidney transplantation.

In vitro tests for responsiveness are of course preferable to challenging by transfusions. The mixed leukocyte culture (MLC) blocking test for enhancing antibodies appears promising (Sengar *et al.*, 1973), but it is not satisfactory as a responsiveness test *before* transfusions or transplants. We have examined the MLC test for this purpose and found it unsatisfactory. Essentially, all cells respond to other unrelated donors; and the distribution of the counts forms a single peak which cannot readily be divided into responders and nonresponders.

(*iii*) *Proposed deliberate transfusions.* To give deliberate transfusions may appear to be an extremely risky undertaking in view of our knowledge of hyperacute rejections in presensitized recipients. However, the actual risk can be broken down as given in Table 4.3. If more than 10 transfusions are given, the patients as a whole would have a one-year survival of 55 per cent, an acceptable rate by current standards. In other words, disregarding the formation of antibodies, 10 transfusions may be better than no transfusions which yield 30 per cent survival rate. Even if this last figure is too low, since it is based on a rather small number of patients, transfusions do not make the situation worse. The potential gain comes from patients who do not develop antibodies and who will have a high probability of success (80 per cent at one year). Among those who develop antibodies, the advances in crossmatching, by more sensitive testings (Ting *et al.*, 1973), and detection of specificities in the serum so that given mismatches can be avoided, should permit successful transplants even in these patients. In other words, as long as the patient who has anti-HL-A2 antibodies is not grafted with a donor with the HL-A2 antigen, he would have a 45 per cent chance of one-year transplant function. Though the data is still insufficient, if such patients with antibodies are grafted with completely compatible grafts, there is no reason to expect success rates which would be any lower than 50 per cent. Thus, following transfusions, it should be possible to rapidly identify the non-responders and among those with antibodies to provide the right type of mismatch so that the overall success rates would be higher than the current 50 per cent rate.

Table 4.3 *Influence of Pretransplant Transfusions on survival of Cadaver Kidney Transplants at one year*

Patients without transfusions = 30 per cent		
Patients with > 10 transfusions = 55 per cent	Patients without antibodies after 10 transfusions = 80 per cent	
	Patients who develop cytotoxic antibodies = 35 per cent	Patients grafted with kidneys mismatched for the same specificity as his antibodies = 20 per cent
		Patients grafted with kidneys mismatched for spceificities other than his antibodies = 45 per cent
		Patients grafted with HL-A compatible kidneys = 75 per cent

Mixed leukocyte culture tests for histocompatibility

There has recently been some tendency to think that the MLC test provides a clearer measurement of histocompatibility than does HL-A (van Hooff *et al.*, 1972; Cochrum *et al.*, 1973; van Rood *et al.*, 1973). It is rare to find a parent-to-child MLC combination which does not stimulate. On this basis, most of such grafts would be expected to fail. Yet the opposite happens. Moreover, 99.9 per cent of unrelated MLC combinations stimulate, yet 50 per cent of transplants survive for one year. No convincing set of MLC data shows that the extent of stimulation is correlated to the time of survival, though some indication of such a correlation has been claimed for skin grafts (Koch *et al.*, 1972) and for bidirectional MLC (Cochrum *et al.*, 1973).

Eijsvoogel has provided evidence from crossover cases that an MLC locus which governs MLC response is adjacent to the second HL-A locus (Eijsvoogel *et al.*, 1972). But even if an MLC locus existed, its alleles could not play a role in kidney transplantation very different from the alleles of HL-A. Since almost all unrelated combinations stimulate, there must be many alleles (as in HL-A); and since many mismatched transplants function, the alleles must be 'intermediate' in strength (as in HL-A).

GENETIC RESPONSIVENESS LOCUS

In mice, the existence of IR (i.e. immune response) genes linked to the histocompatibility locus has been well established (McDevitt and Benaceraff, 1969). We might assume that similar IR genes also exist in man and that they are linked to HL-A. At this point we do not know if response to several HL-A specificities or a single one is coded for. Conceivably, there is a separate allele for response to each specificity.

IR genes to HL-A specificities could go a long way in helping to explain the way in which patients respond to incompatible transfusions and incompatible transplants. Now that some knowledge has been developed on the transplantation antigens acquisition of comparable knowledge on the responsiveness to these antigens should provide the necessary missing half of the information needed to select the proper donors for transplants.

References

Amos, D. B., Anderson, E. E., Glenn, J. F., Gunnells, J. C., Lancaster, S. L., MacQueen J. M., Robinson, R. R., Seigler, J. F., Stickel, D. L. and Ward, F. E. (1971). Selection of donors for kidney transplantation. *Transplant. Proc.*, **3,** 993

Bach, F. H. and Voynow, N. K. (1966). One-way stimulation in mixed leukocyte cultures. *Science*, **153,** 545

Barnes, B. A., Murray, J. E. and Atkinson, J. (1968). In *Advances in Transplantation*, p. 351 (J. Dausset, J. Hamburger and G. Mathé, editors). Copenhagen: Munksgaard)

Beliel, O. M., Mickey, M. R. and Terasaki, P. I. (1972). Comparison of male and female kidney transplant survival rates. *Transplantation*, **13,** 493

Caseley, F., Moses, V. K., Lichter, E. A. and Jonasson, O. (1971), Isoimmunization of hemodialysis patients: Leukocyte-poor versus blood transfusions. *Transplant. Proc.*, **3,** 365

Ceppellini, R., Curtoni, E. S., Mattiuz, P. L., Leigheb, G., Visetti, M. and Colombani, A. (1966). Survival of test skin grafts in man: Effect of genetic relationship and of blood groups in compatibility. *Ann. N.Y. Acad. Sci.*, **129,** 421

Cochrum, K., Kountz, S., Belzer, F., Perkins, H. and Payne, R. (1973). Correlation of MLC with graft survival. *Transplant. Proc.*, **5,** 391

Dausset, J. (1958). Iso-Leuco-anticorps. *Acta Haemat. (Basel)*, **20,** 156

Dausset, J. (1969). Histocompatibility studies in haplo-identical genetic combinations. *Transplant. Proc.*, **1,** 649

Dausset, J. (1971). The genetics of transplantation antigens. *Transplant. Proc.*, **3,** 8

Dausset, J. and Hors, J. (1971). Analysis of 221 renal transplants. Influence of cross-reactions between donor and recipient HL-A antigens. *Transplant. Proc.*, **3**, 1004

Dausset, J. and Hors, J. (1972). L'Association France transplant. II. Les transplantations de reins effectuees entre donneurs et receveurs groupes dans le systeme HL-A. *Presse Med.*, **1**, 1273

Dausset, J., Rapaport, F. T., Ivanyi, P. and Colombani, J. (1965). Tissue allo-antigens and transplantation. *Histocompatibility Testing* 1965, p. 63 (H. Balner, F. J. Cleton, and J. G. Eernisse, editors). Copenhagen: Munksgaard

Dausset, J., Rapaport, F. T., Legrand, L., Colombani, J. and Marcelli-Barge, A. (1970). Skin allograft survival in 238 human subjects. Role of HL-A sub-loci. *Histocompatibility Testing* 1970 (P. I. Terasaki, editor). Copenhagen: Munksgaard

Dossetor, J. B. and Olson, L. A. (1972). Evidence of latent sensitization to HL-A antigens. *Transplantation*, **13**, 576

Eijsvoogel, V. P., van Rood, J. J., du Toit, E. D. and Schellekens, P. Th. A. (1972). Position of a locus determining mixed lymphocyte reaction distinct from the known HL-A loci. *Eur. J. Immunol.*, **2**, 413

Garovoy, M. R., Franco, V., Zschaeck, D., Carpenter, C. B., Strom, T. B. and Merrill, J. P. (1973). Direct lymphocyte-mediated cytotoxicity as an assay of presensitization. *Lancet*, **1**, 573

Halgrimson, C. G., Rapaport, F. T., Terasaki, P. I., Porter, K. A., Andres, G., Penn, I., Putnam, C. W. and Starzl, T. E. (1971). Net histocompatibility ratios (NHR) for clinical transplantation. *Transplant. Proc.*, **3**, 140

Hamburger, J. J. *et al.* (1962). Renal homotransplantation in man after radiation of the recipient: Experience with six cases since 1959. *Amer. J. Med.*, **32**, 854

Hors, J., Feingold, N., Fradeliz, D. and Dausset, J. (1971). Critical evaluation of histocompatibility in 179 renal transplants. *Lancet*, **1**, 609

Hume, D. M., Lee, H. M., Williams, G. M., White, H. J. O., Ferre, H., Wolf, J. S., Prout, G. R., Jr., Slapak, M., O'Brien, J., Kilpatrick, S. J., Kauffman, H. M., Jr., and Cleveland, R. J. (1966). The comparative results of cadaver and related donor renal homografts in man, and the immunological implications of the outcome of second and paired transplants. *Ann. Surg.*, **164**, 352

Kissmeyer-Nielsen, F., Jorgensen, R. and Lamm, L. U. (1972). The HL-A system in clinical medicine. *Johns Hopkins Med. J.*, **131**, 385

Kissmeyer-Nielsen, F., and 35 other authors (1971). Scandiatransplant: Preliminary report of a kidney exchange program. *Transplant. Proc.*, **3**, 1019

Kissmeyer-Nielsen, F. and Thorsby, E. (1970). Human histocompatibility antigens.

Transplant. Rev., **4,** 1

Koch, C. T., van Hooff, J. P., van Leeuwen, A., van den Tweel, J., Frederiks, E., van der Steen, G., Schippers, H. M. A. and van Rood, J. J. (1972). *Histocompatibility Testing* (J. Dausset, editor) (In press)

McDevitt, H. O. and Benacerraf, B. (1969). Genetic control of specific immune responses. *Advances in Immunology*, p. 31 (F. J. Dixon and H. G. Kunkel, editors). New York and London: Academic Press

Mickey, M. R., Kreisler, M., Albert, E. D., Tanaka, N. and Terasaki, P. I. (1971). Analysis of HL-A incompatibility in human renal transplants. *Tissue Antigens*, **1,** 157

Mickey, M. R., Mittal, K. K., Opelz, G. and Terasaki, P. I. (1972). Transplant compatibility predictions based on antibody–antigen profile relationships. *Histocompatibility Testing* 1972 (J. Dausset, editor). Copenhagen: Munksgaard (In press)

Mittal, K. K. and Tersaki, P. I. (1972). Cross-reactivity in the HL-A system. *Tissue Antigens*, **2,** 94

Morris, P. J., Ting, A. and Stocker, J. (1968). Leucocyte antigens in renal transplantation. I. The paradox of blood transfusions in renal transplantation. *Med. J. Aust.*, **2,** 1088

Morris, P. J. (1971). Analyses of histocompatibility in cadaver renal transplantation. *Transplant. Proc.*, **3,** 1030

Oliver, R. T. D., Sachs, J. A., Festenstein, H., Pegrum, G. D. and Moorehead, J. F. (1972). Influence of HL-A matching, antigenic strength and immune responsiveness on outcome of 349 cadaver renal grafts. *Lancet*, **11,** 1381

Opelz, G., Mickey, M. R. and Terasaki, P. I. (1972a). Identification of unresponsive kidney transplant recipients. *Lancet*, **1,** 868

Opelz, G., Mickey, M. R. and Terasaki, P. I. (1972b). Prolonged survival of second human kidney transplants. *Science*, **178,** 617

Opelz, G., Mickey, M. R. and Terasaki, P. I. (1973). (To be published)

Opelz, G., Sengar, D. P. S., Mickey, M. R. and Terasaki, P. I. (1973). Effect of blood transfusions on subsequent kidney transplants. *Transplant. Proc.*, **5,** 253

Opelz, G. and Terasaki, P. I. (1972a). Histocompatibility matching utilizing responsiveness as a new dimension. *Transplant. Proc.*, **4,** 433

Opelz, G. and Terasaki, P. I. (1972b). Second kidney transplants and presensitization *Transplant. Proc.*, **4,** 743

Overweg, J. and Engelfriet, C. P. (1969). Cytotoxic leucocyte iso-antibodies formed during the first pregnancy. *Vox Sang.* (*Basel*), **16,** 97

Patel, R. and Briggs, W. (1971). Limitation of lymphocyte cytotoxicity crossmatch test in recipients of kidney transplants having preformed antileukocyte antibodies

New Engl. J. Med., **284**, 1016

Patel, R. and Myrberg, S. (1970). Value of prospective tissue typing in kidney transplantation between HL-A identical siblings. *Brit. Med. J.*, **2**, 709

Rapaport, F. T. and Dausset, J. (1970). Ranks of donor–recipient histocompatibility for human transplantation. *Science*, **167**, 1260

Sengar, D. P. S., Opelz, G. and Terasaki, P. I. (1973). Outcome of kidney transplants and suppression of mixed leukocyte culture by plasma. *Transplant. Proc.*, **5**, 641

Simonsen, M. (1965). Strong transplantation antigens in man. *Lancet*, **1**, 415

Starzl, T. E. (1964). *Experience in Renal Transplantation.* W. B. Saunders Co.

Staub Nielsen, L. and Svejgaard, A. (1972). HL-A immunization and HL-A types in pregnancy. *Int. Symp. on Standardization of HL-A Reagents*, Copenhagen, Vol. 18

Stickel, O. L., Seigler, J. F. and Amos, D. B. (1970). Immunogenetics of consanguineous allografts in man. 2. Correlation of renal allografting with HL-A genotyping. *Ann. Surg.*, **172**, 160

Tanaka, N., Takasugi, M. and Terasaki, P. I. (1971). Presensitization to transplants detected by cellular immunity tests. *Transplantation*, **12**, 514

The Tenth Report of the Human Transplant Registry. *J. Amer. Med. Ass.*, **221**, 1495

Terasaki, P. I. and McClelland, J. D. (1964). Microdroplet assay of human serum cytotoxins. *Nature (London)*, **204**, 998

Terasaki, P. I., Mandell, M., van de Water, J. and Edginton, T. S. (1964). Human blood lymphocyte cytotoxicity reaction with allogenic antisera. *Ann. NY Acad. Sci.*, **120**, 332

Terasaki, P. I., Marchioro, T. L. and Starzl, T. E. (1965). Serotyping of human lymphocyte antigens. II. Preliminary trials on long-term kidney homograft survivors. *Nat. Acad. Sci.*, **1229**, 83

Terasaki, P. I. and Mickey, M. R. (1971). Histocompatibility-transplant correlation, reproducibility, and new matching methods. *Transplant. Proc.*, **3**, 1057

Thorsby, E., Sandberg, L., Lindholm, A., Mayr, W., Jorgenson, F. and Kissmeyer-Nielsen, F. (1971). Polymorphism of the HL-A system. *Transplant. Proc.*, **3**, 101

Ting, A., Hasegawa, T., Ferrone, S., Reisfeld, R. A. and Terasaki, P. I. (1973). Presensitization detected by sensitive crossmatch tests. *Transplant. Proc.*, **5**, 813

van Hooff, J. P., Schippers, H. M. A., van der Steen, G. J. and van Rood, J. J. (1972). Efficacy of HL-A matching in Eurotransplant. *Lancet*, **II**, 1385

van Rood, J. J. (1971). The (relative) importance of HL-A matching in kidney transplantation. *Progress in Immunology*, p. 1027 (B. Amos, editor). Copenhagen: Munksgaard

van Rood, J. J., Koch, C. T., van Hooff, J. P., van Leeuwen, A., van den Tweel, J. G., Frederiks, E., Schippers, H. M. A., Hendriks, G. and van der Steen, G. J. (1973).

Graft survival in unrelated donor-recipient pairs matched for MLC and HL-A. *Transplant. Proc.*, **5**, 409

van Rood, J. J. and van Leeuwen, A. (1963). Leucocyte grouping. A method and its application. *J. Clin. Invest.*, **42**, 1382

van Rood, J. J., van Leeuwen, A., Schippers, A., Ceppellini, R., Mattiuz, P. L. and Curtoni, S. (1966). Leukocyte groups and their relation to homotransplantation. *Ann. NY Acad. Sci.*, **129**, 467

Walford, R. L., Gallagher, R. and Staarda, J. R. (1964). Serologic typing of human lymphocytes with immune sera after homografting. *Science*, **144**, 868

Wonham, V. A., Winn, J. H. and Russell, P. S. (1971). Serotyping and genetic analysis in the selection of related renal allograft donors. *New Engl. J. Med.*, **284**, 509

5

Mixed Leukocyte Culture and Cell-Mediated Lympholysis Assays: Models of Allograft Rejection

F. H. Bach and Marilyn L. Bach*

One approach to match donor and recipient for transplantation involves the use of *in vitro* models for study of the different phases of the homograft reaction. By far the most common one which has been used in this regard is the mixed leukocyte culture (MLC) test. The MLC test (Bain *et al.*, 1964; Bach and Hirschhorn, 1964) serves as an *in vitro* model of the recognition phase of the homograft reaction. As such it is useful for the study of histocompatibility and cellular mechanisms of graft rejection. More recently the MLC test has been combined with *in vitro* assays for cell-mediated lympholysis (CML). Lymphocytes sensitized in MLC are, after a number of days, cytotoxic to chromate (^{51}Cr) labeled target cells carrying histocompatibility antigens to which the lymphocytes are sensitized. This allows the *in vitro* study of the effector phase of the homograft reaction. Since the techniques used for the studies reported herein have been published, we will simply refer to the appropriate papers for the methodological details.

Stimulation in MLC tests (Bach and Voynow, 1966; Bach *et al.*, 1970; Hartzman *et al.*, 1971) is for the most part dependent on differences for the major histocompatibility complex (MHC). To the extent that it can be critically determined, this is

---

Supported by NIH grants AI 08439 and GM 15422; National Foundation-March of Dimes grant CRBS 246; and ONR grant N00014-67-A-0128-0003.

*MLB is a recipient of the Faculty Research Award of the American Cancer Society.
This is Paper No. 1637 from the Laboratory of Genetics, University of Wisconsin, Madison, Wisconsin 53706.

true in man (HL-A) (Bach and Amos, 1967), mouse (H-2) (Dutton, 1965; Dutton, 1966) and rat (AgB) (Silvers *et al.*, 1967), although exceptions have been reported in the mouse (Festenstein, 1972). In mouse the MHC includes two serologically defined (SD) loci, H-2K and H-2D, the immune response (Ir) loci and the Ss-Slp locus (loci). In man only the two SD loci (LA and FOUR of the HL-A system) have been identified to date. The finding in man that cells of siblings fail to stimulate each other in MLC approximately 25 per cent of the time, whereas cells of virtually all unrelated individuals tested stimulate, suggests that differences of a single genetic region control reactivity in MLC (Bach, 1966). In collaboration with Amos (Bach and Amos, 1967) it was possible to show that this genetic region was either the same as or closely linked to that controlling the SD antigens of the LA and FOUR loci.

In those initial studies, Amos and Bach (Amos and Bach, 1968) suggested that the genetic region may be more complex than would be suggested by the serological studies alone. Whereas in the great majority of cases cells of two siblings who had inherited the same MHC chromosomes as defined serologically did not stimulate in MLC, we studied two siblings who had inherited the same SD loci antigens (a finding that has since been confirmed with the much more sophisticated serology now available) but whose cells did stimulate in MLC. We suggested that 'a discrepancy of this kind might be expected if crossing-over had occurred and the part of the HL-A chromosome associated with the cross-over had no detectable antigens associated with it' (Bach *et al.*, 1969). The suggestion was that the two SD loci identical siblings were different for a locus which can be defined by a lymphocyte response (a lymphocyte defined—LD-difference) secondary to a recombinational event in one of the parents. This suggestion has received support from the studies of Plate *et al.* (Plate *et al.*, 1970), the more informative family study of Yunis and Amos (Yunis and Amos, 1971), and the extensive studies of Eijsvoogel, van Rood and their colleagues (Eijsvoogel *et al.*, 1972b). This hypothesis is diagrammed in Figure 5.1 (Yunis and Amos, 1971). Each bar represents the chromosomal region containing the MHC in man. Numbers refer to existing HL-A (SD) antigen specificities. Each individual (father, mother, and their offspring A, B, C, D, E) contains two homologous MHC regions. Sibs A, B, C, and D represent the standard Mendelian segregation pattern of this genetic region. Sib E contains HL-A specificities from the white paternal chromosome and the LD specificity fiom the darkened paternal chromosome. Such an event would be the product of a genetic recombination (chromosomal breakage and reunion) in one of the paternal spermatogonia. Note that sibs A and E are identical in SD antigens, yet sib A will recognize LD specificity X on E as foreign, and E will recognize the LD antigen W as foreign cells from sib A, thereby explaining MLC stimulation despite HL-A identity. Note also that sibs C and E are only haploidentical

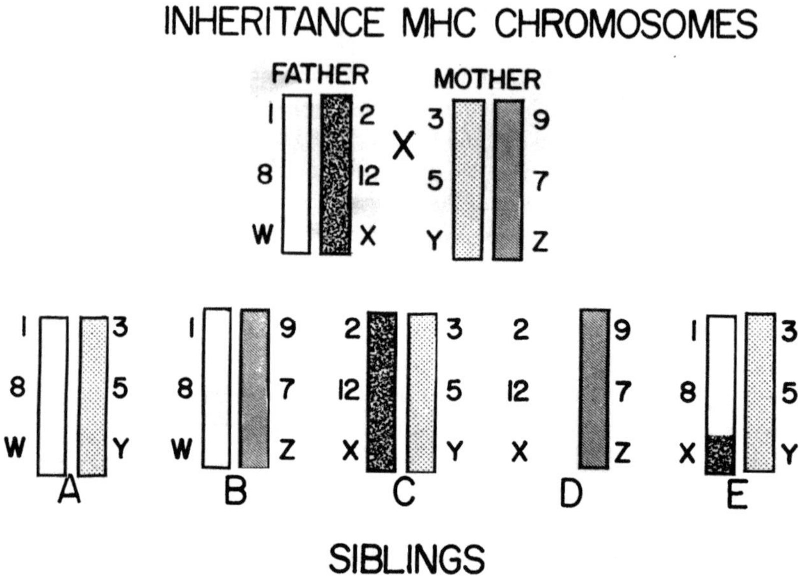

Figure 5.1 *Inheritance of MHC chromosomes in a family. The Figure is explained in the text.*

with respect to HL-A antigens, while both carry X and Y LD specificities. In such cases there is either little or in some cases no MLC stimulation (Yunis and Amos, 1971; Eijsvoogel *et al.*, 1972b). These findings could be explained either by weak stimulation caused by the SD antigen in some cases or by an additional LD locus between the FOUR and LA loci (Bach, 1972).

Studies in mouse give further information in this regard. The elegant and pioneering studies of Snell, Gorer, and many others for the past several decades defining the mouse MHC make this an ideal animal species for further study. A simplified genetic map of the mouse MHC is given in Figure 5.2. The H-2K locus is proximal to the

————H-2K————Ir-1————Ss-Slp————H-2D————

Figure 5.2 *A map of the mouse MHC showing the two SD loci, H-2K and H-2D, with the Ir and Ss-Slp loci in between. The map is discussed in the text.*

centromere and thus written to the left of H-2D (Klein and Shreffler, 1972). (These two SD loci are analogous to the LA and FOUR loci of HL-A.) Between these loci

Table 5.1 *MLC studies in C57BL/6 and H(zl) Mice*

AA_m	3755 ± 812	BB_m	9338 ± 1404	CC_m	3731 ± 741
AB_m	17 007 ± 2198 $P < 0.001$	BA_m	17 058 ± 1307 $P < 0.001$	CA_m	28 099 ± 2310 $P < 0.001$
AC_m	38 420 ± 2619 $P < 0.001$	BC_m	69 223 ± 5222 $P < 0.001$	CB_m	24 871 ± 2245 $P < 0.001$

A C57BL/6
B H(zl)
C B10.BR

are the Ir (immune response) loci (McDevitt and Benacerraf, 1972) as well as the Ss-Slp locus (Passmore and Shreffler, 1970). The Ss locus controls the quantitative level of a serum protein; the Slp locus (which may be the same as the Ss locus) controls the presence of a serum antigen. This antigen is expressed only if the Slp^a gene is present and then only in males.

Our initial studies, in collaboration with Dr Donald Bailey, were designed to obtain evidence for the existence of LD differences in the MHC, i.e. those which are not detected serologically with the usual method of immunization and testing but which can cause stimulation in MLC. Bailey *et al.* had discovered a spontaneous mutation in the MHC in C57BL/6 mice (Bailey *et al.*, 1971). The mutant mice, H(zl), are genetically identical (including serological identity at H-2K and H-2D) to C57BL/6 mice except for a mutation in the MHC which results in H(zl) skin graft rejection by C57BL/6 mice and vice versa. It is not clear whether the mutation in the H(zl) mice is between H-2K and Ss-Slp, within the H-2K locus or to the left of H-2K. Despite extensive immunization schedules these workers have been unable to obtain agglutinating or cytotoxic antisera against the 'difference'. There is stimulation in both directions in MLC experiments. One representative experiment including cells of a third mouse strain differing from C57BL/6 and H(zl) at the MHC is shown in Table 5.1. In each case a significantly higher number of counts per minute is incorporated in the allogenic mixtures than into the control isogeneic ones. There is thus reciprocal MLC stimulation as there is reciprocal skin graft rejection (Plate *et al.*, 1970; Widmer *et al.*, 1972).

Further experiments involving C57BL/6 and H(zl) were designed to determine

Table 5.2 *CML in C57BL/6 and H(zl)*

MLC sensitization			*CML destruction*		
Mixture	*Mean c.p.m. ± SD of [³H] thymidine incorporation*	*Target*	*Mean c.p.m. ± SD*	*Mean minus spontaneous release*	*Per cent ⁵¹Cr release*
H(zl)[H(zl)]$_m$	10 615 ± 1449	H(zl)	1329 ± 62*	−419	−42.5
		B6†	1256 ± 89	−289	−33.6
		BR	1515 ± 63	−452	−38.3
H(zl)(B6)$_m$	22 713 ± 968	B6	2243 ± 161	698	81.1
		H(zl)	1695 ± 198	− 53	− 5.4
		BR	2028 ± 107	61	5.2
B6(B6)$_m$	13 117 ± 470	B6	1142 ± 22	−403	−46.8
		H(zl)	1254 ± 12	−494	−50.1
		BR	1475 ± 66	492	−41.6
B6[H(zl)]$_m$	73 083 ± 2522	H(zl)	2617 ± 84	869	88.1
		B6	1499 ± 78	− 46	− 5.3
		BR	2448 ± 83	481	40.7

*c.p.m. of ^{51}Cr released
†C57BL/6 is referred to as B6; B10.BR as BR

Lymph node cell suspensions from the same animals used for MLC sensitization were cultured in RPMI containing 5% human plasma at 5 × 10^6 cells/ml, in metal-closed glass tubes (1 ml per tube). After 24 h of incubation 25 μl of PHA-M (Difco) were added to each tube. PHA stimulated lymph node cells harvested at the end of culture (day 4) were incubated in 0.5 ml autochthonous media containing 250 μCi

$^{51}Cr(Na_2CrO_4$—New England Nuclear) at 37 °C for 60 min. Labeled cells were washed 3 times in ice cold phosphate buffered saline (PBS) and suspended in 5% RPMI. Target cell concentration was adjusted to give 1×10^4 viable cells per 0.1 ml of suspension. 7.5×10^5 viable effector cells from MLC were combined with 10^4 labeled target cells in a final volume of 0.2 ml in Linbro (IS-MRC-96TC) microtiter plates and incubated for 4 h in 5% CO_2 and air at 37 °C. Aliquots of released ^{51}Cr removed from triplicate cultures were counted in a Nuclear Chicago gamma counter. Per cent CML is calculated as follows:

$$\frac{\text{c.p.m. (released in CML)} - \text{c.p.m. (spontaneous release)}}{\text{c.p.m. (freeze-thaw release)} - \text{c.p.m. (spontaneous release)}} \times 100$$

Spontaneous release of target: H(zl) = 1748 ± 215; C57BL/6 = 1545 ± 15;
B10.BR = 1967 ± 1
Maximum release of target: H(zl) = 2734 ± 32; C57BL/6 = 2406 ± 40;
B10.BR = 3148 ± 61

---

whether differences existing between them, in addition to their ability to produce an MLC, are also functional in allowing the effector phase of the homograft reaction as measured by CML.

Effector lymphocytes sensitized *in vitro* were tested for the ability to mediate specific killing of ^{51}Cr-labeled target lymphocytes (Widmer *et al.*, 1972). Table 5.2 shows the results of an experiment representative of the three experiments performed. Cells from H(zl) animals sensitized to C57BL/6 in MLC caused 81% lysis of C57BL/6 target cells. Specificity of the reaction is demonstrated by the release of only 5% of the ^{51}Cr from B10.BR target lymphocytes and −5% from control H(zl) target lymphocytes. The cytotoxicity between C57BL/6 and H(zl), like the graft rejection and MLC, is reciprocal. C57BL/6 cells sensitized to H(zl) cause 88% ^{51}Cr release from H(zl) target cells, with 41% killing of B10.BR, and −5% of control C57BL/6 target cells. Killing of B10.BR target cells by C57BL/6 cells sensitized to H(zl) is probably explained by sharing of target antigens by H(zl) and B10.BR.

The findings discussed above from man, as well as this finding in the mouse, forced a re-evaluation of the genetic and immunological complexity of the MHC as forcefully dictated by the work of Yunis and Amos (Yunis and Amos, 1971). We have, in collaboration with Dr Jan Klein (Bach *et al.*, 1972a; 1972b), studied a large number of congenic strains of mice carrying recombinant MHC chromosomes—strains that are genetically identical except for certain regions of the MHC. The MHC genotype for any given mouse strain is identified by the H-2 chromosome from which each of the four regions (H-2K, Ir, Ss-Slp, and H-2D) is derived. Several different mouse

Table 5.3 *Strains used in mouse MHC studies*

Strain	*H-2*	*K*	*Ir-1*	*Ss-Slp*	*D*
C57BL/6	b	B	B	B	B
B10.BR	k	K	K	K	K
B10.D2	d	D	D	D	D
B10.A	a	K	K	D	D
B10.A(1R)	h-Sg	K	K	D	B
B10.A(2R)	h-2Sg	K	K	D	B
B10.A(3R)	i-Sg	B	B	D	D
B10.A(4R)	h-3Sg	K	K	B	B
B10.G	q	Q	Q	Q	Q
B10.AKM	m	K	K	K	Q
AQR	y-Klj	Q	K	D	D
B10.T(6R)	y-Sgi	Q	Q	Q	D

strains will be referred to in these studies. The MHC genotypes are given in Table 5.3. This allows us to test two animals differing for only some segments of the MHC. Our results indicate that the strongest MLC activation is associated not with MHC SD loci incompatibility but rather with differences for the Ir region. H-2K and H-2D differences without Ir region differences results in relatively weak MLC stimulation. In some cases we have found mouse strain combinations that have, as in the study with Bailey, only LD differences (with SD loci identity) whose cells likewise stimulate in MLC. In at least two of these cases the LD loci can be more specifically localized.

Stimulation in allogeneic mixtures is expressed and evaluated in two ways. First, to test whether stimulation exists in a given allogeneic mixture, a *t*-test is performed on the log converted c.p.m. of the allogeneic mixture compared to the log c.p.m. in the isogeneic control mixture (the same responding cells with isogenic or syngeneic mitomycin C treated 'stimulating cells'). The significance of stimulation is then expressed with a p value. Second, to compare the response of cells of one strain to a number of different stimulating cells, for instance differing from the responding cells by different regions of the MHC, results in each combination are expressed as a ratio of c.p.m. in the allogeneic mixture divided by c.p.m. in the isogeneic control. Whereas there are probably drawbacks to the use of the ratio method, it is one way to pool results from several experiments testing the same combinations. It also permits some measure of the relative strength of stimulation in the MLC; for instance, the average ratio of stimulation observed in strain combinations that differ for all four of the MHC regions is 7.2.

Whereas some mouse strain combinations that differ for only the H-2D region fail to stimulate, other such combinations do show significant, although relatively weak, stimulation. The results shown in Table 5.4 are from an experiment in which we noted one of the stronger stimulating combinations with only an H-2D region difference. B10.AKM cells are included as control cells. Response of B10.G cells to B10.T(6R) mitomycin C treated stimulating cells is significantly stronger than the response in the opposite direction at all four times that this combination has been tested. In fact, the response of B10.T(6R) cells to B10.G stimulating cells was not significant in some of the experiments.

We have tested one combination which differs only for the H-2K region, B10.A

Table 5.4 *MLC studies in B10.G and B10.T(6R) mouse strains*

	Stimulators		
	B10.G	*B10.T(6R)*	*B10.AKM*
Responders:			
B10.G	3512 ± 983*	10 434 ± 1300 $P < 0.005$†	25 388 ± 3286 $P < 0.001$
B10.T(6R)	7348 ± 720 $P < 0.025$	3440 ± 1409	44 151 ± 1472 $P < 0.001$
B10.AKM	23 627 ± 4298 $P < 0.001$	39 535 ± 3982 $P < 0.001$	3727 ± 1068

*counts per minute (c.p.m.) ± standard deviation
†probability that c.p.m. in allogeneic mixture differs from the c.p.m. in isogeneic control mixture using the same responding cell

versus AQR. This combination differs for minor loci segregating independently of the MHC as well as the MHC. The results obtained in four separate experiments involving these two strain combinations, tested in both directions in each experiment, also suggest that there is little stimulation in this combination. One example of an MLC test in this combination is given in Table 5.5. Experiments involving B10.T(6R) will be discussed below.

Table 5.5 *MLC studies in AQR, B10.T(6R) and B10.A mouse strains*

	Stimulators		
	B10.A	*B10.T(6R)*	*AQR*
Responders:			
B10.A	(6856 ± 1416)*	25 823 ± 1583 $P < 0.001$†	8425 ± 722 $0.1 < P < 0.2$
B10.T(6R)	52 402 ± 4292 $P < 0.001$	(3440 ± 1409)	44 181 ± 2071 $P < 0.001$
AQR	7869 ± 439 $0.01 < P < 0.025$	32 087 ± 1900 $P < 0.001$	(3567 ± 1190)

*counts per minute (c.p.m.) ± standard deviation
†probability that c.p.m. in allogeneic mixture differs from the c.p.m. in isogeneic control mixture using the same responding cell

One would thus have to conclude that H-2D region differences and H-2K region differences alone are only weakly stimulatory and in some cases not at all stimulatory. It cannot be ruled out that the failure to obtain stimulation in some cases represents insensitivity of the MLC method being used.

Most interesting are those MHC differences with SD loci identity. One set of three strains, B10.A(1R), B10.A(2R), and B10.A(4R), is of special interest since these strains were derived from different cross-overs from the same F_1 genotype. The genotypes of the $H\text{-}2^a/H\text{-}2^b$ F_1 heterozygote and three resultant recombinant chromosomes are given in Figure 5.3. Since the 1R, 2R and 4R strains are derived in this manner and are on a congenic background, they differ only for the portion of the MHC between the two SD loci as indicated. 1R and 2R are, with respect to the markers available to us, identical, although the recombinational events may, and quite likely did, take place at different positions. Both 1R and 2R cells reproducibly and significantly stimulate the cells of the 4R strain; however, there is either very weak or no response of 1R or 2R cells to 4R stimulating cells if compared in the same experiment (Table 5.6). Since this unidirectional response is an unusual finding we have tested the cells

$H\text{-}2K^k$	$Ir\text{-}1^k$	$Ss\text{-}Slp^d$	$H\text{-}2D^d$	H-2 a/b heterozygote
$H\text{-}2K^b$	$Ir\text{-}1^b$	$Ss\text{-}Slp^b$	$H\text{-}2D^b$	
$H\text{-}2K^k$	$Ir\text{-}1^k$	$Ss\text{-}Slp^d$	$H\text{-}2D^b$	B10.A(1R) chromosome
$H\text{-}2K^k$	$Ir\text{-}1^k$	$Ss\text{-}Slp^d$	$H\text{-}2D^b$	B10.A(2R) chromosome
$H\text{-}2K^k$	$Ir\text{-}1^k$	$Ss\text{-}Slp^b$	$H\text{-}2D^b$	B10.A(4R) chromosome

Figure 5.3 *The strains B10.A(1R), B10.A(2R) and B10.A(3R) were all derived from a H-2 a/b heterozygote. The genotype of the heterozygote as well as the recombinant chromosomes are shown in this Figure. 1R and 2R were derived by a recombinational event between Ss-Slp and H-2D; 4R by a recombinational event between Ir-1 and Ss-Slp. 2R and 4R differ for an Ir locus* (R. Liebermann, *Fed. Proc.*, 31, 777, 1972).

of these strains at multiple concentrations of stimulating and responding cells assayed on several days to maximize response using this MLC method. Whereas we have obtained an occasional stimulation value where cells of 1R or 2R respond weakly but significantly to stimulating cells of 4R, for the most part MLC tests in this direction have failed to stimulate. Although in this particular combination the Slp antigen is present in mice of the 1R and 2R genotype but absent from mice of the 4R genotype, our studies suggest that stimulation is not due to the Slp antigen, but to LD loci of the MHC (Bach *et al.*, 1972a; 1972b).

The other strain combination of great interest is that of AQR-B10.T(6R). This combination differs not only for the MHC genotypes as shown in Table 5.3 but also for minor loci. Our studies indicate, however, that the minor loci differences either

Table 5.6 *MLC studies in B10.A(1R), B10.A(2R) and B10.A(4R) mouse strains*

	Stimulators			
	B10.A(1R)	*B10.A(2R)*	*B10.A(4R)*	*B10.D2*
Responders:				
B10.A(1R)	5500 ± 1100*	5058 ± 1517 $0.5 < P$†	5081 ± 1410 $0.5 < P$	27 691 ± 3080 $P < 0.001$
B10.A(2R)	5590 ± 1045 $0.2 < P$	5644 ± 1816	5947 ± 1316 $0.5 < P$	25 462 ± 1457 $P < 0.001$
B10.A(4R)	5976 ± 1412 $P < 0.001$	5472 ± 201 $P < 0.001$	1926 ± 304	22 952 ± 2487 $P < 0.001$
B10.D2	49 868 ± 8010 $P < 0.001$	41 911 ± 11 244 $P < 0.001$	23 918 ± 5667 $P < 0.001$	3898 ± 472

*counts per minute (c.p.m.) ± standard deviation
†probability that c.p.m. in allogeneic mixture differs from the c.p.m. in isogeneic control mixture using the same responding cell

do not lead to MLC activation or are extremely weak in doing so. This is based on the finding already discussed above (Table 5.5). In those examples cells of AQR were tested with the cells of B10.A which differ from AQR at H-2K as well as the same two minor loci by which AQR and B10.T(6R) differ. [B10.A and B10.T(6R) are genetically identical except for the MHC]. Since there was repeatedly very little stimulation in the AQR-B10.A combination, it must be concluded that, even if the H-2K difference does not lead to any MLC activation, stimulation due to minor loci differences is very weak.

Stimulation in the mixture of AQR-B10.T(6R) cells is strong and highly significant. The results in one experiment are shown in Table 5.5. There is stimulation in both directions in one-way MLC tests and this is highly significant in both directions. We must therefore again conclude that stimulation is associated with LD differences of the MHC, although in this particular case we cannot conclude whether MLC stimulation is due to LD differences located between the two SD loci and/or outside the SD loci.

Since so few strain combinations are available which differ for only one of the four regions of the MHC, it is worthwhile to analyze strain combinations that differ for two or more of the MHC regions as well as to obtain an indication of which of the regions is the most important for MLC stimulation. An example of an experiment providing this type of data is given in Table 5.7. In this particular case, B10.A(2R) cells are used as responding cells and a number of other strains, congenic with the B10.A(2R) cells,

Table 5.7 *Response of B10.A(2R) to various stimulators*

Stimulating cells	*K*	*Ir-1*	*Ss-Slp*	*D*	*Ratio*
B10.G	Q	Q	Q	Q	5.93
B10	B	B	B	B	5.81
B10.A(3R)	B	B		D	9.71
B10.A(4R)			B		1.75
B10.BR			K	K	1.89
B10.A				D	1.74

are used as stimulating cells. For each combination those regions of the MHC which are carried by the stimulating cells and which are different from the responding cells are designated. Thus, for instance, B10.A(2R) cells differ from B10.BR cells for the Ss-Slp and H-2D regions but are identical for the H-2K and Ir regions. Stimulation in each combination is indicated by the ratio method. This experiment is chosen to demonstrate what is the general pattern of stimulation we have found in the 173 different strain combinations we have tested in one-way mixed leukocyte culture involving 15 different strains: if there is an Ir region difference, there is strong stimulation; if there is no Ir region difference, the stimulation is relatively weaker.

All data we obtained in collaboration with Dr Jan Klein are summarized in this manner in Table 5.8. For those combinations in which the Ir region differs, the average ratio of stimulation varies from 5.8 to 8.3; in those cases where there is no Ir difference, it varies from 1.4 to 3.4.

Table 5.8 *MLC stimulation in strain combinations differing for various regions of the MHC*

MHC regions which are different	*Range**	*Ratio of stimulation (average)*
K, Ir-1, Ss-Slp, D	1.2–33.6	7.2
K, Ir-1, Ss-Slp	1.4–15.7	6.1
K, Ir-1, D	3.3–20.5	7.0
K, Ss-Slp, D	1.5– 8.6	3.3
Ir-1, Ss-Slp, D	2.7–15.1	8.3
K, Ir-1	3.2–18.3	6.6
K, Ss-Slp	no experiments	
Ir-1, Ss-Slp	2.7–12.8	5.8
K, D	3.0– 3.8	3.4
Ir-1, D	no experiments	
Ss-Slp, D	0.7– 4.7	2.0
K	0.8– 2.2	1.4
Ir-1	no experiments	
D	0.8– 5.4	1.8
Ss-Slp	0.6– 4.9	2.0
none	0.6– 1.9	1.2

*These numbers represent the lowest and highest ratios of stimulation noted

We must thus reevaluate our concept about the stimulatory molecules which are important for lymphocyte activation in MLC.

In vitro studies by Eijsvoogel and his colleagues (Eijsvoogel *et al.*, 1972a) showed that in a family in man, LD differences alone led to MLC activation without subsequent CML and that SD differences were needed for CML. Similarly, the work of Trinchieri, Ceppellini and their colleagues suggests a correlation between the SD phenotype and CML (Trinchieri, 1972). We have obtained similar results (Alter *et al.*, 1973) in certain mouse strain combinations, including the B10.A(4R)—B10.A(2R) combination mentioned above. (These results are given below.) In both human and mouse studies the differences needed for CML are either the SD antigens themselves or a presumed cell surface component determined by genes very closely linked to those determining the SD antigens.

Table 5.9 *MLC and CML studies in HL-A SD-identical unrelated individuals*

MLC	*Mean c.p.m. ± SD of [^3H] thymidine incorporated*	*Per cent CML ± SD target cells**			
		A	*B*	*C*	*X*
AA_m	293 ± 97	− 1.0 ± 4.8†			
AB_m	61 703 ± 5868	0.6 ± 4.6	4.1 ± 3.6	5.6 ± 1.0	5.4 ± 2.7
AC_m	48 213 ± 5202	8.1 ± 4.0	11.9 ± 2.7	13.4 ± 2.0	12.2 ± 3.1
BB_m	1424 ± 1470		−2.5 ± 3.2		
BA_m	75 983 ± 10 616	12.5 ± 4.0	3.8 ± 3.5	6.5 ± 1.4	5.4 ± 1.5
BC_m	58 121 ± 7099	9.6 ± 4.5	−0.4 ± 3.6	2.3 ± 1.4	0.0 ± 1.9
CC_m	1027 ± 119			0.6 ± 1.8	
CA_m	91 792 ± 4369	26.6 ± 5.4	5.0 ± 3.1	7.0 ± 1.9	12.6 ± 2.0
CB_m	72 305 ± 3490	13.5 ± 3.8	6.7 ± 3.0	6.4 ± 2.2	7.0 ± 2.7
AX_m	92 575 ± 883	4.7 ± 4.3			26.1 ± 2.4
BX_m	98 307 ± 6058		0.5 ± 3.5		35.4 ± 6.2
CX_m	117 408 ± 8881			4.2 ± 1.7	27.8 ± 2.7
XX_m	708 ± 472				0.5 ± 3.7
XA_m	84 422 ± 7787	52.7 ± 6.3	34.3 ± 4.4	33.5 ± 3.0	8.3 ± 7.2
XB_m	82 677 ± 2506	30.6 ± 7.5	19.7 ± 3.7	18.7 ± 2.3	5.5 ± 2.4
XC_m	84 681 ± 7447	59.1 ± 3.1	42.6 ± 4.4	38.8 ± 2.0	12.2 ± 4.1

*Cells A, B and C are HL-A 1, 2, 8, 12. Cell X is HL-A 10, 11. Effector to target cell ratio in CML is 70:1.

†The % CML is calculated by the following formula:

$$\frac{\text{experimental release} - \text{spontaneous release}}{\text{maximum release} - \text{spontaneous release}} \times 100$$

The dichotomy between MLC and CML holds not only in a family study in man and in inbred mouse strains, but also in unrelated human subjects.

We have studied MLC and CML reactions in five unrelated individuals having the same four HL-A antigens, 1, 2, 8, 12 (Bach *et al.*, 1973). Results of one experiment involving three of these individuals (A, B and C) are shown in Table 5.9. MLC activation assessed by tritiated thymidine incorporation is positive in all combinations as shown in column 2, yet there is little or no CML in combinations involving donor X (HL-A 10, 11) where cells A, B and C can either provoke (as stimulators in MLC) or provide (as effectors in CML) a good CML reaction.

The only case of markedly positive CML among the HL-A identical combinations is combination No. 8: C cells sensitized to A_m stimulating cells, tested on A target cells. This does not appear to be due to a greater non-specific 'lysability' of A targets since A effector cells do not cause significant lysis of A targets (combination No. 1) nor do effector cells not sensitized to antigens of A as seen in other experiments. We have previously reported that cells of A (donor K.M.) are significantly higher stimulators than other HL-A 1, 2, 8, 12 cells with an HL-A 1, 2, 8, 12 responder (Segall *et al.*, 1972). The biological significance, if any, of this conjunction of exceptions is unknown.

These findings give further support to the concept that the LD differences which result in MLC stimulation do not necessarily serve as targets for CML. The significant CML occurring on at least one target cell (Table 5.9, No. 8) despite apparent SD antigenic identity could be explained either by heterogeneity of the antigens (i.e. the cells do differ for SD) or by lympholysis directed against antigens other than SD. We have discussed this problem in the past in relation to a similar finding in two LD different mouse strains which are SD-identical, but give positive MLC and CML (Widmer *et al.*, 1972). In addition, the results presented here provide new and stronger evidence that the SD antigens, or the phenotypic product of a locus very closely linked to SD are the targets for CML. If the products of alleles at such a hypothetical locus are the CML targets, the alleles must be in marked linkage disequilibrium with those of the SD loci.

Our studies in mouse (referred to above) further investigate the rôle of LD and SD differences in CML. In certain strain combinations which are SD identical but different for LD (i.e. there is MLC reactivity) there is no CML. However, the presence of either an H-2K or an H-2D region difference (thus including an SD difference) is sufficient for significant CML to occur.

The two strain combinations (AQR-B10.T(6R) and B10.A(4R)-B10.A(2R)) of greatest interest in these studies have LD differences associated with MLC activation (Bach *et al.*, 1972a; 1972b) and graft versus host reactions (Livnat *et al.*, 1972), but are

SD identical. Table 5.10 shows the results of MLC and CML tests in these combinations. Despite significant CML activation, AQR effector cells do not lyse B10.A(6R) target cells nor do B10.T(6R) effector cells lyse AQR target cells. Both AQR and B10.T(6R) cells are capable of mediating CML when sensitized and tested against target cells which differ in several regions of the MHC: likewise these cells are extensively lysed when used as target cells in combinations differing in all four regions of the MHC. Similar results are obtained when B10.A(4R) cells are tested in combination with B10.A(2R) cells. Despite MLC activation there is no CML.

Table 5.11,A shows the results of experiments testing whether differences at either end of the MHC can lead to CML. In the first combination (B10.A-AQR) the effector and target cells differ for the H-2K region, but are identical for the Ir, Ss, and H-2D regions. There is no MLC activation nor CML in this combination. However, when B10.A is sensitized against B10.T(6R) which differs for the H-2K, Ir, and Ss regions one finds strong MLC activation and significant CML directed at the B10.T(6R) target cell. These B10.A effector cells are also cytotoxic to AQR target cells. Therefore, if the effector cells are properly activated the H-2K region difference alone is a sufficient target for CML.

Similarly when one sensitizes the effector cell population against only an H-2D region difference (B10.A(2R)–B10.A) there is neither MLC activation nor CML (Table 5.11,B). The B10.A(2R)–B10.D2 combination leads to strong MLC activation and CML; CML occurs also on the B10.A target cells which differ from the B10.A(2R) effector cells at only the H-2D region. Less CML occurs if the effector cell is confronted with a target cell carrying a different H-2K or H-2D region.

These studies (Alter *et al.*, 1973) confirm the observation in man that in some instances an LD difference is sufficient to give MLC activation but not sufficient to allow CML. Those combinations with SD differences and MLC activation lead to CML whether the SD differences are associated with the H-2K region or the H-2D region. This contrasts with the reported findings in one family in man where differences at one of the two SD loci appear to play the predominant role in CML (Eijsvoogel, 1972a).

Whether it is the serologically defined antigens themselves which are the targets for CML must be left open for further investigation. We have noted that significant CML occurs in the C57BL/6-H(zl) combination (Widmer *et al.*, 1972). These strains differ by a spontaneous mutation in the MHC which leads to reciprocal MLC activation, skin graft rejection and CML. Although it is possible that C57BL/6 and H(zl) differ by antigens that can be defined serologically, no such differences have been detected to date (Bailey *et al.*, 1971).

Table 5.10 *Results of MLC and CML tests*

	MLC (mean c.p.m. ± SD)	*MLC sensitization*		*CML assay*		
		Responding cell (effector)	*Stimulating cell (sensitizing)*	*Target cell*	*^{51}Cr released (mean c.p.m. ± SD)*	*% CML*
A†	45 841 ± 1921	AQR (QKDD)*	B10.T(6R) (QQQD)	AQR (QKDD)	489 ± 51	− 5.1
				B10.T(6R) (QQQD)	558 ± 50	2.2
	63 491 ± 4511	B10.T(6R) (QQQD)	AQR (QKDD)	B10.T(6R) (QQQD)	471 ± 7	5.0
				AQR (QKDD)	475 ± 23	− 6.0
	49 763 ± 1726	AQR (QKDD)	C57BL/10 (BBBB)	AQR (QKDD)	690 ± 41	9.5
				C57BL/10 (BBBB)	1158 ± 66	66.9
	70 687 ± 3425	B10.T(6R) (QQQD)	B10.A(2R) (KKDB)	B10.T(6R) (QQQD)	716 ± 18	15.3
				B10.A(2R) (KKDB)	2004 ± 58	74.5
	64 048 ± 1846	C57BL/10 (BBBB)	AQR (QKDD)	C57BL/10 (BBBB)	709 ± 20	7.3
				AQR (QKDD)	1749 ± 114	86.5
	52 782 ± 1534	C57BL/10 (BBBB)	B10.T(6R) (QQQD)	C57BL/10 (BBBB)	706 ± 6	7.0
				B10.T(6R) (QQQD)	1565 ± 151	85.4
	12 327 ± 1901	AQR (QKDD)	AQR (QKDD)	AQR (QKDD)	436 ± 31	8.9

	15 101 ± 529	B10.T(6R) (QQQD)	B10.T(6R) (QQQD)	B10.T(6R) (QQQD)	488 ± 35	− 3.6
	14 843 ± 3858	C57BL/10 (BBBB)	C57BL/10 (BBBB)	C57BL/10 (BBBB)	438 ± 14	− 28.5
B‡	18 729 ± 3810	B10.A(4R) (KKBB)	B10.A(2R) (KKDB)	B10.A(4R) (KKBB)	468 ± 25	− 4.6
				B10.A(2R) (KKDB)	469 ± 8	− 5.5
	98 911 ± 2753	B10.A(4R) (KKBB)	C57BL/10 (BBBB)	B10.A(4R) (KKBB)	747 ± 62	27.0
				C57BL/10 (BBBB)	1345 ± 30	74.1
	44 163 ± 5606	C57BL/10 (BBBB)	B10.A(2R) (KKDB)	C57BL/10 (BBBB)	679 ± 38	3.8
				B10.A(2R) (KKDB)	1184 ± 17	62.2
	6430 ± 2204	B10.A(4R) (KKBB)	B10.A(4R) (KKBB)	B10.A(4R) (KKBB)	437 ± 52	− 8.2
	18 057 ± 2815	C57BL/10 (BBBB)	C57BL/10 (BBBB)	C57BL/10 (BBBB)	578 ± 45	− 9.1

*The four capital letters (i.e. QKDC) refer to the various regions of the MHC as explained in the text

†The % CML is based on the following spontaneous release (SR) and maximum release (MR) values (mean of triplicates ± SD) for each target cell: AQR SR = 558 ± 6 MR = 1935 ± 53; B10.T(6R) SR = 531 ± 35 MR = 1742 ± 94; C57BL/10 SR = 653 ± 56 MR = 1408 ± 81; B10.A(2R) = 621 ± 77 MR = 2476 ± 179

‡The % CML is based on the following spontaneous release (SR) and maximum release (MR) values (mean ± SD of triplicates for each target cell: B10.A(4R) SR = 509 ± 42 MR = 1388 ± 116; B10.A(2R) SR = 527 ± 29 MR = 1582 ± 11; C57BL/10 SR = 662 ± 28 MR = 1585 ± 83

Table 5.11

		MLC sensitization		*CML assay*		
	MLC (mean c.p.m. ± SD)	*Responding cell (effector)*	*Stimulating cell (sensitizing)*	*Target cell*	*^{51}Cr released (mean c.p.m. ± SD)*	*%CML*
A*	14 819 ± 1406	B10.A (KKDD)	AQR (QKDD)	B10.A (KKDD)	469 ± 11	− 4.6
				AQR (QKDD)	372 ± 36	− 3.6
	44 777 ± 5237	B10.A (KKDD)	B10.T(6R) (QQQD)	B10.A (KKDD)	484 ± 21	− 1.4
				B10.T(6R) (QQQD)	534 ± 19	37.5
				AQR (QKDD)	623 ± 19	42.6
				C57BL/10 (BBBB)	383 ± 33	13.8
	14 487 ± 846	B10.A (KKDD)	B10.A (KKDD)	B10.A (KKDD)	417 ± 54	− 15.4

B†	13 725 ± 2236	B10.A(2R) (KKDB)	B10.A (KKDD)	B10.A(2R) (KKDB)	532 ± 142	– 4.9
				B10.A (KKDD)	552 ± 13	5.3
	79 236 ± 6902	B10.A(2R) (KKDB)	B10.D2 (DDDD)	B10.A(2R) (KKDB)	889 ± 67	24.9
				B10.D2 (DDDD)	1541 ± 140	72.3
				B10.A (KKDD)	1041 ± 32	78.5
				C57BL/10 (BBBB)	1232 ± 43	40.6
	10 423 ± 623	B10.A(2R) (KKDB)	B10.A(2R) (KKDB)	B10.A(2R) (KKDB)	434 ± 7	– 13.1

*The % CML is based on the following spontaneous release (SR) and maximum release (MR) values (mean of triplicates ± SD) for each target cell:

B10.A SR = 491 ± 20 MR = 974 ± 61; AQR SR = 391 ± 24 MR = 935 ± 45; B10.T(6R) SR = 328 ± 25 MR = 877 ± 66; C57BL/10 SR = 721 ± 73 MR = 1978 ± 30

†B10.A(2R) SR = 591 ± 23 MR = 1786 ± 60; B10.A SR = 516 ± 14 MR = 1184 ± 59; B10.D2 SR = 684 ± 47 MR = 1869 ± 34; C57BL/10 SR = 721 ± 73 MR = 1978 ± 30

SUMMARY

Evidence from both mouse and man thus suggests that the genetic elements of the major histocompatibility complex which are important in the activation of presumed T cells in the mixed leukocyte culture are genetically separable from those important in determining the serologically defined antigens. The importance of these lymphocyte defined (LD) components of the MHC is suggested by the following lines of investigation. First, there are the *in vitro* studies which suggest that differences for the LD components are important in generating cytotoxic cells active in the cell-mediated lympholysis assay. Second, there is the evidence that the MLC test is predictive of splenomegaly graft versus host reactions *in vivo* (it cannot be conclusively stated that the same genetic elements control the proliferation of cells in MLC as control the proliferation of cells in the splenomegaly GvHR; this seems like a very reasonable assumption however). Third, there is the evidence that at least in some mouse strains that differ only by LD differences (where no serological differences have been detected to date) there is skin graft rejection. Whether this indicates that in some cases the LD differences which activate cells in MLC are sufficient to lead to graft rejection or whether in these cases there is an additional difference for an LD target is not clear.

The evidence seen that at least in some cases the LD differences do not serve as an adequate target for CML *in vitro* has been discussed above. The *in vivo* significance of these findings has yet to be determined—as has the nature of the cell mediating CML.

From the point of view of transplantation biology these new findings regarding the dichotomy of both the genetic control and the cell populations active in the initial recognitive events versus the destructive phase as studied in CML provide new ways for dissecting the events leading to allograft rejection. From the point of view of histocompatibility testing the above findings, as well as the preliminary correlations which have been suggested by some between MLC reactivity and graft survival (Bach *et al.*, 1970; Koch *et al.*, 1972; Kountz *et al.*, 1972) makes it reasonable to suggest that evaluation of MLC reactivity should be included in any situation where this is possible. It may be that for allograft survival MLC (LD) identity is sufficient even given SD differences or that MLC disparity is (at least to a given point) acceptable given SD identity.

References

Alter, B. J., Schendel, D. J., Bach, M. L., Bach, F. H., Klein, J. and Stimpfling, J. (1973). Cell mediated lympholysis: importance of serologically defined H-2 regions. *J. Exp. Med.*, **137,** 1303

Amos, D. B. and Bach, F. H. (1968). Phenotypic expressions of the major histocompatibility locus in man (HL-A): Leukocyte antigens and mixed leukocyte culture reactivity. *J. Exp. Med.*, **128,** 623

Bach, F. H. (1966). Lymphocyte reactivity in mixed leukocyte cultures—its assays and genetics. In *In Vitro*, p. 32. Baltimore: Williams and Wilkins

Bach, F. H. (1972). In *Genetic Control of the Immune Response* (H. O. McDevitt and M. Landy, editors). New York: Academic Press

Bach, F. H. and Amos, D. B. (1967). HU-1: Major histocompatibility locus in man. *Science*, **156,** 1506

Bach, F. H. and Hirschhorn, K. (1964). Lymphocyte interaction: a potential *in vitro* histocompatibility test. *Science*, **143,** 813

Bach, F. H., Segall, M., Zier, K. S., Sondel, P. M., Alter, B. J. and Bach, M. L. (1973). Cell mediated immunity separation of cells involved in recognitive and destructive phases. *Science*, **180,** 403

Bach, F. H. and Voynow, N. K. (1966). One-way stimulation in mixed leukocyte culture. *Science*, **153,** 545

Bach, F. H., Widmer, M. B., Bach, M. L. and Klein, J. (1972a). Serologically defined and lymphocyte defined components of the major histocompatibility complex in the mouse. *J. Exp. Med.*, **136,** 1430

Bach, F. H., Widmer, M. B., Segall, M., Bach, M. L. and Klein, J. (1972b). Genetic and immunological complexity of major histocompatibility regions. *Science*, **176,** 1024

Bach, J. F., Debray-Sachs, M., Crosnier, J., Kreis, H. and Dormont, J. (1970a). Correlation between MLC performed before renal transplantation and kidney function. *Clin. Exp. Immunol.*, **6,** 821

Bach, M. L., Solliday, S. and Stambuk, M. (1970b). Detection of disparity in the mixed leukocyte culture test: a more rapid assay. In *Histocompatibility Testing 1970* (P. I. Terasaki, editor). p. 643. Copenhagen: Munksgaard

Bailey, D. W., Snell, G. D. and Cherry, M. (1971). Complementation and serological analysis of an H-2 mutant. In *Proc. Symp. Immunogenetics of the H2 System*, p. 155. Basel: S. Karger

Bain, B., Vas, M. R. and Lowenstein, L. (1964). The development of large mononuclear cells in mixed leukocyte cultures. *Blood*, **23,** 108

Dutton, R. W. (1965). Further studies of the stimulation of DNA synthesis in cultures of spleen cell suspensions by homologous cells in inbred strains of mice and rats. *J. Exp. Med.*, **122,** 759

Dutton, R. W. (1966). Spleen cell proliferation in response to homologous antigens studied in congenic resistant strains of mice. *J. Exp. Med.*, **123,** 655

Eijsvoogel, V. P., du Bois, M. J. G. J., Melief, C. J. M., de Groot-Kooy, M. L., Koning, C., van Leeuwen, A., van Rood, J., du Toit, E. and Schellekens, P. Th. A. (1972a). *Histocompatibility Testing* 1972. Proceedings of the Fifth International Histocompatibility Workshop Conf., Evian (In press)

Eijsvoogel, V. P., Koning, L., Groot-Kooy, L., Huismans, L., van Rood, J. J. and Schellekens, P. Th. A. (1972b). HL-A and MLC. *Transplantation Proc.*, **4** (In press)

Festenstein, H., Abbasi, K., Sachs, J. A. and Oliver, R. T. D. (1973). Serologically undetectable immune responses in transplantation. *Transplant. Proc.*, Vol. IV, No. 2, 219

Hartzman, R. J., Segall, M., Bach, M. L. and Bach, F. H. (1971). Histocompatibility Matching. VI. Miniaturization of the mixed leukocyte culture test: a preliminary test. *Transplantation*, **11,** 268

Klein, J. and Shreffler, D. C. (1972). Evidence supporting a two-gene model for the H-2 histocompatibility system in the mouse. *J. Exp. Med.*, **135,** 924

Koch, C. T., Frederiks, E. and van Rood, J. J. (1972). HL-A Identical Donor-Recipient Pairs. *Transplantation Proc.* (In press)

Perkins, H. A., Kountz, S. L., Belzer, F. O., Kidd, K. K. and Payne, R. O. (1973). Selection of Cadaver Kidney Donors with HL-A Phenotypes Identical to those of potential recipients. *Transplantation Proc.*, *V*, No. 1, 237

Livnat, S., Klein, J. and Bach, F. H. (1972). Graft versus host reactions in strains of mice identical for the serologically defined H-2 antigens. Submitted for publication.

McDevitt, H. O. and Benacerraf, B. (1972). Histocompatibility-linked immune response genes. *Science*, **175,** 273

Passmore, H. C. and Shreffler, D. C. (1970). A sex-linked serum protein variant in the mouse: inheritance and association with the H-2 region. *Biochem. Genet.*, **4,** 351

Plate, J. M., Ward, F. E. and Amos, D. B. (1970). The mixed leukocyte culture response between HL-A identical siblings. In *Histocompatibility Testing* 1970 (P. I. Terasaki, editor). p. 531. Copenhagen: Munksgaaard

Segall, M., Omodei-Zorini, C., Bach, F. H., Jorgensen, F. and Kissmeyer-Nielsen, F. (1973). HL-A antigens and mixed leukocyte culture (MLC) reactivity. *Transplantation Proc.*, *V*, No. 1, 338

Silvers, W. K., Wilson, D. B. and Palm, J. (1967). Mixed leukocyte reactions and histocompatibility in rats. *Science*, **155,** 703

Trinchieri, G., Bernoco, D., Curboni, S. E., Miggiano, V. C. and Ceppellini, R. (1972). Cell mediated lympholysis in man: relevance of HL-A antigens and antibodies. In *Histocompatibility Testing* 1972 (J. Dausset, editor). Copenhagen: Munksgaard (In press)

Widmer, M. B., Alter, B. J., Bach, F. H. and Bach, M. L. (1973). Lymphocyte reactivity to serologically undetected components of the major histocompatibility complex. *Nature*, **242**, 239

Yunis, E. J. and Amos, D. B. (1971). Three closely linked genetic systems relevant to transplantation. *Proc. Nat. Acad. Sci. (Wash.)*, **68**, 3031

6
Human Renal Allografts: The Significance of Blocking Factors

G. E. Striker, L. J. Quadracci, and T. L. Marchioro

INTRODUCTION

Many factors influence the duration and quality of organ homograft survival and function. Significant advances have been made in surgical technical skills and of the condition of the organ at the time of grafting. Similarly, recognition and delineation of the HL-A system and improved immunosuppressive regimens have significantly increased overall renal allograft survival. In the individual patient, however, it is often difficult or impossible to predict renal allograft survival even among patients with apparently similar histocompatibility matches and drug regimens. This observation prompted us to postulate that the host response to the grafted organ plays a decisive role in graft survival. We have used a lymphocyte microcytotoxicity assay or cell inhibition (CI) test (Hellström and Hellström, 1971) to assess the potential significance of this response in allograft function and survival.

The CI test measures the presence or absence of cellular immunity to donor tissue and serum blocking factors. This technique has been used in studies of animal (Hellström *et al.*, 1969) and human (Hellström *et al.*, 1968) tumors, tetra-parental mice (Wegmann *et al.*, 1971), pregnancy (Hellström *et al.*, 1969) and rats' tolerance to renal homografts (Stuart *et al.*, 1971). This chapter is concerned with our analysis and interpretation of cellular immunity and serum blocking factors in 36 recipients of renal homografts obtained from related living donors studied at intervals from 3 weeks

---

Supported in part by U.S. Public Health Service Grant AI 10494, AM 15867, RR-37.
Dr Quadracci was supported by U.D. Public Health Service Special Fellowship AM 50678.

to 37 months after operation. In addition, 5 patients have been studied sequentially from 22 days to 37 months after operation.

The CI assay

The target cells, fibroblasts, are derived from skin biopsies taken at the time of transplantation. They are allowed to grow from skin explants to confluency, are trypsinized and then subcultured. Cells from the second or third passage were used in the assay or frozen cryogenically and stored at − 70 °C for future use

Lymphocytes are separated from whole blood using a silica-sol gradient. They are collected and used on the day of the test or are isolated, frozen cyrogenically and stored for future use. Lymphocytes stored in this manner remain viable for extended periods as measured by vital dye exclusion or incorporation of ^{3}H–thymidine following PHA stimulation.

The CI assay is performed as follows: Single cell suspensions of fibroblasts are added to each of the 96 wells of a Falcon Microtiter II^R plate so that approximately 100 cells are plated per well (Figure 6.1). The plates are allowed to incubate in a CO_2 gassed incubator overnight to allow the cells to adhere to the bottom of the wells. The media is decanted, and a 1:5 dilution of control serum and recipient serum is

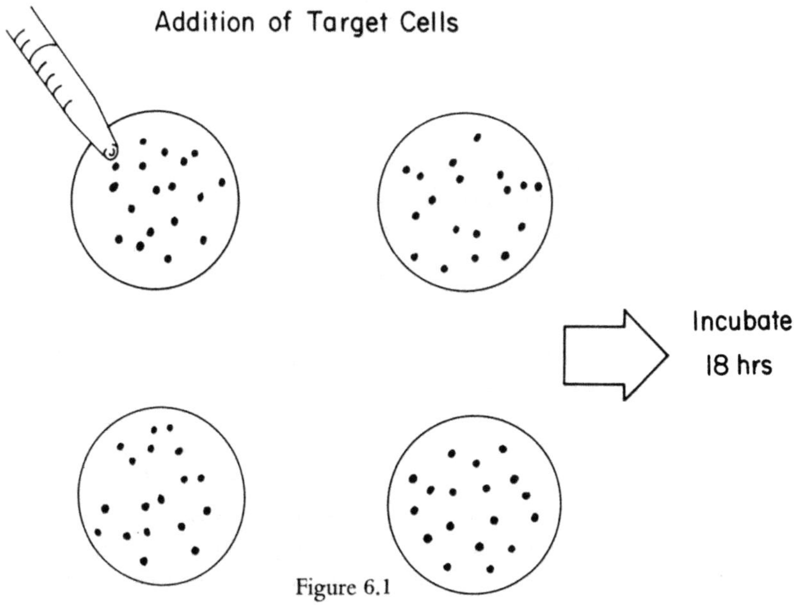

Figure 6.1

added to each of a series of wells (Figure 6.2). The culture plates are then incubated for 45 minutes. The serum is decanted and a suspension of control or test lymphocytes

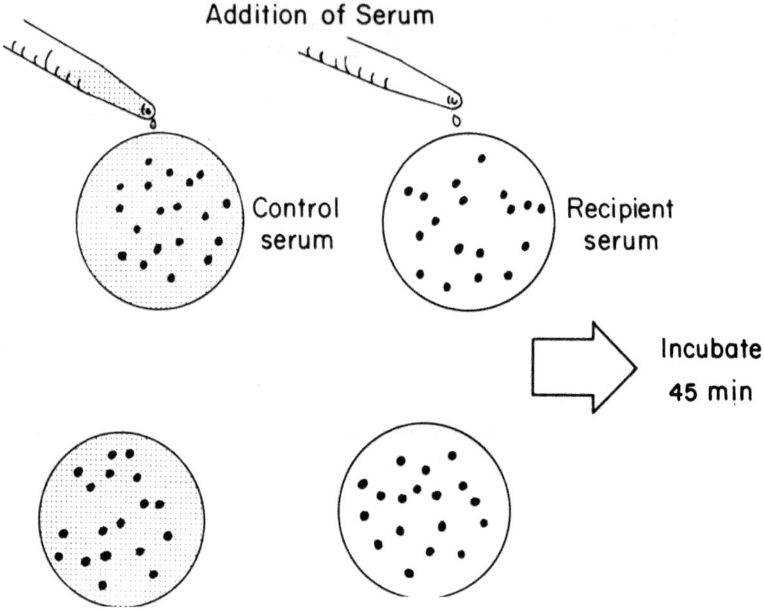

Figure 6.2

are added to a series of wells which previously had been exposed to control or test serum (Figure 6.3). One hour after the addition of lymphocytes, fetal calf serum is added to make a final dilution of 20% serum. The plates are incubated for 48 hours, fixed and stained with crystal violet. The number of fibroblasts remaining in each well is counted with the aid of a dissecting microscope. In these studies, control serum is obtained from the recipient prior to transplantation, and the recipient test serum during the post-transplant period on the date that the test lymphocytes are obtained. Control lymphocytes are obtained from random donors.

The combinations of control and test serum and lymphocytes are duplicated in at least eight wells of the test plates and mean cell counts are used in the comparisons. Cell counting is done without knowledge of the experimental design or clinical status of the patients. Cellular immunity is interpreted as present when the test lymphocytes cause a significant decrease in cell number (Student's *t*-test, $P < 0.05$) as compared to the cell count in the presence of control lymphocytes and control

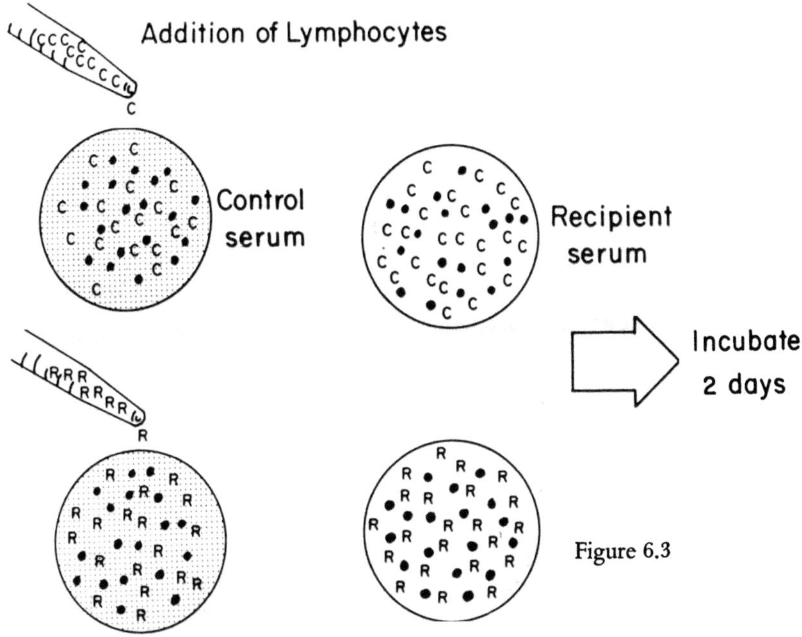

Figure 6.3

serum (Figure 6.4). The ability of the test serum to abrogate the inhibitory effect of the test lymphocytes is used to determine the presence of blocking. A 30% increase in cell survival when comparing the effect of test lymphocytes in the presence of test serum to the effect of test lymphocytes in the presence of control serum is considered significant.

Non-specific reactivity or toxicity of the test and control serum or lymphocytes are assessed using a second source of fibroblasts. In the majority of tests the recipient's skin fibroblasts are used in this capacity.

Patients studied

Thirty-six recipients of renal homografts from related living donors at the University of Washington were studied on one or more occasions post-operatively. All are ABO compatible and lack preformed cytotoxic antibodies to donor antigens.

Immunosuppression is provided with azathioprine, prednisolone, variable courses of equine anti-human lymphocyte globulin (ALG) and local irradiation to the kidney. A rejection episode is considered to have occurred clinically if and when the serum creatinine rose and the prednisolone dose is increased. Rejection episodes within 30 days before or after a given CI assay are considered to be related to that particular test.

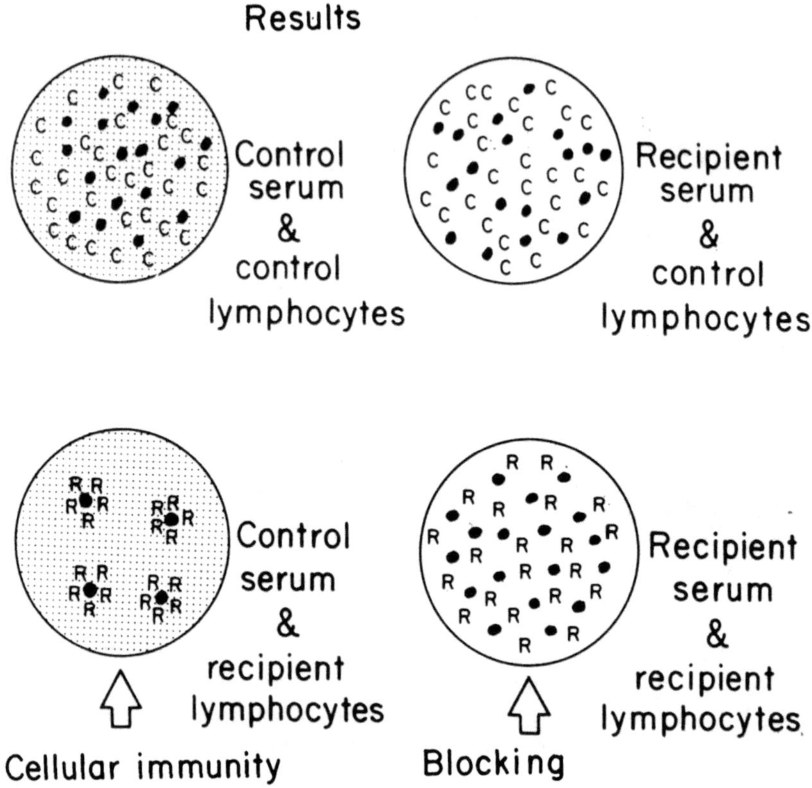

Figure 6.4

Patients are assigned a clinical grade at the time of the assay using the following criteria: Grade A: normotensive, serum creatinine under 1.4 mg/100 ml, no proteinuria (0.0 g/24 h); Grade B: hypertension easily controlled, serum creatinine 1.4–2.0 mg/100 ml, urine protein $<$ 1 g/24 h; Grade C: hypertension controlled with large doses of drugs, serum creatinine 2.0–4.0 mg/100 ml, urine protein 1–4 g/24 h.

RESULTS

The results of 97 C1 assays in 36 patients from 22 days to 37 months after transplantation are shown in Figure 6.5. Most patients were studied at least twice, and five had a total of 37 assays. Reactive lymphocytes with or without serum blocking were found

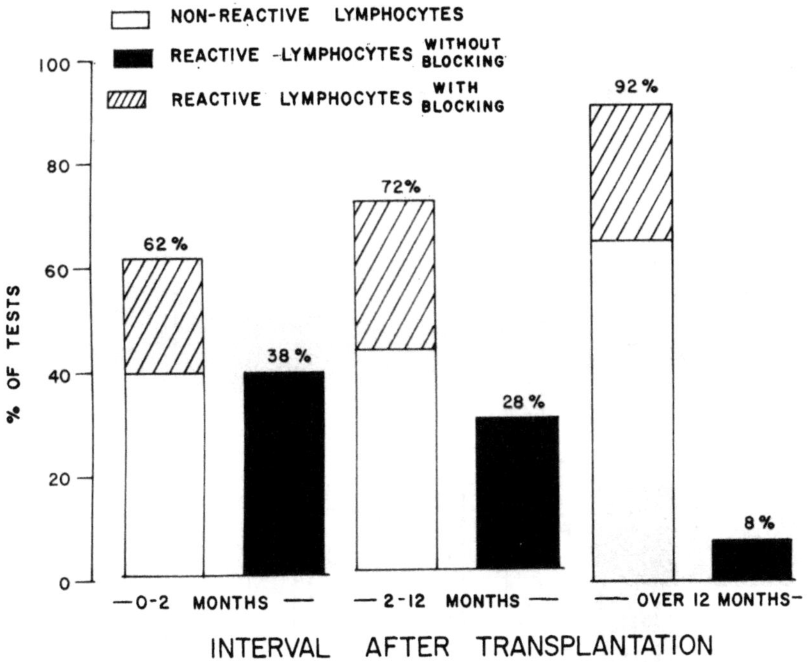

Figure 6.5 *Percentage of CI tests showing reactive lymphocytes as compared to blocked or non-reactive lymphocytes during three intervals after transplantation. There is a progressive decline in the percentage of immune lymphocytes and a corresponding increase in the incidence of blocked and non-reactive lymphocytes with increasing time after operation.*

in 38% of assays performed in the first two months, 28% from 2 to 10 months, and 8% over one year (Figure 6.5). There was a steady decline in the number and frequency of reactive lymphocytes with a parallel increase in blocked or non-reactive lymphocytes during the same intervals.

Rejection episodes were more frequently encountered in patients with reactive lymphocytes than in those with non-reactive or blocked lymphocytes (Figure 6.6). Non-reactive or blocked lymphocytes were found most commonly in patients with the best clinical grade (Figure 6.7).

The temporal relations among cellular immunity, serum blocking factor and loss of immunity were studied in five patients (Figures 6.8 and 6.9). In every case but one (patient 53) cellular immunity developed early in the post-transplant period. Patient 52 had a rejection episode at 4 weeks and had cellular immunity without blocking at

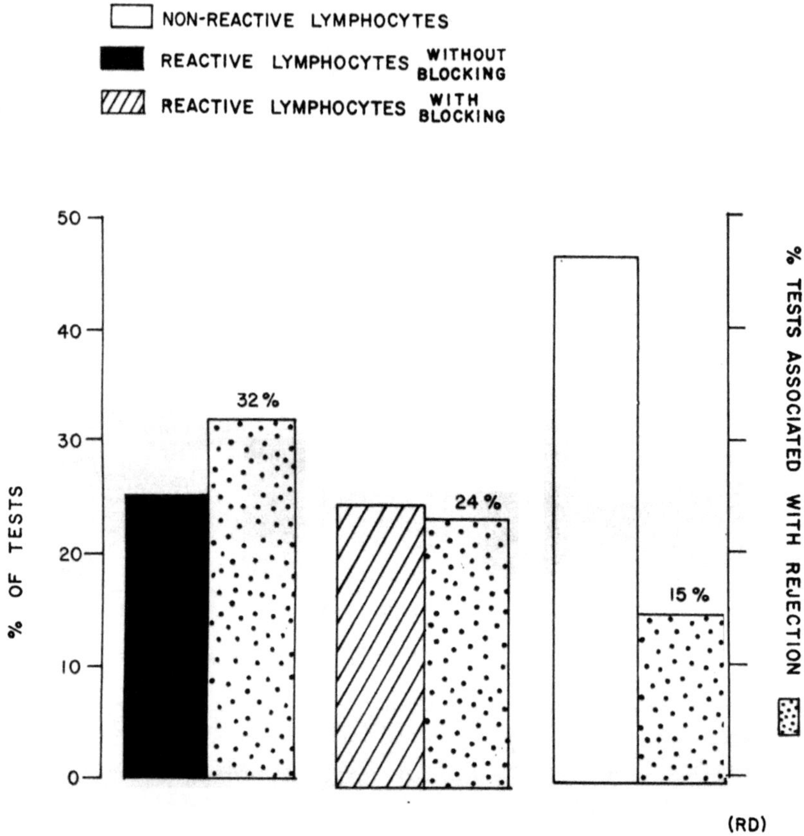

Figure 6.6 *Relationship of rejection episodes to results of the CI assay. A higher percentage of rejection episodes were diagnosed and treated one month before or after tests showing reactive lymphocytes without blocking.*

5 weeks. With reversal of the rejection episode renal function improved. When re-tested at 7 weeks blocking was evident. The blocking effect had disappeared when tested at 11 weeks, and a clinical rejection was evident at 12 weeks. Again with stabilization of the clinical course the blocking effect was present at 17 weeks.

Patients 54 and 31 had benign clinical courses. They had reactive lymphocytes when first tested, developed blocking in the next tests, and subsequently have had non-reactive lymphocytes except for one probably aberrant assay in patient 54 at 25 weeks.

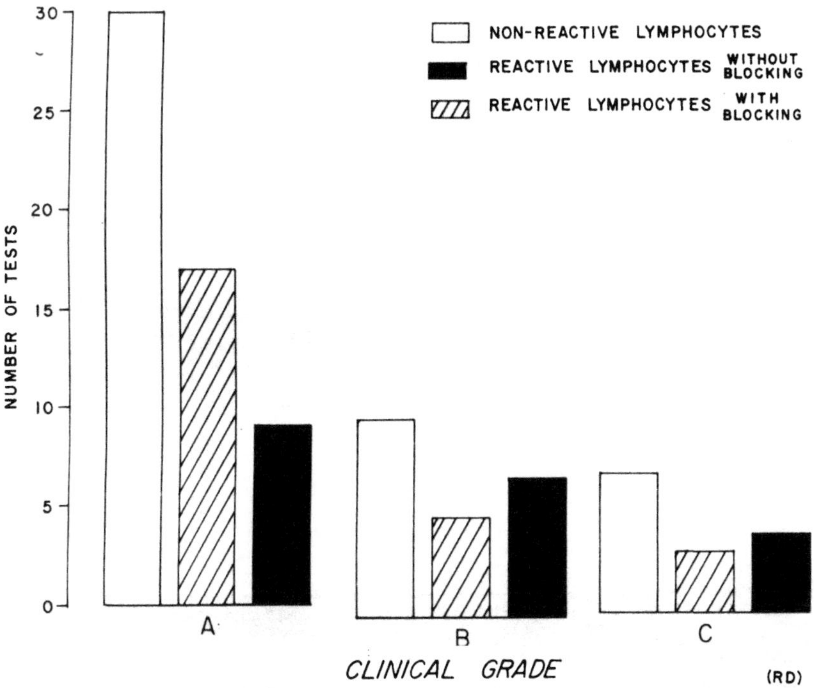

Figure 6.7 *Correlation of clinical grades with results of 97 CI assays in 36 patients. Grade A patients had a higher number of non-reactive or blocked lymphocytes. Grade B and C patients conversely had proportionately more tests demonstrating cellular immunity without blocking.*

Although patient 53 had a definite rejection episode at 5 weeks, reactive lymphocytes could not be demonstrated until 31 weeks.

The CI assays on patient 51 have demonstrated reactive lymphocytes in every instance except one, even though he has not had a definite clinical rejection episode. Blocking effect was present at 19 and 27 weeks, and cellular immunity could not be demonstrated at 50 weeks.

One pattern was common to all patients studied sequentially. The loss of cellular immunity was preceded by the development of serum blocking factors.

Relationship between the CI assay and allograft histology

During the early phase of these studies on renal allograft recipients, percutaneous renal biopsies were obtained at 6 weeks, 3 months, 6 months, one year, and yearly

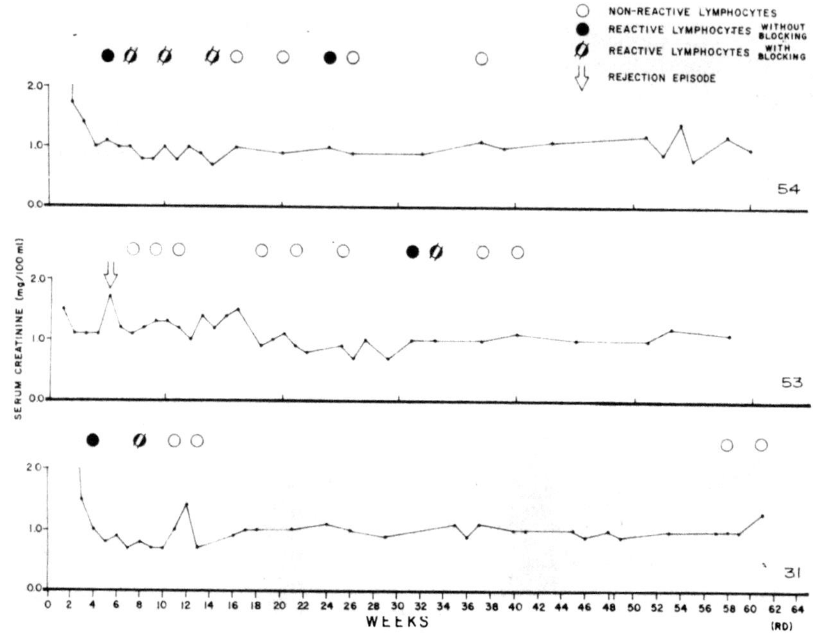

Figure 6.8 *Temporal relationship among the development of cellular immunity, serum blocking and non-reactive lymphocytes in three individual patients. The elevation of serum creatinine of patient 31 at the 12th week was a laboratory error.*

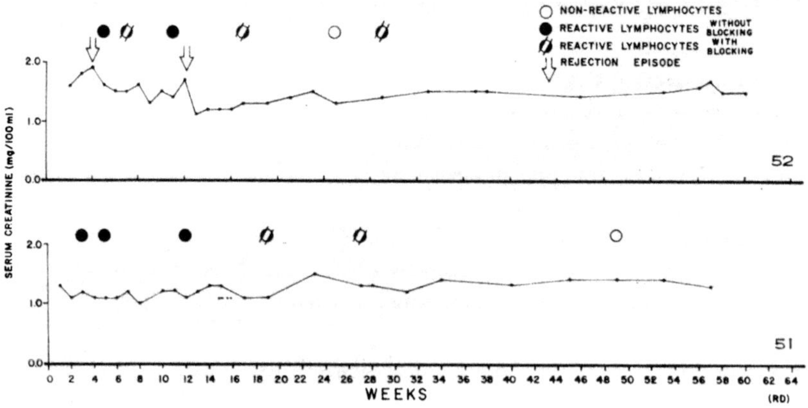

Figure 6.9 *Same data as shown in Figure 6.8 for two additional patients.*

thereafter. Patients who developed cellular immunity also had lymphocytic and plasma cell infiltrates in the renal interstitium. In those who subsequently developed serum blocking factor(s) the infiltrates were or became focal aggregates (Figure 6.10).

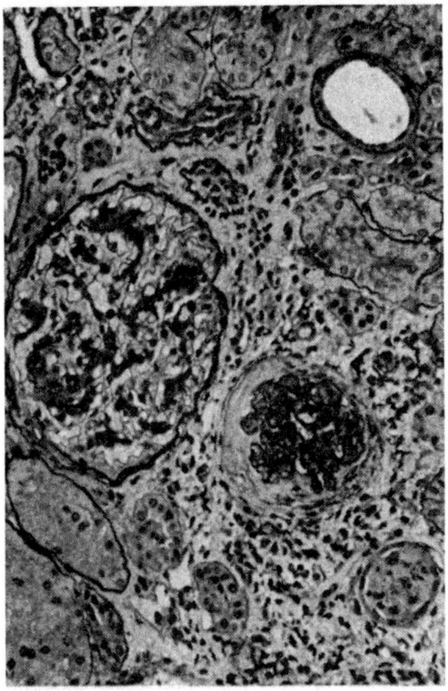

Figure 6.10 *Renal biopsy demonstrating focal areas of mononuclear infiltration and tubular atrophy. Other areas demonstrating normal tubular profiles.*

However, in those patients who had cellular immunity and either never developed blocking factor(s) or in whom it disappeared the cellular infiltrates were scattered diffusely throughout the interstitium (Figure 6.11). In this group neutrophilic infiltration and tubular necrosis were commonly present. When unresolved, interstitial fibrosis and tubular atrophy resulted.

Several patients who had cellular immunity for a short period of time never had significant interstitial infiltration. Glomeruli, tubules and vessels also remained normal in these patients.

Technical factors influencing interpretation of the CI assay

The CI assay appears to be an indicator of the immunological status of the recipients; in fact, the test results correlate with various clinical parameters. However, the assay

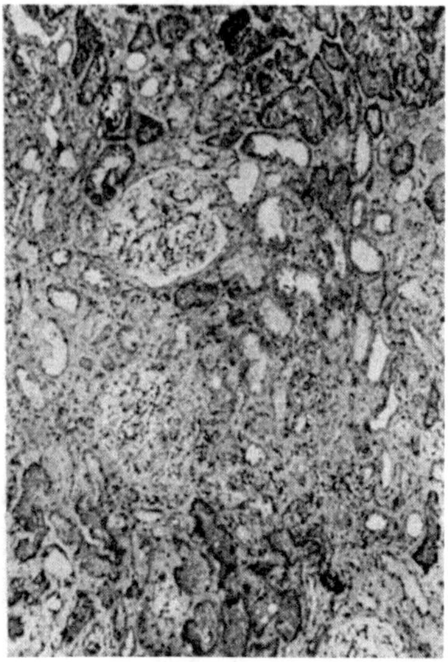

Figure 6.11 *Renal biopsy demonstrating diffuse interstitial cellular infiltration and tubular nephrosis.*

is technically difficult and the results subject to misinterpretation.

The experimental design must adequately test the various combinations of control and test serum and lymphocytes within the rather limited confines of the microtiter test plate. Comparisons cannot be made across plates as we have shown in previous studies (Quadracci *et al.*, 1971a). If the same target cell is pipetted into two different rows of wells of a group of test plates, allowed to attach and incubate for two days, then stained and counted, an unexpected result is obtained. As shown in Table 6.1, the difference in cell counts from row to row in the same plate is not significant. However, the counts from plate to plate are quite variable. Therefore, if the control combinations were on one plate and the test on another, accurate interpretation of the results would be impossible. Eight experimental replicates of each combination appear to be optimal for proper interpretation.

The conditions under which the assay is done are crucial. The target cells must be in excellent condition and actively dividing. If the cells have been passaged too many times or are in poor condition, it is impossible to predict plating efficiency, and the number of cells which survive in each individual well can be quite variable. The cells should not have gone past the log phase of growth prior to trypsinization but should

Table 6.1 *Cell growth reproducibility within and between plates*

Plate		*Mean* ± *S.E.*	*Plate*		*Mean* ± *S.E.*
1.	Row A	31.8 ± 2.3	5.	Row A	15.1 ± 1.6
	Row B	30.0 ± 4.7		Row B	16.9 ± 2.2
2.	Row A	39.9 ± 3.0	6.	Row A	21.6 ± 2.4
	Row B	31.8 ± 4.4		Row B	23.9 ± 2.4
3.	Row A	29.8 ± 3.9	7.	Row A	40.8 ± 2.4
	Row B	28.8 ± 2.2		Row B	41.9 ± 2.8
4.	Row A	54.8 ± 4.0	8.	Row A	33.8 ± 2.6
	Row B	44.3 ± 4.2		Row B	28.8 ± 2.8

have reached confluency. Sufficient trypsinization to provide an unicellular suspension free of clumps but not so vigorous as to cause cellular injury is desirable. One hundred cells are pipetted into each well to yield a final number of 60–80 cells. This number is easy to count reproducibly and lymphocyte/target cell ratio appears ideal to demonstrate cellular immunity and blocking. Final cell counts in excess of 150 are difficult to count accurately, while numbers less than 20 will often fail to show significant differences between control and test lymphocytes.

Various methods for lymphocyte separation can be used effectively in the CI assay. Sedimentation of red cells followed by removal of polymorphonuclear leukocytes (PMN) using the nylon wool or density gradient methods are currently used with good results. PMN in excess of 20% or heavy RBC or hemoglobin contamination may have direct cytotoxic effects and interfere with interpretation of the results. The lymphocytes should have a degree of viability in excess of 90%.

The selection of appropriate control lymphocytes is difficult in the outbred human population. In this case cross reactivity (? cross immunity) of both recipient and control to the same antigen(s) would make interpretation of the test impossible. Multiple controls are therefore mandatory and the limitations of the test plate size are often difficult to overcome.

In the tumor system serum blocking factors have been shown to be quite sensitive and can be removed by freeze-thawing more than once and possibly by prolonged storage at −20 °C. Ideally, serum should be fresh or stored at −70 °C and not refrozen.

The variable which is impossible to control is the test subject, the transplant recipient. Each patient receives different doses of immunosuppressive agents and responds to them in a unique manner. Many also are taking numerous antihypertensives to maintain normal blood pressure. The direct or indirect influence of this on the results of the assay are unknown. Although we were unable to correlate the dose of immunosuppression to the results of the assays (Pierce *et al.*, 1971), our experience is limited and the effect may be hidden, since immunosuppression is known to influence other *in vitro* assays.

A further difficulty arises from the fact that a clinical rejection episode is defined by changes in organ function. At best, this is an indirect measure of immunological events in the host. Under such circumstances specific therapy is imprecise and frequently may even be unnecessary. For these reasons, correlation of the results of the CI test and the patients' clinical course is imperfect.

If the CI test can be modified so that results are rapidly and repeatedly available, this measure of immunologic activity may be a more precise means of determining the presence of rejection as well as of relative stability.

Correlations in University of Washington patients

These data extend our previous observations on patients with renal transplants using the CI assay as a means of assessing immune response to donor tissue. We continue to find a high incidence of patients with sensitized lymphocytes in the early post-transplant period. There also is a progressive increase in serum blocking factors and non-reactive lymphocytes (Figure 6.5). The clinical correlations between rejections and clinical grades remain comparable to that previously described (Figures 6.6 and 6.7).

In addition, we have now documented the evolution of sensitized lymphocytes, serum blocking factors and non-reactivity in five patients tested sequentially (Figures 6.8 and 6.9). In four of the five patients studied cellular immunity was present in the early phase after transplantation. Subsequently, blocking factors appeared and ultimately non-reactivity occurred in all five. Furthermore, rejection episodes, although infrequent in these five patients, were correlated in all but one instance with reactive lymphocytes without serum blocking.

Although limited by relatively short-term observations, numbers of patients, and the fact that these five patients fortuitously had good clinical courses, inspection of the data reveals that any given immunological state as defined by the CI assay is not necessarily stable. Additional support for this comes from our study of a patient

(Springberg, 1973) from Harbor General Hospital in Los Angeles, California. The patient, a 21-year-old white female, received a renal allograft from her mother. In the early post-transplant period she had several rejection episodes, one of which occurred after she independently discontinued her drugs. These rejections were successfully reversed and renal function became normal. The patient again discontinued drug therapy. Renal function remained stable for 18 months. During this period she had cellular immunity to maternal fibroblasts and her serum contained blocking substance(s). Thirty-two months after transplantation and 22 months after discontinuing drug treatment she was found to be severely azotemic. There was no response to therapy, and she returned to a chronic dialysis program. During the final episode she continued to demonstrate cellular immunity to donor antigens, but serum blocking substance(s) were no longer found (Figure 6.12).

Demonstration of blocking by the MLC assays

Recent studies in humans using the mixed leukocyte culture (MLC) assay tend to support the theory that serum blocking factors may play an important role in allograft survival. Ceppellini *et al.*, 1971, and Revillard *et al.*, 1972, have demonstrated the inhibition of the MLC by ALG, multiparous woman's sera placental extracts and renal allograft recipient's serum. Shons *et al.*, 1972, have shown a similar effect in a large group of allograft recipients and Miller *et al.*, 1971 and 1972, have followed up their excellent studies in dogs with human observations (Miller and Hattler, 1972). In a recent report by Hattler and Miller, 1972, three patients were studied with stable renal allografts whose serum blocked the MLC reaction. Antibody eluate from a biopsy of these grafts also blocked.

SPECULATIONS

The obvious question to be asked of the demonstration of cellular immunity and blocking factor(s) is their clinical significance. Are they an indicator of a stable state, the cause, or a spurious observation? These questions would be much easier to answer if the blocking factor(s) could be isolated. Hellström and Hellström (1969) reported that the blocking factor(s) were contained in a serum fraction eluting in the region of IgG. Work is in progress to assess this in humans.

For the present the evidence that blocking factors are of primary significance in clinical transplantation is indirect. Stable renal function resulted in those patients who had an orderly progression from reactive lymphocytes with blocking factor(s) to non-reactive lymphocytes. The opposite was true also, i.e. those patients who did not develop or lost serum blocking factor(s) had deterioration of renal function rejection episode(s). The presence or absence of serum blocking factor(s) was not related to drug therapy or antilymphocyte globulin administration. There was a positive correlation between allograft histology and results of the CI assay. Those patients with serum blocking factors or who no longer had reactive lymphocytes demonstrated few or no inflammatory cells in the interstitium. However, those who had reactive lymphocytes without blocking had inflammatory cells in the interstitium and tubular and vascular changes. Thus, the CI assay appears to provide a reasonable assessment of the status of the balance between the host and the allograft. The current technical demands make it presently unusable as a technique for routine monitoring of renal allograft recipients.

Our observations and those of others (Batchelor *et al.*, 1970) in humans and in experimental animals (French and Batchelor, 1969; Batchelor *et al.*, 1972; Gordon *et al.*, 1971; Miller *et al.*, 1971 and 1972; Lucas *et al.*, 1970; Stuart *et al.*, 1968; French *et al.*, 1971; Kim *et al.*, 1972; Fabre and Morris, 1972) clearly establish the presence of blocking factors in transplant recipients. These data raise the hope that serum containing enhancing antibody or blocking factor(s) might be therapeutically useful when passively administered.

References

Batchelor, J. R., Ellis, F., French, M. E., Bewick, M. and Cameron, J. S. (1970). Immunological enhancement of human kidney graft. *Lancet*, **2**, 1007

Batchelor, J. R., Fabre, J. and Morris, P. J. (1972). Passive enhancement of kidney allografts. *Transplantation*, **13**, 610

Ceppellini, R., Bonnard, G. D., Coppo, F., Miggiano, V. C., Pospisil, M., Curtoni, E. S. and Pellegrino, M. (1971). Mixed leukocyte cultures and HL-A antigens. I. Reactivity of young fetuses, newborns and mothers at delivery. *Transpl. Proc.*, **3**, 58

Fabre, J. W. and Morris, P. J. (1972). The mechanism of specific immunosuppression of renal allograft rejection by donor strain blood. *Transplantation*, **14**, 634

Falk, R. E., Guttmann, R. D., Beaudoin, J. G., Morehouse, D. D. and Oh, J. H. (1972). Leukocyte migration in vitro and its relationship to human renal allograft rejection and enhancement. *Transplantation*, **13**, 461

French, M. E. and Batchelor, J. R. (1969). Immunological enhancement of rat kidney grafts. *Lancet*, **2**, 1103

French, M. E., Batchelor, J. R. and Watts, H. G. (1971). The capacity of lymphocytes from rats bearing enhanced kidney allografts to mount graft-versus-host reactions.

Transplantation, **12,** 45

Gordon, R. O., Stinson, E. B., Souther, S. G. and Oppenheim, J. J. (1971). Inhibition of the mixed leukocyte reaction as an assay for enhancing alloantisruem. *Transplantation*, **12,** 484

Hattler, B. G., Jr. and Miller, J. (1973). Blocking antibody in the sera and on the kidneys of successful human transplants. *Transpl. Proc.* (In press)

Hattler, B. G., Jr., Miller, J. and Johnson, M. C. (1972). Cellular and humoral factors governing canine mixed lymphocyte cultures after renal transplantation. II. Cellular. *Transplantation*, **14,** 47

Hellström, I., Hellström, K. E., Evans, C. A., Heppner, G. A., Pierce, G. E. and Yang, J. P. S. (1969). Serum-mediated protection of neoplastic cells from inhibition by lymphocytes immune to their tumor specific antigens. *Proc. Nat. Acad. Sci.*, **62,** 362

Hellström, K. E., Hellström, I. and Brown, J. (1969). Abrogation of cellular immunity to antigenically foreign mouse embryonic cells by a serum factor. *Nature (London)*, **224,** 914

Hellström, I. Hellström, K. E., Pierce, G. E. and Yang, J. P. S. (1968). Cellular and humoral immunity to different types of human neoplasma. *Nature (London)*, **220,** 1352

Hellström, I. and Hellström, K. E. (1971). Colony inhibition and cytotoxicity assays, in *in vitro methods in cell-mediated immunity* (B. R. Bloom and P. R. Glade, editors). pp. 409-414 New York: Academic Press

Hornung, M. O., Layne, E. and McDonald, J. C. (1971). The use of human $F(ab^1)_2$ fragments as blocking agents in the mixed lymphocyte reaction. *J. Immunol.*, **107,** 979

Kim, J., Shaipanich, T., Sells, R. A., Maggs, P., Lukl, P. and Wilson, R. E. (1972). Active enhancement of rat renal allografts with soluble splenic antigen. *Transplantation*, **13,** 322

Lucas, Z. J., Markley, J. and Travis, M. (1970). Immunologic enhancement of renal allografts in the rat. I. Dissociation of graft survival and antibody response. *Fed. Proc.*, **29,** 2041

Miller, J. and Hattler, B. G., Jr. (1972). Reactivity of lymphocytes in mixed culture in response to human renal transplantation. *Surgery*, **72,** 220

Miller, J., Hattler, B., Davis, M. and Johnson, M. C. (1971a). Cellular and humoral factors governing canine mixed lymphocyte cultures after renal transplantation: I. Antibody. *Transplantation*, **12,** 65

Miller, J., Hattler, B. G., Jr. and Johnson, M. C. (1972b). Cellular and humoral factors governing canine mixed lymphocyte cultures after renal transplantation: III.

Further studies with antibody. *Transplantation*, **14**, 57

Pierce, G. E., Quadracci, L. J., Tremann, J. A., Moe, R. E., Striker, G. E., Hellström, I., Hellström, K. E. and Marchioro, T. L. (1971). Studies on cellular and humoral immune factors in human renal transplantation. *Ann. Surg.*, **174**, 609

Quadracci, L. J., Cambi, V., Christopher, T. G., Harker, L. A. and Striker, G. E. (1971a). Assay of serum abnormalities in uremic and dialysis patients; evidence for depletion of vital substances in hemodialysis. *Trans. Amer. Soc. Artificial Internal Organs*, **17**, 96

Quadracci, L. J., Hellström, I., Striker, G. E., Marchioro, T. L. and Hellström, K. E. (1971b). Immune mechanisms in human recipients of renal allografts. *Cellular Immunol.*, **1**, 561

Quadracci, L., Pierce, G., Striker, G., Tremann, J. and Marchioro, T. (1973). Homograft survival and serum blocking factors. *Transpl. Proc.* (In press)

Quadracci, L. J., Striker, G. E., Tremann, J. A., Pierce, G. E. and Marchioro, T. L. (1973). Serum blocking factors in human renal allograft recipients. (Submitted for publication)

Revillard, J. P., Robert, M., Betuel, H., Latour, M., Bonneau, M., Brochier, J. and Traeger, J. (1972). Inhibition of the mixed lymphocyte reaction by antibodies. *Transpl. Proc.*, **4**, 173

Shons, A. R., Etheredge, E. E. and Najarian, J. S. (1973). The mixed leukocyte response in human transplantation. *Transpl. Proc.* (In press)

Springberg, P., Striker, G. E., Glassock, R., Siegler, H. F., Ward, F., Moore, T. and Quadracci, L. J. (1973). Prolonged function of a human renal allograft after discontinuation of immunosuppressive therapy: report of a case. (Submitted for publication)

Stuart, F. P., Fitch, F. W., Rowley, D. A., Biesecker, J. L., Hellström, K. E. and Hellström, I. (1971). Presence of both cell-mediated immunity and serum blocking factors in rat renal allografts 'enhanced' by passive immunization. *Transplantation*, **12**, 331

Stuart, F. D., Saitoh, T. and Fitch, F. W. (1968). Rejection of renal allografts: Specific immunological suppression. *Science*, **160**, 1463

Wegmann, T. G., Hellström, I. and Hellström, K. E. (1971). Immunological tolerance: 'Forbidden clones' allowed in tetraparental mice. *Proc. Nat. Acad. Sci.*, **68**, 1644

7

Immunological Tolerance: The Chimeric State: The Difference Between Full Tolerance and Partial Tolerance

Elizabeth Simpson

INTRODUCTION

Acquired tolerance is defined as immunological non-reactivity specific for the inducing antigen. According to Burnet's theory of clonal elimination (Burnet and Fenner, 1949), natural tolerance to self antigens develops during ontogenesis, all self-reacting clones being eliminated. The mechanism of the induction of acquired and natural tolerance may be very similar. The early work on transplantation tolerance (Billingham *et al.*, 1956) in which antigen in the form of living allogeneic cells was introduced into fetal or neonatal mice, indicated that the resulting tolerance to appropriate skin grafts was due to central failure of the immune response. This was consistent with clonal elimination theories.

Since then a mass of data has accumulated confirming the lack of peripheral reactivity both in transplantation tolerance, and in tolerance to protein and red cell antigens (see section on full tolerance). However, there is another body of data relating to transplantation, protein and polysaccharide antigens, suggesting that peripheral reactivity is indeed present in some measurable form, but that the immunological response is held at negligible or low levels by other factors (see section on partial tolerance). I do not propose to provide a unifying concept to consider forms of tolerance and specific hyporeactivity because it seems likely that several mechanisms are at work. The interpretation of one set of data on the subject is frequently irreconcilable with that of other data using an apparently similar system. Much of the conflict can be resolved if tolerance is subdivided into two main categories. The first, which I shall call 'full tolerance', is marked by a complete lack of peripheral activity; that is using such criteria as antigen binding cells, antibody producing cells, and the various manifestations of T cell activities, no antigen reactive cells can be found. The sections devoted to full tolerance will select examples of tolerance to various antigens in which the specific loss of such peripheral activities has been demonstrated. The implication is that full tolerance is associated with clonal elimination. The second main category will be called 'partial tolerance' and will include specific hyporeactive states in which various types of peripheral activity can be detected. These will be detailed in the sections on partial tolerance, and there will be a discussion of the various possible mechanisms whereby the hypo-reactive state is induced and maintained. There will be a bias towards presenting data and discussing tolerance to transplantation antigens, since it is the reactivity to these that transplanters would wish to abrogate or modify. Tolerance to other types of antigen, protein, erythrocyte and polysaccharide, will be discussed where they throw light on the subject and provide relevant information which is not available for transplantation antigens, but which may be applicable to them.

TARGET CELLS FOR TOLERANCE INDUCTION; THE LYMPHOCYTES

T and B

Before pursuing the analysis any further, it will be necessary to consider the various subpopulations of lymphoid cells which comprise the immune system because they each have somewhat different rôles to play in immunity and tolerance. Lymphocytes can be categorized according to their developmental pathways as 'B' (bursa equivalent) cells and 'T' (thymus processed) cells (Warner, 1967; Raff, 1970).

In mammals, B cells arise from stem cells in the bone marrow, from where they migrate to some organ or tissue (the equivalent of the bursa of Fabricius of birds) where they undergo maturation. This involves the appearance of immunoglobulin on the cell surface, and the ability to proliferate into a clone of cells capable of manufacturing immunoglobulin when stimulated to do so by reaction with antigen via the cell surface immunoglobulin receptors. Such mature B cells are found in the thymus independent areas of lymph nodes and spleen (Parrott *et al.*, 1966) and as a proportion of the recirculating pool of lymphocytes, in blood and lymph (for review, see Metcalf and Moore, 1971; Cooper *et al.*, 1972). Once stimulated by antigen to form a clone of antibody producing cells, further differentiation to plasma cells takes place, and these cells do not recirculate but remain within lymph nodes or spleen or within lesions such as grafts and granulomas. B cells can be further subdivided into cells which make different classes of antibody, each class having different biological activities (Fahey *et al.*, 1964a and b; Ovary *et al.*, 1965).

Antibody responses to a number of antigens appear to require the presence of 'helper' T cells which bear surface receptors that recognize a determinant on the antigen (see Mitchell *et al.*, 1971 for review). Antigens which require T cells to co-operate with B cells prior to antibody production are known as 'thymus dependent antigens'. The manner in which co-operation takes place has been a matter of speculation and controversy, but there is now good evidence to suggest that for some antigens at least, the T cell has a receptor for a carrier determinant of the antigen, and that on contact with antigen, the receptor is shed and the receptor–antigen complex then becomes attached to macrophages. From this location it inter-reacts with B cells having receptors for the haptenic determinant of the antigen in such a way that the B cell is 'turned-on', and produces antihapten antibody (Feldmann and Basten, 1972a). Antibodies which elicit antibody responses without the need for T cell help are known as 'thymus independent antigens' and seem to be able to interact directly with B cells to turn them on to antibody production. It is characteristic of thymus independent antigens that they are composed of many repeating units, for example, the pneumococcal polysaccharide SIII (for review see Ivanyi and Howard, 1971).

In both birds and mammals, T cells arise from stem cells in the bone marrow and migrate to the thymus, where they further divide and differentiate within the thymic cortex and may then travel to the medulla of the thymus (Owen and Raff, 1970). From the thymus T cells migrate to the peripheral lymphoid organs, primarily to the spleen, where they may undergo a further maturational step before becoming recirculating T cells (Raff and Cantor, 1971; Cantor, 1972a). These mature T cells now pass between the thymus dependent areas of lymph nodes and spleen (Parrott *et al.*, 1966) and the lymph and blood.

The immunological capabilities of T cells at the different stages of maturation listed above, namely, cortical thymocytes, medullary thymocytes, spleen seeking T cells and recirculating T cells, do differ. In the mouse, cortical thymocytes bearing the differentiation antigens TL (Old *et al.*, 1963; Leckband, 1970) and theta (θ) (Reif and Allen, 1964; Raff, 1969) are not competent to function as graft-versus-host (GVH) reactive cells, 'helper' cells or cytotoxic cells (Asofsky *et al.*, 1971; Raff and Cantor, 1971; Wagner *et al.*, 1972). In contrast, medullary thymocytes, which have lost TL, have less θ on their surface but are rich in H-2 surface antigens (Raff and Cantor,

1971). These cells can mediate GVH and MLR reactions (Asofsky *et al.*, 1971; Mosier and Cantor, 1971) and on contact with antigen, can develop helper activity (see Raff and Cantor, 1971, for review) and cytotoxic activity (Wagner *et al.*, 1972). Although it is clear that the thymus seeds cells to the periphery in neonatal and adult life, it is not established whether thymic emigrants leave at different stages of thymic maturation. There is evidence that immature and spleen seeking T cells that are diminished by adult thymectomy can act as 'regulator cells' (for review, see Gershon, 1973; Cantor and Simpson, 1973), but this function will be discussed later in some detail. By contrast, the recirculating T cells appear long lived in the absence of the thymus in adult life (Raff and Cantor, 1971); they play a rôle as 'amplifier' cells in the GVH reaction (Cantor and Asofsky, 1972); are probably the cytotoxic precursor cells (Cantor and Simpson, 1973) and represent the bulk of memory T cells (Cantor, 1971; Cantor and Simpson, 1973). It is not known whether the different rôles (helper, cytotoxic, memory, amplifier, suppressor) within any one compartment are played by different cell populations within that compartment, or whether the same cell is capable of playing several rôles. The sub-populations of T cells and their different biological functions can be preferentially affected by various drugs and maneuvers. Cortical thymocytes are very sensitive to cortisone *in vivo* and the thymuses of mice given cortisone contain only medullary, cortisone resistant, thymocytes (Jacobssen and Blomgren, 1972). Medullary thymocytes have H-2 on their surface, and can therefore be selectively removed from suspensions of thymocytes by treatment with alloantisera and complement, leaving the cortical cortisone sensitive thymocytes, which bear little H-2 antigen (Mosier and Pierce, 1972). Spleen-seeking T cells (Cantor, 1972a; Stobo and Paul, 1973) appear to be inactivated in the absence of the thymus in adult life (Kerbel and Eidinger, 1972; Cantor and Simpson, 1973). Unlike adult thymectomy, which spares the more mature, long lived recirculating T cell in the periphery, antilymphocyte serum (ALS) *in vivo* has a preferential effect when given in low doses on the recirculating lymphocytes (Raff and Cantor, 1971; Cantor and Simpson, 1973). Spleens of mice so treated are enriched for the non-recirculating probably less mature, spleen-seeking T cells, and thus provide a source for investigating the functions of this sub-population.

Tolerance in T and B cells

It has been necessary to describe the various sub-populations of lymphocytes in some detail, because not only do the functions of B cells in antibody production, and T cells in cell mediated immunity have different rôles in graft rejection, but they have different sensitivities to tolerance induction. T cells can be readily tolerized by low doses of protein antigen, whereas B cells can only be tolerized by very high doses (see Mitchison, 1971b; Weigle *et al.*, 1971). Using the appropriate antigen, dose and regime, it is possible to tolerize either T cells, or T and B cells, in a manner which appears to result in the elimination or peripheral inactivation of appropriate antigen reactive cells (see section on full tolerance). This has been called 'central failure' (Billingham *et al.*, 1956) and is only reversible when the concentration of tolerizing antigen falls to levels which allow newly maturing T and or B cells to emerge from precursor cells, and function in the periphery. It is to this form of tolerance that the term 'full tolerance' has been given for the purposes of this review.

However, it would be unwise to ignore the various states of hyporeactivity, to which the term 'partial tolerance' has been given, since in the event of failure to induce full tolerance, partial tolerance may well supervene. It is therefore important to attempt to understand what factors control such partial tolerance or hyporeactivity since this state may be a useful clinical achievement in the face of the difficulty of producing full tolerance. As will be seen later, it is for the better understanding of partial tolerance that a knowledge of the various sub-populations of B and T cells may be important, since regulatory mechanisms may well involve certain of them.

FULL TOLERANCE

In cell mediated immunity

Chimerism

Techniques for inducing chimerism. The earliest systematic work on tolerance was done by Sir Peter Medawar and his colleagues (Billingham *et al.*, 1956). They worked on transplantation tolerance in inbred strains of mice in which they attempted to analyze in detail the finding of Owen (1945) that twin cattle which had had a shared placental circulation *in utero* were red blood cell chimeras, and would accept skin grafts from one another (Billingham *et al.*, 1952). Following Burnet's theory of clonal elimination (Burnet and Fenner, 1949) it was postulated that if foreign antigens were introduced to fetuses during or before the stage at which clones of self-reacting cells were eliminated, they would accept the foreign antigen as 'self' and develop tolerance to it in the same way. The early work on tolerance induction in mice was therefore carried out by injecting fragments of tissue and cell suspensions of various tissues from adult allogeneic donors into fetuses during the later stages of pregnancy, or into newborns. Using the techniques then available, it was not easy to measure the dose of antigen, nor to be accurate as to the exact site of injection in fetuses. However, it was quite clear that a proportion of the mice after such treatments were tolerant of skin grafts from the allogeneic donor and that this tolerance was specific, inasmuch as third party grafts were promptly rejected. It was also found that tolerance could be abrogated by the injection of syngeneic lymphoid cells from either normal mice, or mice presensitized by skin grafting with skin of the appropriate strain. This finding argued for a mechanism of tolerance induction involving central failure in the original host, inasmuch as the deficit could be made good by normal peripheral lymphocytes. Had an efferent block or enhancement been responsible for the state of tolerance, one should expect the normal lymphoid cells injected to have been likewise blocked.

Subsequent work on tolerance induction to transplantation antigens showed clearly that tolerance could be induced in mice in the early postnatal period, as well as in fetal life (Billingham and Brent, 1959). Lymphoid cells were the best tolerance inducing inoculum, probably because they continued to live and divide within the host, rendering it a chimera with respect to the lymphoid tissues (Silobrcic, 1971). In this way, throughout the life of the host newly emerging immunocompetent cells are confronted by antigens of donor origin, and thus tolerance, induced originally in the very young animal, can be maintained in the adult.

The fact that tolerance to transplantation antigens can be induced more readily in the neonate than in the adult is probably due to the smaller number of peripheral antigen reactive cells and their relative immaturity in the neonate. In the chimeric adult, tolerance is maintained by exposing immature antigen reactive cells as they emerge along the differentiation pathway to doses of antigen which are tolerogenic to them, i.e. clonal elimination is a life long process. Such doses of antigen would probably not be tolerogenic to the mature recirculating population of lymphocytes, hence the relative difficulty of tolerance induction in the adult, especially where major transplantation antigens are concerned.

Later work showed that tolerance to strong histocompatibility antigens could be induced in mice up to 6 days after birth by weight adjusted doses of allogeneic or semi-allogeneic lymphoid cells, but that thereafter the young mouse was extremely resistant to tolerance induction by single large doses of lymphoid cells (Brent and Gowland, 1961). In adult mice heroic multiple injections of semi-allogeneic lymphoid cells could lead to tolerance induction associated with chimerism in a proportion of mice, and could be abrogated by injection of normal syngeneic cells, thus bearing the same hallmarks as neonatally induced tolerance (Brent and Gowland, 1962).

A number of early improvements in the techniques of tolerance induction have facilitated later studies. It had been discovered in the early stages of this work that injection of immunocompetent allogeneic cells could lead to graft-versus-host (GVH) disease. This troublesome complication was avoided by using semi-allogeneic, or F_1 cells, which were genetically incapable of reacting against the host (Billingham and

Brent, 1959). It was found that the intravenous route was the most effective for tolerance induction, and although the intraperitoneal route could be used, larger numbers of F_1 cells had to be injected (Brent *et al.*, 1962). The number of F_1 cells needed to induce tolerance depended on the strength of the histocompatibility barrier between donor and recipient. Thus for strongly incompatible combinations, differing at the H-2 locus, larger numbers were necessary than weaker combinations in which the incompatibility lay only at non-H-2 loci (Brent and Gowland, 1961). For very weak antigenic differences such as the HY antigen carried by males (but not females), tolerance induction in females could be achieved by injections of syngeneic male lymphoid cells either in neonatal or adult females, although the dose for adult induction was much higher (Billingham *et al.*, 1963).

Strong histocompatibility antigens are characterized by there being large numbers of antigen reactive cells to such allogeneic antigens present in the peripheral lymphoid tissue of normal, unimmunized mice and rats (Wilson *et al.*, 1967). In contrast, there are very few peripheral antigen reactive cells to weak histocompatibility antigens in non-immunized mice and rats, although their number can be increased by immunization (for discussion, see Raff and Cantor, 1971; Cantor, 1971). One of the reasons for the difficulty in inducing tolerance to strong histocompatibility antigens in adults may lie in the large number of these peripheral immunocompetent cells, and therefore any treatment which reduces their number should help in subsequent attempts at tolerance induction and the establishment of chimerism. Various methods have been attempted, amongst them x-irradiation (Koller *et al.*, 1961) and antilymphocyte serum (Lance and Medawar, 1969). In irradiation induced chimeras, the host hematopoietic and lymphoid tissues are totally replaced by donor cells, so that the tolerance induction proceeds in the opposite direction, i.e. the engrafted allogeneic cells must become tolerant of recipient antigens or the recipient will die of graft-versus-host disease. In the case of inbred mice, it has been shown that the donor cells from tolerant mice become completely depleted of antigen reactive cells towards the host (Grant *et al.*, 1972) and so in this case the criteria for full tolerance would appear to be met. In dogs, among the long term survivors of such radiation chimeras, evidence for reactivity of donor versus host has been found and this will therefore be discussed under partial tolerance (Hellström *et al.*, 1970).

The use of ALS to aid tolerance induction, and to help establish chimerism has been explored in mouse (Lance and Medawar, 1969), monkey, and dog (Lance, 1971a). In mouse, the timing of ALS in relation to the injection of semi-allogeneic lymphoid cells was found to be critical. ALS given 9 days before the first injection of lymphoid cells was found to give the best results, and both the chimeric state and tolerance could be maintained for longer if further injections of semi-allogeneic cells were given periodically. However, eventually chimerism did wane, and shortly thereafter the previously tolerated grafts were rejected. It is interesting that this type of full tolerance, albeit of limited duration, could also be achieved in presensitized mice.

The mechanism of full tolerance

The main evidence for central failure of the immune response in fully tolerant, chimeric animals was originally the observation that it could be abrogated by the injection of normal lymphoid cells syngeneic with the recipient. Further evidence on this point has been accumulating over the past few years, as new and more sensitive techniques for measuring the activity of antigen reactive cells in the periphery have been devised. The easiest reactivity to measure is antibody production against the foreign histocompatibility antigens of the engrafted chimeric cells. Attempts to detect cytotoxic or hemagglutinating antibody have been negative in chimeric mice, but it is interesting that whenever chimerism wanes, hemagglutinating antibodies appeared preceding graft rejection by a short interval (Lance and Medawar, 1969). However, perhaps the most relevant reactivity to measure in the case of transplantation tolerance is that of the T cells, since it is predominantly by cell mediated immunity that allografts are rejected (Billingham *et al.*, 1954).

The work of Wilson (Wilson *et al.*, 1967) on the mixed lymphocyte reaction (MLR) gave a useful measure of the potential reactivity of peripheral T lymphocytes, as the MLR measures stimulation of a non-sensitized T lymphocyte population against histocompatibility antigens on allogeneic or F_1 lymphoid cells (Mosier and Cantor, 1971). When the one-way MLR was used to assess the peripheral reactivity of lymphocytes from normal and tolerant rats, it became clear that tolerant rats were incapable of producing an MLR against F_1 cells bearing the antigen to which the rats were tolerant, but were fully capable of an MLR to F_1 cells carrying a third party antigen. The specificity of this reactivity exactly paralleled the specificity of tolerance towards skin grafts which had been shown in mice (Billingham *et al.*, 1956). Subsequently it has been shown that MLR in tolerant chimeric mice shows an identical pattern of non-reactivity to the tolerated antigen, and reactivity to a third party antigen (Beverley *et al.*, 1973).

Simonsen's work on the graft-versus-host reaction (GVHR) (Simonsen. 1962) has provided another tool for examining the potential reactivity of peripheral T cells. In this test, immunocompetent lymphoid cells are injected into F_1 hosts. An increase in size of one or other of their lymphoid organs (spleen in the case of neonatal F_1 mice injected intraperitoneally with allogeneic cells, popliteal lymph nodes in the case of adult rats injected into the foot pad with allogeneic cells) in comparison with the appropriate control is taken as a measure of the graft-versus-host reactivity of the injected cells. Using this test, Atkins and Ford (1972) failed to find GVH reactive cells in either lymph nodes or thoracic duct of neonatally induced tolerant, chimeric rats, in respect to the AgB antigen to which the animals were tolerant, although their reactivity to third party antigens was normal. Furthermore, these workers found that when either these non-reactive cells or serum from the same animals were added to normal cells prior to the GVH test, the performance of the normal cells in the GVHR was not affected, suggesting that there had been no efferent blockade. Using a slightly different GVH assay, involving injection of putatively reactive cells under the kidney capsule of F_1 rats and then measuring the increase in size of that kidney, Elkins (1972) has confirmed the findings of Atkins and Ford (1972). Moreover, studies in mice by Brent *et al.* (1972) have also shown that lymphoid cells from tolerant mice are specifically non-reactive in the GVHR, and that when cells or serum from tolerant mice are admixed with normal cells, the GVH reactivity of normal cells is not affected. This study has also reconfirmed earlier work demonstrating that in mice tolerant across this strong H-2 barrier (CBA/A) tolerance cannot be transferred to normal mice by parabiosis, and that such tolerance can be abrogated by normal cells (Billingham *et al.*, 1956 and 1963). Comparable findings have been made by Hamilton (1973) using a different assay. He made 'B' mice by adult thymectomy, followed by sub-lethal irradiation and restoration with bone marrow. Such mice are deprived of T cells, and cannot reject allogeneic grafts. However, they can be induced to reject such grafts if adoptively transferred with normal syngeneic lymphoid cells. Lymphoid cells from mice made tolerant by neonatal injection of F_1 cells will not cause graft rejection in B mice, and if tolerant cells are mixed with normal cells, the graft rejecting capacities of the normal cells are not decreased. These results and those of Brent *et al.* (1972) argue for the absence of both antigen reactive cells and peripheral blocking factors in the tolerant mice.

In an elegant study using karyotype analysis of reacting cells in the GVH lesion, Elkins (1973) has investigated the GVH reactivity in cells from initially tolerant rats of one sex, whose tolerance has been abrogated by injection of normal syngeneic cells from a rat of the opposite sex. Such cells provoke a GVHR within the first month after abrogation; all the reactive cells initially bear the sex chromosome of the non-tolerant donor, whereas subsequently cells of the initially tolerant rat appear, although they can be prevented from appearing by thymectomizing the rat following the adoptive transfer of normal cells. This important study makes two clear points: (1) antigen reactive cells are absent in the periphery of tolerant rats and (2) once tolerance has been broken, the antigen reactive cells which emerge are newly formed, coming into the periphery via the thymus, so that if this pathway is cut by removing the thymus in the adult tolerant rat, no antigen reactive T cells from that rat appear.

Another form of antigen reactive T cell is the cytotoxic cell, which is found in the periphery of animals sensitized by allogeneic skin grafts (Canty and Wunderlich, 1971). The finding of such cells in neonatally induced tolerant mice has been a matter of some controversy: Hellström *et al.* (1971) demonstrated a low level of cytotoxic cells, and serum blocking factors which abrogated their *in vitro* cytotoxicity, in nine mice of the CBA and A strains given F_1 cells at birth, but these mice were not grafted and it was not established whether or not they were chimeras at the time of the cytotoxicity testing. In a study involving the same strains of mice, in which graded numbers of F_1 cells were given at birth and the mice were subsequently tested for tolerance as measured by skin graft survival, degree of chimerism, the presence of cytotoxic cells and serum blocking factors, Beverley *et al.* (1973) found that high doses of F_1 cells (50×10^6) at birth were associated with permanent acceptance of skin grafts, high levels ($>10\%$) of chimerism and the absence of cytotoxic cells and blocking factors. However, when fewer F_1 cells were given at birth (25×10^6 or 12.5×10^6) the degree of skin graft tolerance was variable, some grafts being rejected by 50 days by a chronic process of rejection, and others being maintained for longer periods but without normal hair growth, suggesting that they too were under some form of immunological attack. In these mice, the degree of chimerism when tested at 6–8 weeks of age was much lower (1–5%) than in the fully tolerant group which received 50×10^6 F_1 cells at birth, and both cytotoxic cells and blocking factors were found in some mice in these lower groups. It was therefore argued that such groups of mice were 'partially tolerant' and they will be discussed later under that heading. It was concluded that the mice in the group receiving the highest number of F_1 cells, and showing the highest levels of chimerism, were fully tolerant, and had no antigen reactive cells or peripheral blocking factors.

Full tolerance to transplantation antigens has been achieved in bursectomized chickens (Rouse and Warner, 1972) which cannot make antibody, thus confirming that a humoral response is not a necessary prerequisite for tolerance induction and maintenance.

The absence of tolerance in chimeric animals

Under certain circumstances a mouse may be a lymphoid chimera, and yet at presumably fairly high levels of chimerism, may fail to show tolerance to transplanted skin. One example of this is where the skin carries an antigen not present on lymphoid cells. A careful analysis of this situation is described by Lance (1971b). Adult C57BL mice were irradiated and given (C57 × A)F_1 bone marrow or spleen cells, and then subsequently grafted with A skin, which was rejected. Antibodies were found which were cytotoxic to A epidermal cells, but not to A lymphoid cells. Back cross experiments indicated that the newly described SK allele and H-2 segregated independently. This seems to be an example of sensitization and rejection due to an organ specific antigen, and it is not known how many more of such antigens exist. SK is apparently not limited in its distribution to skin, as it also appears on brain. Tolerance can only ensue when the antigens on the grafted organ or tissue are all represented on the lymphoid cells with which the recipient is made chimeric. H-2 antigens are present on lymphoid cells and most tissues, including skin, and in the case of the early experiments of Medawar and his colleagues (Billingham *et al.*, 1956; Billingham and Brent, 1959; Brent and Gowland, 1961; 1962) using the A and CBA strains, it was indeed fortunate that both strains share the same SK allele, for in this case, the H-2 antigens and whatever other antigens are present on lymphoid tissue as well as skin, are responsible for tolerance induction, which can be measured by skin graft survival.

Transplantation tolerance in the absence of chimerism

The attempt to induce transplantation tolerance with soluble and semi-soluble antigens prepared from lymphoid tissues has met with limited success. In fact in most cases the limited prolongation of graft survival achieved is perhaps better not described as tolerance, since it is merely a delay in the manifestation of immunization, or, in some cases, an alteration in the manifestation of immunity.

In 1963 Medawar reported on the use of soluble and semi-soluble extracts to weaken the immunological reaction against skin grafts. He found that it was easier to prolong grafts differing only at non-H-2 loci, and that the intravenous route of administering his extract was better than the intraperitoneal for graft prolongation. The combination of antigen extracts with immunosuppressive agents such as irradiation or methotrexate produced better prolongation than when either was used alone. More recently Law *et al.* (1972) have demonstrated the complications of using pure solubilized H-2 antigens in an attempt to produce tolerance. Their mice were injected from birth until they were several weeks of age with high doses of antigen. They were bled for antibody determinations and skin grafted to test their cell mediated immunity towards the antigen under test. Whereas there was a specific depression of antibody formation, the skin grafts were rejected normally, indicating no suppression of this cell mediated arm of the response.

A more successful attempt at tolerance induction in adult mice with antigen extract and ALS has been made by Brent *et al.* (1971). In this system antigen is given 16 days prior to ALS and skin grafting, and a high proportion of the resulting mice retain skin grafts indefinitely, and have no measurable antibody. It has proved easier to induce tolerance across a non-H-2 than an H-2 barrier, and this is in line with the induction of neonatal tolerance in mice with semi-allogeneic cells. The specific unresponsiveness produced by Brent and his colleagues with antigen and ALS can be abrogated by sensitized cells but the results with normal cells were equivocal (report by Brent, 1971) and so the exact nature of the tolerance is not clear. It might fall into the category of partial tolerance, where antigen reactive cells are found in the periphery but held in check by factors which will be discussed later.

In humoral responses

Full tolerance to protein antigens

The measure of an immune response to protein antigens, or to haptenic determinants attached to proteins, is usually antibody formation. A great deal of the literature on tolerance to such antigens is limited to consideration of antibody. However, as T cells need to co-operate with B cells in the production of antibody to most of these and erythrocyte antigens (Claman *et al.*, 1966; Taylor, 1968) the production of antibody is an indication of both T and B cell function, and its absence can indicate a lesion in one or both of these cell populations.

For the strict definition of 'full tolerance' given in the introduction, it would be necessary to demonstrate that there were neither T or B antigen reactive cells present, and this has been done in several instances. For bovine serum albumin (BSA), Dresser and Mitchison (see Dresser and Mitchison, 1968; Mitchison, 1971a) have shown there are two zones of tolerance; low zone, produced by small amounts of antigen, in which only the T cells are tolerized, and high zone, produced by much larger doses of antigen, in which both T and B cells are tolerized. In both zones, tolerance can be abrogated by the injection of normal lymphoid cells. For bovine gamma globulin (BGG), Weigle *et al.* (1971) have demonstrated specific unresponsiveness in B cells from bone marrow and T cells from thymus, and in T and B cells in the periphery (spleen). They have confirmed that T cells are rendered tolerant at much lower dose levels of antigen than B cells. They have also shown that the time course of tolerance induction is different for thymic T cells, which become tolerant in 2 to 5 days, and B cells from the bone marrow, which take 8 to 21 days to be rendered tolerant, although B cells in the spleen do not apparently take as long. The recovery from tolerance (in the absence of injection of further antigen to maintain a tolerogenic concentration) is faster in bone marrow (being complete by 49 days) than in thymus, where tolerance lasts over 100 days. This may reflect the more rapid turnover of B cells in comparison with T cells.

Further proof that B cells can be made tolerant comes from studies of tolerance induction to haptenic determinants, which normally elicit only a B cell response (with T cell help) to a protein carrier. Such studies have been made by Mitchison

(1971b) and Davie *et al.* (1972). In Mitchison's system, the antigen BSA-NIP is used to induce tolerance at the high zone level by injecting large doses intraperitoneally three times a week for ten weeks into mice that have been previously irradiated. At the end of this procedure the mice are unresponsive to test doses of BSA-NIP, producing neither anticarrier antibody (anti-BSA) nor antihapten antibody (anti-NIP). Moreover, when NIP is introduced on another carrier, e.g. chicken gamma globulin (CGG) CGG-NIP, the mouse makes a negligible response at day 10, when a response would be expected, a very low response at day 20, and a somewhat diminished response at day 40 post-challenge. This initial non-reactivity is attributed to the absence of hapten-specific cells in the tolerant mouse; the breaking of tolerance eventually seen is probably due to the introduction of a new carrier, stimulating an existing population of T cells to respond (only the BSA responsive T cells having disappeared due to tolerance induction) and help newly emerging B cells to respond to the NIP determinant.

In tolerance to protein antigens, tolerance is maintained only so long as antigen remains above a certain concentration. When the concentration of retained antigen falls (cf. when a previously chimeric animal loses chimerism, Lance and Medawar, 1969), newly emerging T and B cells are no longer exposed to a tolerizing dose of antigen, and the animal regains the ability to respond to that antigen again. Early work by Claman and Talmage (1963) and Taylor (1964) showed that if a mouse was made tolerant to BGG or BSA, and was then thymectomized, its recovery from tolerance was greatly impaired. This was attributed to the failure of thymectomized animals to provide new antigen reactive cells as the antigenic concentration fell below tolerogenic levels. This result is entirely analogous with that of Elkins's (1973) study of tolerance to transplantation antigens, already discussed, in which antigen reactive cells of recipient type could not be detected after adult thymectomy, even after tolerance had been broken by adoptively transferred cells. Both results point to the importance of cell turnover in restoring the previously tolerant animal, and argue against the idea that recovery from tolerance may reflect recovery of tolerant peripheral T cells. Experiments in which tolerance was induced to HSA in chickens, reported by Ivanyi and Howard (1971) give further weight to this view, and produce evidence that normal B cell turnover as well as T cell turnover is important in recovery from tolerance. They found that both bursectomy and thymectomy impaired recovery from tolerance induced by HSA.

Recovery from full tolerance, with disappearance of the antigen, is followed in some cases by a variable period of hyporeactivity (Mitchison, 1962; Humphrey, 1964). Initially this may be due to the presence of only small numbers of antigen reactive cells, due to slow cell turnover, but when hyporeactivity is maintained for long periods in the absence of antigen (Humphrey, 1964) active processes such as those discussed under 'partial tolerance' may be operating.

Full tolerance to erythrocyte antigens

There is still some controversy as to whether sheep red blood cells (SRBC) can induce tolerance in mice at both the B and T cell level. Playfair (1969) and Gershon and Kondo (1970) have shown that B cells can be made tolerant, although tolerance induction in at least a portion of B cells probably requires the presence of T cells (Gershon and Kondo, 1970). In contrast, Miller and Mitchell (1970) demonstrated tolerance at the level of the T cell but failed to show it at the level of the B cell. In these experiments the activities of putatively tolerant and normal T cells were compared by injecting them into neonatally thymectomized mice which have a greatly diminished number of T cells. Such mice have a normal B cell component capable of co-operating with adoptively transferred T cells and producing an antibody response, but cannot by themselves respond to SRBC. When given the antigen, neonatally thymectomized mice receiving normal T cells in the form of thoracic duct lymphocytes (TDL) made a good anti-SRBC antibody response, whereas B mice given TDL from tolerant mice were unable to respond. From this it was concluded that tolerance was present at the level of the T cell. To examine whether it was present at the level of the B cell, irradiated recipients, which had no functional B or T cells, were injected with SRBC and normal T cells, and B cells from either tolerant or normal donors. In every case there was restoration of the co-operative response, i.e. the B cells were not demonstrated to be tolerant. However, it was not excluded that the B cell response might have come from recently matured B cells in the irradiated recipients. Attempts were therefore made to induce tolerance in B mice, i.e. mice with no T cells, and these were unsuccessful. But as Gershon and Kondo (1970) have shown that the presence of T cells are required for the induction of tolerance to SRBC in B cells, this is not altogether surprising.

PARTIAL TOLERANCE

In cell mediated immunity

Examples where the mechanism is not clear

Voisin (1971 for review) was the first to suggest that transplantation tolerance was an example of a state of balance between an immune responsive state, which he termed 'rejection reaction' and a suppressive state, which he called 'facilitation reaction'.

He produced evidence that antibodies which would enhance the growth of allogeneic tumors were present in the serum of mice made tolerant by neonatal injection of F_1 cells, and suggested that these antibodies were the mediators of the suppressed state. The presence of an antibody response to the putatively tolerated antigen places these tolerant mice of Voisin in the partially tolerant category in this review, since full tolerance has been defined as the absence of any antigen reactive cells.

Following their work on enhancing antibody in mice and in patients with progressively growing tumors (Hellström and Hellström, 1969), Hellström *et al.* (1971) examined the reactivity of mice injected neonatally with F_1 spleen cells and found low levels of cytotoxic cells as measured by *in vitro* tests using a lymphocyte : target cell ratio of 4000:1, and serum blocking factors, which could abrogate this presumed T cell activity. Beverley *et al.* (1973) were able to repeat these results, but only when smaller numbers of F_1 cells were given at birth, in comparison with the larger numbers of F_1 cells which induced a state of complete tolerance. In this study the prolonged (now $>$200 days) acceptance of skin grafts was present in all the fully tolerant mice, but in only about 50% of mice in the partially tolerant groups in which a low level of chimerism had been demonstrated at 50 days of age. The possibility was therefore raised that the mechanism of maintaining partial tolerance might be different from that of full tolerance and involve control factors present in the serum of such mice, which interfered with the activity of cytotoxic or potentially cytotoxic T cells. Because of the length of the *in vitro* assay, 48 hours, it cannot be determined whether the block is afferent, i.e. blocking the induction or maturation of cytotoxic T cells, or efferent, i.e. coating the target cells with antibody and thus rendering them no longer vulnerable to cytotoxic T cell attack. In recent work involving injection of 20 to 40 million allogeneic bone marrow cells intravenously into neonatal rats, Bansal *et al.* (1973) have shown that a high proportion of the recipients maintain skin grafts for at least 50 days, and that when tested within 2 months of birth, both rats with intact skin grafts, and those which had rejected their grafts, had cytotoxic cells in their peripheral blood lymphocytes (PBL). It was also noted that PBL from purposely immunized rats had activity at lower lymphocyte : target cell ratios than the partially tolerant rats, i.e. they were more active. When tested later (84 or more days after skin grafting), a smaller proportion of rats with intact skin grafts showed cytotoxic cells (8/13) and those which did, showed it at lower levels. Blocking factors were demonstrated only in the serum of rats with intact grafts, and when individual rats which eventually rejected grafts were examined serially, it was found that the blocking factors disappeared 3–10 days prior to rejection. There was thus a high degree of correlation between *in vivo* graft survival and *in vitro* detected blocking factors in these experiments, and it is therefore not unreasonable to speculate that they may be causally related. The numbers of allogeneic cells given at birth were lower than those reported by Billingham *et al.* (1963), in which the recipient rats had evidence of central failure as a cause of the induced tolerance, by virtue of the abrogation of tolerance by adoptive transfer of normal lymphocytes. It may therefore be that in the studies of Bansal *et al.* (1973), it might have been possible to induce full tolerance, with elimination of antigen reactive cells, if higher numbers of cells had been given at birth. Nevertheless, their findings indicate a mechanism of suppression in partial tolerance.

Mouse radiation chimeras have been shown to lack graft-versus-host reactivity, having no measurable cytotoxic cell activity or serum blocking factors (Grant *et al.*, 1972, and see section on full tolerance associated with chimerism). In contrast, a series of long term surviving canine radiation chimeras were shown to have cytotoxic cells of donor origin active against host skin fibroblasts, and serum factors which would specifically block this reactivity (Hellström *et al.*, 1970).

Another situation in which low levels of both cytotoxic and MLR reactive cells have been found is in allophenic mice (Wegman *et al.*, 1971; Phillips *et al.*, 1971). This, at first glance is rather surprising, since these animals grow as chimeras from the blastocyst stage, a situation which should be optimal for the induction of full tolerance. However, it is well known that the level of chimerism in the various organs of allophenic mice is very unstable, and subject to wide variation during postnatal life (Mintz and Silvers, 1967), and this might go some way towards explaining the findings, which otherwise throw doubt on the hypothesis that full tolerance reflects central failure.

Suppression by antibody (immune deviation)

Crowle and Hu (1969) have shown that the development of delayed hypersensitivity (DH), a manifestation of T cell reactivity, towards BSA and OVA can be prevented by prior injection of the antigen in water-in-oil emulsion. They also showed that this hyporeactive state, as far as DH was concerned, could be terminated by injection of spleen cells presensitized to the antigen in question, but not by normal spleen cells. The partial tolerance, i.e. inactive T cells but active B cells, could be transferred from tolerant mice to normal mice, either with serum or spleen cells, and the suggestion was that the spleen cells were active by virtue of the antibody they were producing. This sort of partial tolerance, which has also been called 'immune deviation' (Asherson and Stone, 1965) would therefore appear to be antibody mediated in a manner rather similar to immunological enhancement (Kaliss, 1966), except that in this case the afferent arc of induction appears to be affected rather than the effector stage since normal cells cannot abrogate tolerance, but immune cells can. This is one of the few examples of modification of induction of the T cell response by humoral antibody. It also suggests that the T cells responsible for DH are different from those which act as helpers, as the former are absent or inactivated, whilst the latter must be present to get the antibody response to these thymus dependent antigens.

Suppression by antigen

Following the injection of protein antigens in adjuvant into guinea pigs, an early delayed hypersensitivity (DH) response is seen. This response can be temporarily abrogated for 3–10 days by injecting large doses of antigen intravenously or intraperitoneally. Schlossmann *et al.* (1971) reported that the abrogation or desensitization was antigen specific, and was accompanied by disappearance from the peritoneal cavity of lymphocytes which could respond to antigen by DNA synthesis or the production of macrophage inhibitory factor. In contrast, lymph node cells from desensitized guinea pigs, like those from control immunized animals, did respond to antigen *in vitro* by DNA synthesis. Schlossmann *et al.* (1971) suggested that the abrogation of skin reactivity and the *in vitro* findings were due to a selective disappearance from the recirculating lymphocyte pool of antigen reactive cells (ARC), and that recovery from desensitization was due to the reappearance in the periphery of ARC from the lymph nodes. Using a similar system, but different antigens, Dwyer and Cantor (1973) reported that following immunization with two or more protein antigens, marked decrease in DH reactions to all of them could be induced by intravenous or subcutaneous injection of large doses of one or more of the immunizing antigens. These authors found that transfer of peritoneal exudate cells from these desensitized animals into syngeneic unimmunized guinea pigs resulted in the appearance in the recipients of DH, which though of lesser magnitude than in recipients of peritoneal exudate cells from sensitized donors, was greater than that in the desensitized donors themselves, before transfer. They postulated a non-specific humoral factor as the cause of desensitization following antigen administration to guinea pigs.

It seems that in both these examples of temporary abrogation of cell mediated immunity, some sort of control mechanism is limiting the presence or activity of antigen reactive cells in the periphery.

Partial tolerance via suppressor cells

A finding which may throw some light on another mechanism of partial tolerance has been that of Elkins (1972), who found that he could inhibit the induction of a GVHR by normal rat spleen cells by mixing them in a 1:2 ratio with cells from the spleens of previously fully tolerant rats whose tolerance had been abrogated by an adoptive transfer of normal cells. Suppressor cells could not be obtained from the spleens of tolerant rats unless tolerance had been broken by adoptive transfer. The suppressive effect was maximal shortly after the adoptive transfer, and thereafter began to wane. The active component in these suppressor spleens has not yet been identified as to type of cell or cell product. Conventional antibody has not been ruled out in the experiments reported, but for reasons to be discussed, would seem an unlikely candidate.

An example of partial tolerance to a transplantation antigen not associated with chimerism, in which suppressor cells may be active, has been reported by Goldberg *et al.* (1972). Different strains of inbred mice differ in the extent to which females will react to the male HY antigen by rejecting syngeneic male skin. Almost all females of the C57B1/6 strain reject such skin grafts, whereas only a proportion of DBA/2 females do, and C3H females normally do not reject male C3H skin. However, the HY antigen is recognized by each of these strains because all females grafted with male skin, whether they reject it or not, produce anti-HY antibody, as demonstrated by its cytotoxicity towards sperm and male epidermal cells. The female mice that maintain syngeneic male skin grafts could therefore be described as partially tolerant, as they are operationally tolerant although they respond to antigens of the graft by making antibody. The fact that they retain their grafts argues either for a complete lack of reactivity on the part of T lymphocytes, whose activities rather than that of antibody, seem to be at least in part responsible for skin graft rejection (Billingham *et al.*, 1954; Davies, 1969), or a blockade of this activity by some factors. In the experiments reported by Goldberg *et al.* (1972), presumed T cell reactivity to male grafts could be elicited in otherwise unreactive C3H mice either by grafting a second skin graft 3 weeks or more after the first, or by splenectomizing the mice before the first graft. These results could argue for a 'blocking' of the T cell response being lessened or removed by these procedures; in the case of the second graft, by increasing the antigen dose, and in the case of splenectomy, removing a population of cells that was responsible for the blocking, either directly, or via some cell product. As will be argued later, it is in spleen that a sub-population of T lymphocytes which can regulate certain responses can be found, and it may well be that these 'suppressor cells' are active in the situation described above, in which reactivity to a very weak transplantation antigen is held in check. However, as with the experiments of Elkins (1972), there is nothing reported in these latter experiments to eliminate the possibility of control via a B cell product, although it is unlikely to be cytotoxic antibody, since all the female mice, whether they rejected the male skin grafts or not, seemed to make it.

In the experiments on the HY antigen reported by Billingham (Billingham *et al.*, 1965) in which he describes 9 ways in which female C57BL/6 mice can be made to accept syngeneic skin grafts, there are two in which chimerism is not a feature; one, 'old breeder' C57BL/6 mice, which have presumably been tolerized by repeated exposure to the HY antigen from male fetuses, and two, female mice given an injection of small numbers of allogeneic male lymphoid cells at birth; these mice ultimately reject the allogeneic lymphoid cells and will not accept skin grafts from mice of that allogeneic strain, but will accept syngeneic male skin grafts. Moreover, when normal C57BL/6 female mice are parabiosed to such 'tolerant' mice, a proportion of them also become tolerant; i.e. this is an example of transfer of tolerance to the normal partner, rather than abrogation of tolerance by the normal mouse, and as such does not fit into the theory of central inhibition, but is a peripheral inactivation. It might be that in this very weakly antigenic system, in addition to the more normal 'full tolerance' induced by chimerism, there can exist under other circumstances a partial tolerance, in which small amounts of inducer antigen have activated a 'suppressor system' and this is capable of suppressing the response of normal mice. A completely different interpretation can be given to experiments involving small antigenic differences in which chimerism is present in tolerant mice (Billingham *et al.*, 1965; Martinez *et al.*, 1959). In this case parabiosis with normal mice results in the normal mice becoming tolerant, possibly because the normal animal is being constantly transfused with small numbers of allogeneic cells, resulting in active tolerization and chimerism; it has been shown that for weak antigens of this sort, even adult mice can be made tolerant by injection of allogeneic or semi-allogeneic cells (Billingham *et al.*, 1965).

There is evidence that even in the cell mediated response evoked in normal animals by alloantigens, suppressor T cells act to limit the extent of the response (Cantor and Simpson, 1973; Simpson, 1973). When spleen cells from mice which have been adult thymectomized three weeks previously are sensitized *in vitro* against alloantigens, their cytotoxic response is considerably greater than that of spleen cells from normal mice. The only T cells missing from the adult thymectomized mouse spleens are the recently migrated spleen seeking thymocytes, which do not recirculate, and are therefore not sensitive to small doses of ALS (Raff and Cantor, 1971; Cantor and Simpson, 1973). When small numbers of these ALS resistant splenic T cells are added back to cultures of hyperactive adult thymectomized spleen cells during *in vitro* induction of a cytotoxic response to alloantigens, the response is reduced to normal levels, thus indicating the suppressor rôle of this population in the normal response, and suggesting the possible rôle of suppressor T cells in initiating or maintaining some types of tolerance in cell mediated responses.

In humoral responses

Examples where the mechanism is not clear

Ada (1970) has described antigen binding cells (ABC) in various lymphoid organs, using a technique in which the antigen is radio-iodinated, and then subsequently visualized on the cell surface by radio autography. This method also enables the morphology of the antigen binding cell to be observed. Antigen binding cells, present at a low level in the unimmunized animal, increase following immunization. Also if bacterial antigens are used, a proportion of the antigen binding cells as demonstrated by radio autography will be found to bind bacteria, suggesting a functional relationship. The immune function of these antigen binding cells can also be demonstrated by measuring the adoptive antibody response of lymphoid populations which have been exposed to very highly radio labeled antigen, a procedure resulting in specific killing of ABC. The antibody response to the antigen with which the cells were preincubated is abolished, whilst the response to other antigens remains. The binding of radio labeled antigen to cells can be inhibited by anti-immunoglobulin sera with specificity against μ chains and light chains. This might suggest that the ABC are B cells, but does not exclude the possibility that they are also T cells (Marcholonis *et al.*, 1972). The subsequent experiments of Basten *et al.* (1971) suggest that both T and B cells can be specifically inactivated by high specific activity radio labeled antigen. The finding that ABC in rats tolerant to flagellin (Ada, 1970) are not fewer than in normal rats suggests that in tolerance to this antigen, there are antigen reactive cells in the periphery. In view of the difficulty commonly found in observing antigen binding T cells, it seems more likely that these ABC are B cells and that this 'partial tolerance' is maintained by tolerant T cells, i.e. there is no antigen reactive T clone. There is, however, no direct evidence on this point.

Benhamin and Weigle (1970) have shown that tolerance induced in neonatal rabbits by bovine serum albumin (BSA) can be broken by giving cross reacting antigens, such as equine serum albumin (ESA) and human serum albumin (HSA). The spectrum of antibodies produced to the cross reacting antigen and to BSA appear to be identical in terms of affinity, to antibodies elicited by the cross-reacting antigen given to normal non-tolerant rabbits. From this it is concluded that the B cells are not tolerized following neonatal antigen administration but that the appropriate T cell clone is, and is probably eliminated. This would therefore be an example of partial tolerance, in that the tolerance resided in the T cell population but not the B cells. Weigle argues that when a cross-reacting antigen is introduced, it stimulates a new clone of T cells, which can act as helper cells for B cells already present. He attributes the lack of success in abrogating tolerance with cross-reacting antigens reported by some to the accidental inclusion of the tolerogen BSA as a contaminant in the cross-reacting antigen used, and in this work reproduces the effect by purposely including BSA in some injections of the cross-reacting antigen. It seems therefore that 'tolerance', resulting in inability to respond with antibody to the homologous antigen, can be induced by merely making the T cell population tolerant, leaving B cells unaffected.

Somewhat different results were obtained by Paul *et al.* (1967), who induced tolerance to BSA in adult rabbits by small doses of BSA, and then broke tolerance with a cross-reacting antigen, $DNP_{10}BSA$. They found that the population of antibodies produced as a result of this maneuver had quite different binding characteristics to the antibodies produced in rabbits given immunogenic doses of BSA alone. The antibodies of the previously tolerant rabbits bound preferentially to $DNP_{10}BSA$, i.e. had a low affinity for BSA. They suggest that in this system, during tolerance induction B cells are affected, and that those with the highest affinity receptors for BSA become irreversibly 'turned off' first, leaving the B cells with low affinity receptors to be stimulated by the later introduction of the cross-reacting antigen, $DNP_{10}BSA$. In their view, partial tolerance is the selective removal or inactivation of cells with high affinity receptors for the antigen.

Suppression by antibody

Rowley and Fitch (1965a and b) reported partial tolerance to srbc in rats, associated with antibody. They injected neonatal rats with multiple tolerogenic doses of srbc and found very low levels of hemolysin antibody and small numbers of plaque forming cells (PFC) in comparison with control rats. This low level of antibody and PFC could be maintained as long as antigen administration continued and could be mimicked by giving anti-srbc antibody to normal growing rats. They argue that in the neonatally induced tolerant rats, PFCs are held at a low level by the small amounts of antibody produced acting (perhaps in conjunction with antigen) to block the induction of further PFC, and that the similar result obtained with passively administered antibody confirms this. That passively administered antibody, especially of the IgG class, can act to regulate antibody production, especially IgM, has been amply confirmed by Moller (for review, see Uhr and Moller, 1968) and more recently Kappler *et al.* (1971) has shown that anti-srbc antibody can inhibit priming for srbc PFC but in contrast to this, the induction of T helper cells cannot be inhibited by antibody. It has been shown by others that antibody does not inhibit the induction of delayed hypersensitivity very effectively (see Uhr and Moller, 1968). This preferential effect of antibody on the afferent arc, i.e. induction of B and T cells, implies that while antibody feedback is probably an important mechanism for control of the B cell response, it is unlikely to be a mechanism for T cell responses.

In a study by Tong and Boose (1970) mice were made tolerant to ultracentrifuged BGG and the immunological response was measured by the elimination of ^{125}I labeled BGG, a more rapid elimination of ^{125}I BGG indicating immunity. They found that in mice which were tolerant as measured by these criteria, tolerance could not be abrogated by the transfer of either normal or immune cells, but that transfer of serum from tolerant mice to normal mice prevented the induction of immunity by immunogenic doses of BGG. No analysis of the serum factors was given, but if it was conventional antibody preventing induction of immunity in T and/or B cells, and preventing expression of immunity by presensitized B cells, it is an antibody which does not result in the elimination of ^{125}I labeled antigen.

Suppression by antigen, or antibody-antigen complexes

Polysaccharide antigens

Polysaccharide antigens are thymus independent, that is, they do not require the co-operation of T cells to provoke an antibody response (see Ivanyi and Howard, 1971). The antibodies elicited are limited to the IgM class. This class of antigens are composed of multiply repeating determinants and are not biodegradable, so they persist in the body for long periods, of the order of months, following injection.

When a tolerizing dose of SIII is injected into a mouse, there is a transitory immune response, followed by a period during which neither circulating antibody or plaque forming cells (PFCs) can be detected. During this period it is possible to detect rosette forming cells, that is, lymphocytes capable of binding erythrocytes coated with the antigen (see Ivanyi and Howard, 1971). The finding of peripheral antigen reactive cells places this type of tolerance in the 'partial tolerance' category, as defined in this review. A similar finding has been made for another thymus independent antigen, lipopolysaccharide (LPS) by Sjöberg (1971).The first appearance of PFCs following a tolerizing dose of SIII depends on the size of the dose: with 50 μg, PFCs first appear between day 40 and 80, whereas with 250 μg, none is detectable in the tolerized mouse by day 150 (see Ivanyi and Howard, 1971). However, if washed spleen cells are transferred from the tolerant mouse into irradiated recipients, large numbers of PFCs rapidly appear, suggesting that antigen reactive B cells in the tolerant mouse are prevented from differentiating into antibody secreting cells by the presence of excess antigen in the circulation, i.e. B cells are being reversibly 'turned off' by antigen —or perhaps by antigen–antibody complexes, if under these circumstances minute amounts of antibody are in fact being formed. This may be analogous to the *in vitro* findings of tolerance induction of B cells by antigen or antigen–antibody complexes, of Diener and Feldmann (see Diener, this volume).

Another phenomenon seen during recovery from tolerance to SIII in the mouse is 'treadmill neutralization'. This occurs once PFCs are detectable, but before serum antibody can be detected. In this case, hyporeactivity is maintained by circulating antigen neutralizing antibody as it is formed. The antigen–antibody complexes formed in this way are subsequently removed from the circulation by the RE system, and broken down, but the SIII, being non-catabolizable, can be returned once again to the circulation to neutralize further antibody (see Ivanyi and Howard, 1971). Thus, in tolerance to the polysaccharide SIII, antigen acts in three ways. Firstly, it induces tolerance in a manner not completely understood, but which involves a transitory immune response. Secondly, it maintains partial tolerance by blocking the differentiation of antigen reactive cells to antibody producing cells, and thirdly, maintains the hyporeactive state by neutralizing antibody formed by newly emerging plaque forming cells.

Protein antigens

Feldmann (1971) has demonstrated in an *in vitro* system, that induction of antibody production or of tolerance can, depending on the chemical form of the antigen, be achieved in B cells. Parish (1971) showed that flagellin could be chemically altered by acetoacetylation, thus altering the antigenicity in such a way that when used to immunize adult rats, the acetoacetylated derivatives suppressed antibody formation, while inducing an increased delayed hypersensitivity. In neonatal rats, the acetoacetylated derivatives produced tolerance both in terms of antibody and delayed hypersensitivity.

Suppression by T cells

Data suggesting the possible rôle of suppressor cells in inducing and/or maintaining partial tolerance in the T cell, or cell mediated response has already been presented. The evidence that the suppressor cell is itself a T cell rests more strongly on partial tolerance in B cells to a variety of antigens, both thymus dependent and thymus independent.

Polysaccharide antigens

Baker and his associates have uncovered an extremely interesting phenomenon relating to a possible suppression by T cells of antibody formation to immunogenic doses of SIII. Their findings are that small doses of ALS, which remove peripheral T cells, enhance the antibody response (Baker *et al.*, 1970a) whilst injection of thymocytes decreases the response (Baker *et al.*, 1970b). Complementary findings have been obtained by Kerbel and Eidinger (1972), who investigated the effect of adult thymectomy on the response to PVP, another thymus independent antigen. Adult thymectomy appears to inactivate a population of non-recirculating T cells which may migrate from thymus to spleen (Raff and Cantor, 1971; Cantor, 1972a; Cantor and Simpson, 1973). Kerbel and Eidinger (1972) found that mice immunized 3 weeks or more after adult thymectomy gave enhanced antibody responses to PVP. These findings could mean that, even in the case of thymus-independent antigens, while T cells are not required for a maximum antibody response, they can nevertheless regulate antibody production by decreasing it. The implications of a suppressor rôle for a sub-population of T cells are important and will be further discussed later.

Erythrocyte antigens

McGregor *et al.* (1967) found that thoracic duct lymphocytes (TDL) from rats made tolerant to srbc would not restore the response of irradiated rats, as would TDL from normal rats, but that if the 'tolerant' TDL were incubated *in vitro* prior to injection, a proportion of the irradiated recipients were able to respond, i.e. tolerance had been broken by the *in vitro* incubation. This implied that potentially responsive cells were present in the periphery in these tolerant rats, but held in check by some factors. Later, McCullagh (1970a) found that the tolerance of rats to srbc could not be abrogated by the injection of normal lymphoid cells unless the recipients were irradiated, which argued either for a 'space effect', i.e. that the injected cells could not function unless space was made for them, implying either that they were crowded out by the lymphoid cells of the tolerant rat, or that an active mechanism on the part of the tolerant rat in induced tolerance in the transferred normal population. This second interpretation is more likely in view of the fact that the normal functions of the transferred cells can be rescued if the cells are removed from the tolerant recipient up to 3 days after transfer, but not thereafter (McCullagh, 1970b). One of the reasons for placing this srbc tolerance in rats in the 'partial tolerance' category is the fact that B cells capable of producing anti-srbc antibody are present in the tolerant rats, and can be turned on within 72 hours by the transfer of allogeneic lymphocytes (McCullagh, 1970c). An allogeneic graft-versus-host or host-versus-graft effect seems to be crucial to this turning on, but it can occur even when the transferred cells are themselves from rats tolerant of srbc, though not when the transferred cells are from rats tolerant of the recipient. This analysis has been made by (1) breaking tolerance to srbc in F_1 rats by the injection of normal parental cells, thus producing a graft-versus-host reaction, (2) breaking tolerance to srbc in parental strain rats by injecting normal F_1 cells, producing a host-versus-graft reaction, and (3) doing (1) or (2) above with cells from srbc tolerant donors. There is no evidence as to the state of tolerance of the T cell population in the srbc tolerant rats, since the allogeneic cells could be acting non-specifically, and during the ensuing GVH or HVG producing non-specific B cell 'helper' substances which can turn on primed B cells (Katz *et al.*, 1971; Kreth and Williamson, 1971). However, the apparent induction of tolerance in normal syngeneic cells transferred to tolerant rats is suggestive of some sort of suppressor function in the recipients, and in view of the absence of measurable anti-srbc antibody, it is tempting to speculate about a suppressive T cell, or T cell product.

The work of Gershon and Kondo (1971) on the induction of 'infections tolerance' to srbc in mice points to the influence of T cells in regulating B cell responses, and is analogous to the T cell suppression of antibody responses to thymus independent antigens, already cited (Baker *et al.*, 1970a and b). But srbc is a thymus dependent antigen, and according to Gershon and Kondo (1970), it is necessary to have T cells present, in order to tolerize B cells with T dependent antigens. In the experiments in which they demonstrate 'infections tolerance', adult thymectomized, irradiated and bone marrow restored mice (B mice) are given a tolerizing dose of srbc, together with a small dose of thymocytes. Spleen cells from these mice are transferred to further B mice, together with enough normal T cells that the recipients would be expected to make a 'co-operative' anti-srbc response. It was found that the inclusion of spleen cells from mice that had been tolerized in the presence of thymocytes prevented the recipients from making a normal IgM or IgG response to srbc. The effect was specific, i.e. they could make antibody to an unrelated erythrocyte antigen, horse rbc. If spleen cells from B mice which had been given tolerogenic doses of srbc in the absence of added thymocytes were given to the recipients along with normal T cells, a normal srbc response was obtained. These results suggest that the thymocytes in the tolerized host became capable, perhaps via the production of some factor, of specifically suppressing the response of normal T and B cells, making them tolerant. It appears unlikely that conventional antibody production by the cells transferred from the tolerized donor could be responsible because in experiments in which cells were transferred from donors which had not been rendered tolerant by this procedure, as evidenced by the fact that they were making some anti-srbc antibody, no suppression took place.

The inability of normal lymphoid cells to restore reactivity in mice made tolerant to srbc following treatment with cyclophosphamide is also shown in the experiments of Miller and Mitchell (1970), although they do not comment further on the fact and go on to analyze this srbc tolerance using cell transfer. However, they show that these tolerant mice, with background direct PFC of about 1000/spleen (partial tolerance) when given large numbers of normal TDL and additional B cells from bone marrow or spleen, increase their PFC to 5000–10 000 per spleen, which is only about 10% of the response in either normal mice, or mice given cyclophosphamide alone. This may be another example of partial tolerance in which some sort of suppression is occurring, and may be analogous to that demonstrated by Gershon and Kondo (1971).

The induction of an anti-srbc antibody response *in vitro* in fractionated splenic lymphocytes from mice sensitized 5 days previously with low doses of srbc was studied by Haskell and Axelrad (1972). They fractionated the cells by velocity sedimentation into small lymphocytes (SL), medium lymphocytes (ML), and blast cells and found that the SL give good responses, but that when blasts were added back to the cultures in small numbers, they inhibited the response, and the cells mediating the inhibition were sensitive to anti-θ serum. The inhibiting effect was still shown when the two cell populations were separated by a nucleopore membrane, suggesting that it was due to a T cell product, perhaps analogous with the specific T cell factors described by Feldmann which can help tolerize primed B cells (Feldmann and Basten, 1972a; Feldmann, 1973).

DISCUSSION

An attempt has been made to separate tolerance into full, meaning specific immunological non-reactivity accompanied by an absence of B or T antigen reactive cells, and partial, meaning a state of hyporeactivity in which some measure of response, or the potential to respond, can be detected in either of the two main lymphocyte sub-populations. The implication of this analysis is that full tolerance is due to central inhibition of the response, whilst in partial tolerance the peripheral activities seen are kept below normal by mechanisms which will be discussed. Full tolerance to transplantation antigens is associated with chimerism, except perhaps in the few examples where soluble or semi-soluble antigens have been used to induce tolerance to a skin transplant, which may thereafter be a sufficient source of antigen to maintain the tolerant state. It is noteworthy that it has only been possible to produce tolerance in this way either to very weak antigens (HY) Kelly *et al.*, 1966, or by some treatment of the recipient which temporarily decreases the number of immunocompetent cells (ALS) (Brent *et al.*, 1971). It is nevertheless a hopeful approach, because the induction and maintenance of chimerism in adult animals is much more difficult than in newborns, although production of chimerism can also be aided by procedures which decrease the number of mature peripheral lymphoid cells in the host (Lance and Medawar, 1969). The maintenance of lymphoid chimerism is also beset with difficulties due to GVHR unless F_1 cells can be used, or the sub-population of GVHR cells removed from an allogeneic inoculum. Man is particularly prone to chronic GVH disease

(Graw *et al.*, 1970) even when donor and recipient are HL-A matched siblings. The complexities of the antigens that need to be represented on the chimeric cells in order to induce transplantation tolerance to various organs have been illustrated by the finding of tissue-specific antigens such as the SK antigen (Lance, 1971b), which is present on skin, but not lymphoid cells. Tissue-specific antigens such as TL and θ (see Raff and Cantor, 1971 for review) have long been recognized and characterized, but it is possible that antigens specific for other tissues will be found and need consideration in transplantation.

The finding that full tolerance involving both T and B cells can be induced to a variety of protein, hapten and erythrocyte antigens is encouraging. The findings underline the necessity for the continuous presence of antigen, because of the constant generation of both T and B cells from which clones of antigen reactive cells can appear in the absence of tolerogenic concentrations of antigen.

For many antigens, i.e. thymus dependent antigens, it would appear to be adequate to induce tolerance in the T cell alone, since in the absence of T cell help, no antibody can be formed. However, the thymus dependent response to a variety of antigens can be enhanced by specific (e.g. via cross-reacting antigens) and non-specific (e.g. the allogeneic effect (Kreth and Williamson, 1971; Katz *et al.*, 1971)) factors, themselves T cell products so that partial tolerance of this sort (T but not B) can be more easily broken. It has been suggested that this may be the mechanism of autoimmunity (Taylor, 1971).

It would be useful to understand the mechanisms by which partial tolerance, or specific hyporeactivity, is induced and maintained. In the clinical situation there will be many instances in which full tolerance induction fails and an uneasy balance of hypo- and hyper-reactivity supervenes. Looking at the various examples of partial tolerance given, it would appear that many different mechanisms are acting, although a pattern may be emerging which implicates, in some cases at least, a suppressor cell population. This should be susceptible to manipulation, when more is understood of its basic biology.

Let us first look at those examples where evidence for a suppressor cell or its product is strong, and where there is some indication of whether such a cell is of T or B lineage.

In the case of the control of the B cell response to two thymus independent antigens, SIII (Baker *et al.*, 1970a and b) and PVP (Kerbel and Eidinger, 1971 and 1972), it is quite clear that removal of sub-populations of T cells by ALS or adult thymectomy, or a combination of the two, markedly enhances the 19S response, and that injection of thymocytes can suppress the response. This is a strong argument for the T cell acting as a suppressor, although it could be argued that it was suppressing via a B cell product, conventional antibody. This argument seems a less likely explanation for the heightened reactivity seen in spleen cells from adult thymectomized mice in the response to alloantigens in both the MLR (Mosier and Cantor, 1971) and following *in vitro* sensitization to produce cytotoxic cells (Simpson, 1973; Cantor and Simpson, 1973) because these are both T cell responses, and the induction of T cell reactivity has been shown to be very resistant to the effect of humoral antibody (Uhr and Moller, 1968; Kappler *et al.*, 1971). The sub-population of T cells missing from an adult thymectomized mouse is the short lived, spleen seeking T cells (Raff and Cantor, 1971; Cantor and Simpson, 1973) and it is this sub-population which would seem to be the most likely candidate for the suppressor cell. The concept of a T suppressor or regulator cell is not new; it was originally postulated by Gershon and Kondo (1970) and the idea has been expanded to include such phenomena as antigenic competition and tolerance (for review, see Gershon, 1973).

There are two further crucial pieces of evidence indicating that T cell products can act to suppress B cell activity at least. One is the work of Haskill and Axelrad (1972), already quoted, in which a cell product from T cell blasts could act on a primed population of small lymphocytes and limit their response to srbc. The other is Feldmann's work (1973) in which he used supernatants from educated T cells to specifically suppress the antibody response of primed B cells to DNP *in vitro*. Such supernatants can also contain T helper factors. The dosage response curves of numbers of activated T cells added in this system (Feldmann and Basten, 1972a and b) show that there is a range in which helper function predominates, beyond which the tolerogenic factor appears.

Examples have been given where clearly the hyporeactivity or partial tolerance is mediated by serum factors which are probably antibody. It is well known (for review, see Uhr and Moller, 1968) that B cell responses can be depressed in this way, and the work of Rowley and Fitch (1965a and b), Kappler *et al.* (1971), and Tong and Boose (1970) exemplify this. Antibody suppressing in this way probably acts on the afferent arc of the response, interfering with induction, and is thus probably different from the mode of action of enhancing antibody, which is generally thought to have a strong efferent or peripheral blocking component (Uhr and Moller, 1968). The use of afferent blockade of this sort to maintain hyporeactivity is probably limited to the control of antibody responses, since B cells and not T cells appear to be sensitive. However, there may be some exceptions, such as immune deviation (e.g. Crowle and Hu, 1969) although whether this should be classified as 'partial tolerance' or enhancement is not clear.

Several examples have been given in which the adoptive transfer of normal lymphoid cells into tolerant hosts, or together with previously tolerant cells, have failed to abrogate tolerance and/or have induced tolerance in the normal population towards transplantation and erythrocyte antigens (Billingham *et al.*, 1965; Elkins, 1972; Gershon and Kondo, 1971; McCullagh, 1970a). Such cases of tolerance are unlikely to be due to central inhibition, but there is no evidence for mediation by humoral antibody, although this has not been formally excluded by the experiments of Elkins (1972) or Billingham *et al.* (1965). These may be examples of partial tolerance by suppressor cells of as yet unknown lineage, although in one case (Gershon and Kondo, 1971) the T cell is implicated.

There remains to be discussed that intriguing category of partial tolerance to transplantation antigens exemplified by the findings of Hellström *et al.* (1970), Bansal *et al.* (1973), and Beverley *et al.* (1973) in which mice and rats injected neonatally with F_1 cells show a degrec of tolerance to skin grafts, and have both cytotoxic cells and blocking factors. The suggestion from Beverley *et al.* (1973) is that at 8 weeks of age a degree of chimerism exists, but is lower than that of comparable, fully tolerant mice. There is no evidence as to whether this chimerism persists, and in the Hellström *et al.* (1971) and Bansal *et al.* (1973) experiments, tests for chimerism were not done. In the experiments of Bansal *et al.* (1973), the level of cytotoxic activity appears to decline with time after grafting, and they have suggested that this may be associated with the acquisition in time of a higher degree of tolerance, and the loss of peripherally active clones. Nevertheless, the striking correlation between skin graft survival and blocking factors which they report strongly suggests a causative effect, especially since blocking factors disappear a few days prior to skin graft rejection. There are no studies of the susceptibility of their 'partially tolerant' animals to tolerance abrogation by normal cells, nor is it known whether their cells confer depression of GVHR on normal cells. Such experiments would yield useful information on whether such animals are just slipping from a central inhibition (i.e. slowly recovering from full tolerance) or whether there is an active suppressor mechanism acting. It is not possible to determine from the available data whether this block is afferent or efferent. If afferent, it may be in line with some of the mechanisms discussed above, and it would be of great interest to know more about the origin of the factor involved.

In summary, full tolerance as defined here appears to be associated with central failure of the immune response, and for maintenance requires persisting antigen either in the form of live, chimeric cells or the periodic reintroduction of the antigen. Partial tolerance represents many different degrees of hyporeactivity, and there are probably several mechanisms capable of maintaining the hyporeactive state: (1) antigen, as in the case of polysaccharide tolerance; (2) antibody, or antibody complexed with antigen; and (3) suppressor cells or substances released by such cells, which may be T cells.

Acknowledgements
I thank Dr John Wunderlich for helpful discussions, and Dr Harvey Cantor and Dr Charles Janeway, Jr, for reading the manuscript and for their helpful comments.

References

Ada, G. L. (1970). Antigen binding cells in tolerance and immunity. *Transplant. Rev.*, **5,** 105

Asherson, G. L. and Stone, S. H. (1965). Selective and specific inhibition of 24 hour skin reactions in the guinea pig. I. Immune deviation: description of the phenomenon and the effect of splenectomy. *Immunology*, **9,** 205

Asofsky, R., Cantor, H. and Tigelaar, R. E. (1971). Cell interactions in the graft-versus-host response. In *Progress in Immunology*, p. 83 (B. Amos, editor). New York and London: Academic Press

Atkins, R. C. and Ford, W. L. (1972). The effect of lymphocytes and serum from tolerant rats on the graft-versus-host activity of normal lymphocytes. *Transplantation*, **13,** 442

Baker, J. B., Barth, R. F., Stashuk, P. W. and Amsbaugh, D. F. (1970a). Enhancement of the antibody response to type III pneumococcal polysaccharide in mice treated with antilymphocyte serum. *J. Immunol.*, **104,** 1313

Baker, J. B., Stashuk, P. W., Amsbaugh, D. F., Prescott, B. and Barth, R. F. (1970b). Evidence for the existence of two functionally distinct types of cells which regulate the antibody response to type III pneumococcal polysaccharide. *J. Immunol.*, **105,** 1581

Bansal, S. C., Hellström, K. E., Hellström, I. and Sjögren, H. O. (1973). Cell mediated immunity and blocking serum activity to tolerated allografts in rats. *J. Exp. Med.*, **137,** 590

Basten, A., Miller, J. F. A. P., Warner, N. L. and Pye, J. (1971). Specific inactivation of thymus derived (T) and non-thymus derived (B) lymphocytes by ^{125}I labelled antigen. *Nature New Biol.*, **231,** 104

Benjamin, D. C. and Weigle, W. O. (1970). The termination of immunological unresponsiveness to bovine serum albumin in rabbits. I. Quantitative and qualitative response to cross reacting albumins. *J. Exp. Med.*, **132,** 66

Beverley, P. C. L., Brent, L., Brooks, C., Medawar, P. B. and Simpson, E. (1973). *In vitro* reactivity of lymphoid cells from tolerant mice. *Transplant, Proc.* **5,** 679

Billingham, R. E., Lampkin, G. H., Medawar, P. B. and Williams, H. L. (1952). Tolerance to homografts, twin diagnosis and the freemartin condition in cattle. *Heredity*, **6,** 201

Billingham, R. E., Brent, L. and Medawar, P. B. (1954). Quantitative studies on tissue transplantation immunity. II. The origin, strength and duration of actively and adoptively acquired immunity. *Proc. Roy. Soc. (London) Series B*, **143,** 58

Billingham, R. E., Brent, L. and Medawar, P. B. (1956). Quantitative studies on tissue transplantation immunity. III. Actively acquired tolerance. *Phil. Trans. Roy. Soc. (London) Series B*, **239,** 357

Billingham, R. E. and Brent, L. (1959). Quantitative studies on tissue transplantation immunity. IV. Induction of tolerance in newborn mice and studies on the phenomenon of runt disease. *Phil. Trans. Roy. Soc. (London) Series B*, **242,** 439

Billingham, R. E., Silvers, W. K. and Wilson, D. B. (1963). Further studies on adoptive transfer of sensitivity to skin homografts. *J. Exp. Med.*, **118,** 397

Billingham, R. E., Silvers, W. K. and Wilson, D. B. (1965). A second study on the H-Y transplantation antigen in mice. *Proc. Roy. Soc. (London) Series B*, **163,** 61

Billingham, R. E., Silvers, W. K. and Wilson, D. B. (1963). Further studies on adoptive transfer of sensitivity to skin homografts. *J. Exp. Med.*, **118,** 397

Brent, L. (1971). Immunological tolerance 1951-1971. In *Immunological Tolerance to Tissue Antigens*, p. 49 (N. W. Nisbet and M. W. Elves, editors). Orthopaedic Hospital, Oswestry, England

Brent, L. and Gowland, G. (1961). Cellular dose and age of host in the induction of tolerance. *Nature (London)*, **192,** 1265

Brent, L. and Gowland, G. (1962). Induction of tolerance of skin homografts in immunologically competent mice. *Nature (London)*, **196,** 1298

Brent, L., Medawar, P. B. and Ruszkiewicz, M. (1962). In *Ciba Foundation Symposium*, p. 6 (M. Cameron and G. E. W. Wolstenholme, editors). London: Churchill

Brent, L., Hansen, J. A. and Kilshaw, P. J. (1971). Unresponsiveness to skin allografts induced by tissue extracts and antilymphocytic serum. *Transplant. Proc.*, **3,** 684

Brent, L., Brooks, C., Lubling, N. and Thomas, A. V. (1972). Attempts to demonstrate an *in vivo* role for serum blocking factors in tolerant mice. *Transplantation*, **14,** 382

Burnet, F. M. and Fenner, F. (1949). In *The Production of Antibodies*. Melbourne: MacMillan

Cantor, H. (1971). The differential migration of lymphocytes with helper and precursor activity. *Europ. J. Immunol.*, **1,** 462

Cantor, H. (1972a). T cells and the immune response. In *Progr. Biophys. Mol. Biol.*, **24,** 71 (J. A. U. Butler and D. Noble, editors). Oxford: Pergamon Press

Cantor, H. (1972b). The effects of anti-theta antiserum upon graft-versus-host activity of spleen and lymph node cells. *Cellular Immunol.*, **3,** 461

Cantor, H. and Asofsky, R. (1972). Synergy among lymphoid cells mediating the

graft-versus-host response. *J. Exp. Med.*, **135,** 764
Cantor, H. and Simpson, E. (1973). In preparation.
Canty, T. G. and Wunderlich, J. R. (1971). Quantitative assessment of cellular and humoral responses to skin and tumor allografts. *Transplantation*, **11,** 111
Claman, H. N. and Talmage, D. W. (1963). Thymectomy: Prolongation of immunological tolerance in the adult mouse. *Science*, **141,** 1193
Claman, H. N., Chaperon, E. A. and Triplet, R. F. (1966). Thymus–marrow cell combinations, Synergism in antibody production. *Proc. Soc. Exp. Biol. Med.*, **122,** 1167
Cooper, M. D., Lawton, A. R. and Kinade, P. W. (1972). A two-stage model for development of antibody-producing cells. *Clin. Exp. Immunol.*, **11,** 143
Crowle, A. J. and Hu, C. C. (1969). Adoptive transfer of immunologic tolerance into normal mice. *J. Immunol.*, **103,** 1242
Davie, J. M., Paul, W. E., Katz, D. H. and Benacerraf, B. (1972). Hapten-specific tolerance: Preferential depression of the high affinity antibody response. *J. Exp. Med.*, **136,** 426
Davies, A. J. S. (1969). The thymus and the cellular basis of immunity. *Transplant. Rev.*, **1,** 43
Dresser, D. W. and Mitchison, N. A. (1968). The mechanism of immunological paralysis. *Adv. Immunol.*, **8,** 129
Dwyer, J. M. and Cantor, F. S. (1973). Regulation of delayed hypersensitivity: Failure to transfer delayed hypersensitivity to desensitized guinea pigs. *J. Exp. Med.*, **137,** 32
Elkins, W. L. (1972). Cellular control of lymphocytes initiating graft-versus-host reactions. *Cellular Immunol.*, **4,** 192
Elkins, W. L. (1973). The cellular basis of transplantation tolerance. *Transplant. Proc.* **5,** 685
Fahey, J. L., Wunderlich, J. and Mishell, R. (1964a). The immunoglobulins of mice. I. Four major classes on immunoglobulins: 7Sγ2-, 7Sγ1-, β2A-, and 18SγIM-globulins. *J. Exp. Med.*, **120,** 223
Fahey, J. L., Wunderlich, J. and Mishell, R. (1964b). The immunoglobulins of mice. II. Two sub-classes of mouse 7Sγ2-globulins: γ2a- and γ2b-globulins. *J. Exp. Med.*, **120,** 243
Feldmann, M. (1971). Induction of immunity and tolerance to the dinitrophenyl determinant *in vitro*. *Nature New Biol.*, **231,** 21
Feldmann, M. (1973). Induction of B cell tolerance by antigen specific T cell factor. *Nature (London)*, **242,** 82
Feldmann, M. and Basten, A. (1972a). Cell interactions in the immune response *in*

vitro. III. Specific collaboration across a cell impermeable membrane. *J. Exp. Med.*, **136,** 49

Feldmann, M. and Basten, A. (1972b). Cell interactions in the immune response *in vitro*. IV. Comparison of the effects of antigen-specific and allogeneic thimus-derived cell factors. *J. Exp. Med.*, **136,** 722

Gershon, R. K. (1973). T cell control of antibody production. In *Current Topics in Immunology* (M. Cooper, editor) (in press)

Gershon, R. K. and Kondo, K. (1970). Cell interactions in the induction of tolerance: The role of thymic lymphocytes. *Immunology*, **18,** 723

Gershon, R. K. and Kondo, K. (1971). Infectious immunological tolerance. *Immunology*, **21,** 903

Goldberg, E., Boyse, E. A., Scheid, M. and Bennett, D. (1972). Production of H-Y antibody by female mice that fail to reject male skin. *Nature New Biol.*, **238,** 55

Grant, C. K., Leuchars, E. and Alexander, P. (1972). Failure to detect cytotoxic lymphoid cells or humoral blocking factors in mouse radiation chimeras. *Transplantation*, **14,** 722

Graw, R. G., Herzig, G. P., Rogentine, G. N. Jr, Yankee, R. A., Leventhal, B. G., Wang-Peng, J., Halterman, R. H., Krieger, G., Berard, C. and Henderson, E. S. (1970). Graft-versus-host reaction complicating HL-A matched bone marrow transplantation. *Lancet*, **ii,** 1053

Hamilton, D. N. H. (1973). Quoted by Brent, L. and French, M. E. *Transplant. Proc.*, **5,** 1002

Haskill, J. S. and Axelrad, M. A. (1972). Cell mediated control of an antibody response. *Nature New Biol.*, **237,** 251

Hellström, K. E. and Hellström, I. (1969). Cellular immunity against tumour antigens. *Adv. Cancer Res.*, **12,** 167

Hellström, I., Hellström, K. E., Storb, R. and Thomas, E. D. (1970). Colony inhibition of fibroblasts from chimeric dogs mediated by the dogs' own lymphocytes and specifically abrogated by their serum. *Proc. Nat. Acad. Sci.*, **66,** 65

Hellström, K. E., Hellström, I. and Allison, A. C. (1971). Neonatally induced allograft tolerance may be mediated by serum-borne factors. *Nature (London)*, **230,** 49

Humphrey, J. M. (1964). Immunological unresponsiveness to protein antigens in rabbits. I. The duration of unresponsiveness following a single injection at birth. *Immunology*, **7,** 449

Ivanyi, J. and Howard, J. G. (1971). Comparative aspects of tolerance to protein and polysaccharide antigens. In *Immunological Tolerance to Tissue Antigens*, p. 145 (N. W. Nisbet and M. W. Elves, editors). Orthopaedic Hospital, Oswestry, England

Jacobssen, H. and Blomgren, H. (1972). Changes of the PHA-responding pool of cells in the thymus after cortisone or X-ray treatment of mice. Evidence for an inverse relation between the production of cortical and medullary thymocytes. *Cellular Immunol.*, **4,** 93

Kaliss, N. (1966). Immunological enhancement: Conditions for its expression and its relevance for grafts of normal tissues. *Ann. N.Y. Acad. Sci.*, **129,** 155

Kappler, J. W., Hoffman, M. and Dutton, R. W. (1971). Regulation of the immune response. I. Differential effect of passively administered antibody on the thymus-derived and bone-marrow-derived lymphocytes. *J. Exp. Med.*, **134,** 577

Katz, D. H., Paul, W. E., Gold, E. A. and Benacerraf, B. (1971). Carrier function in anti-hapten antibody responses. III. Stimulation of antibody synthesis and facilitation of hapten-specific secondary antibody responses by graft-versus-host reactions. *J. Exp. Med.*, **133,** 169

Kelly, W. D., McKneally, M. F., Oliveras, F., Martinez, C. and Good, R. A. (1966). Acquired tolerance to skin grafts induced with cell free antigenic material: Further tissue sources, frozen storage, dose duration requirements. *Transplantation*, **4,** 489

Kerbel, R. S. and Eidinger, D. (1971). The variable effects of anti-lymphocyte serum on humoral antibody formation: Role of thymus dependency of antigen. *J. Immunol.*, **106,** 917

Kerbel, R. S. and Eidinger, D. (1972). Enhanced immune responsiveness to a thymus-independent antigen early after adult thymectomy: Evidence for short lived inhibitory thymus derived cells. *Europ. J. Immunol.*, **2,** 114

Koller, P. C., Davies, A. J. S. and Doak, S. M. A. (1961). Radiation chimeras. *Adv. Cancer Res.*, **6,** 181

Kreth, H. W. and Williamson, A. R. (1971). Cell surveillance model for lymphocyte cooperation. *Nature (London)*, **234,** 454

Lance, E. M. and Medawar, P. B. (1969). Quantitative studies on tissue transplantation immunity. IX. Induction of tolerance with antilymphocyte serum. *Proc. Roy. Soc. (London) Series B*, **173,** 447

Lance, E. M. (1971a). The induction of transplantation tolerance within and across species barriers. In *Immunological Tolerance to Tissue Antigens*, p. 101 (N. W. Nisbet and M. W. Elves, editors). Orthopaedic Hospital, Oswestry, England

Lance, E. M. (1971b). Tissue specific transplantation antigens. In *Immunological Tolerance to Tissue Antigens*, p. 291 (N. W. Nisbet and M. W. Elves, editors). Orthopaedic Hospital, Oswestry, England

Law, L. W., Appella, E., Strober, S., Wright, P. and Fischetti, T. (1972). Induction of immunological tolerance to soluble histocompatibility-2 antigens of mice. *Proc.*

Nat. Acad. Sci., **69,** 1858

Leckband, E. (1970). A minor population of immunocompetent cells among mouse thymocytes. *Fed. Proc. Fed. Amer. Soc. Exp. Biol.*, **29,** 621

Marchalonis, J. J., Cone, R. E. and Atwell, J. L. (1972). Isolation and partial characterization of lymphocyte surface immunoglobulins. *J. Exp. Med.*, **135,** 956

Martinez, C., Smith, J. M., Sharpiro, F. and Good, R. A. (1959). Transfer of acquired immunological tolerance of skin homografts in mice joined by parabiosis. *Proc. Soc. Exp. Biol. Med.*, **102,** 413

Medawar, P. B. (1963). The use of antigenic tissue extracts to weaken the immunological reaction against skin homografts in mice. *Transplantation*, **1,** 21

Metcalf, D. and Moore, M. A. S. (1971). In *Haemapoietic Cells*, p. 158. Amsterdam and London: North Holland Publishing Co.

McCullagh, P. J. (1970a). The transfer of immunological competence to rats tolerant of sheep erythrocytes with lymphocytes from normal rats. *Aust. J. Exp. Biol. Med. Sci.*, **48,** 351

McCullagh, P. J. (1970b). The immunological capacity of lymphocytes from normal donors after their transfer to rats tolerant of sheep erythrocytes. *Aust. J. Exp. Biol. Med. Sci.*, **48,** 369

McCullagh, P. J. (1970c). The abrogation of sheep erythrocyte tolerance in rats by means of the transfer of allogeneic lymphocytes. *J. Exp. Med.*, **132,** 916

McGregor, D. D., McCullagh, P. J. and Gowans, J. L. (1967). The role of lymphocytes in antibody formation: Restoration of the haemoysin response in X-irradiated rats with lymphocytes from normal and immunologically tolerant donors. *Proc. Roy. Soc. (London) Series B*, **168,** 229

Miller, J. F. A. P. and Mitchell, G. F. (1970). Cell to cell interaction in the immune response. V. Target cells for tolerance induction. *J. Exp. Med.*, **131,** 675

Mintz, B. and Silvers, W. K. (1967). 'Intrinsic' immunological tolerance in allophenic mice. *Science*, **158,** 1484

Mitchell, G. F., Mishell, R. and Herzenberg, L. A. (1971). Studies on the influence of T cells in antibody production. In *Progress in Immunology*, p. 324 (B. Amos, editor). New York and London: Academic Press

Mitchison, N. A. (1962). Tolerance of erythrocytes in poultry: Loss and abolition. *Immunology*, **5,** 341

Mitchison, N. A. (1971a). Cell interactions and receptor antibodies in immune responses. In *Proc. Third Sigrid Juselius Symposium*, p. 249 (O. Makela, A. Cross and T. U. Kosunen, editors). London and New York: Academic Press

Mitchison, N. A. (1971b). Tolerance in T and B lymphocytes: Evidence from hapten-specific tolerance. In *Immunological Tolerance to Tissue Antigens*, p. 67

(N. W. Nisbet and M. W. Elves, editors). Orthopaedic Hospital, Oswestry, England

Mosier, D. and Cantor, H. (1971). Functional maturation of mouse thymic lymphocytes. *Europ. J. Immunol.*, **1,** 459

Mosier, D. and Pierce, C. W. (1972). Functional maturation of thymic lymphocyte populations *in vitro*. *J. Exp. Med.*, **136,** 1484

Old, L. J., Boyse, E. A. and Stockert, E. (1963). Antigenic properties of experimental leukaemias. I. Serological studies *in vitro* with spontaneous and radiation induced leukaemias. *J. Nat. Cancer Inst.*, **31,** 977

Ovary, Z., Barth, W. F. and Fahey, J. L. (1965). The immunoglobulins of mice. III. Skin sensitizing activity of mouse immunoglobulins. *J. Immunol.*, **94,** 410

Owen, R. D. (1945). Immunogenetic consequences of vascular anastomoses between bovine twins. *Science*, **102,** 400

Owen, J. J. S. and Raff, M. C. (1970). Studies on the differentiation of thymus-derived lymphocytes. *J. Exp. Med.*, **132,** 1216

Parish, C. R. (1971). Immune response to chemically modified flagellin. II. Evidence for a fundamental relationship between humoral and cell mediated immunity. *J. Exp. Med.*, **134,** 21

Parrott, D. M. V., de Sousa, M. A. B. and East, J. (1966). Thymus-dependent areas in the lymphoid organs of neonatally thymectomized mice. *J. Exp. Med.*, **123,** 191

Paul, W. E., Siskind, G. W. and Benacerraf, B. (1967). A study of the 'termination' of tolerance to BSA with DNP-BSA in rabbits: Relative affinities of the antibodies for the immunizing and paralyzing antigens. *Immunology*, **13,** 147

Phillips, M. S., Martin, J. W., Shaw, A. R. and Wegman, T. G. (1971). Serum-mediated immunological non-reactivity between histoincompatible cells in tetraparental mice. *Nature (London)*, **234,** 146

Playfair, J. H. L. (1969). Specific tolerance to sheep erythrocytes in mouse bone marrow cells. *Nature (London)*, **222,** 882

Raff, M. C. (1969). Theta isoantigen as a marker of thymus-derived lymphocytes in mice. *Nature (London)*, **224,** 378

Raff, M. C. (1970). Two distinct populations of peripheral lymphocytes in mice distinguished by immunofluorescence. *Immunology*, **19,** 637

Raff, M. C. and Cantor, H. (1971). Sub-populations of thymus cells and thymus-derived lymphocytes. In *Progress of Immunology*, p. 83 (B. Amos, editor). New York and London: Academic Press

Reif, A. E. and Allen, J. M. V. (1964). The AKR thymic antigen and its distribution in leukaemias and nervous tissues. *J. Exp. Med.*, **120,** 413

Rouse, B. T. and Warner, N. L. (1972). Induction of T cell tolerance in agammaglobulinemic chickens. *Europ. J. Immunol.*, **2,** 102

Rowley, D. A. and Fitch, F. W. (1965a). The mechanism of tolerance produced in rats to sheep erythrocytes. I. Plaque-forming cell and antibody response to single and multiple injections of antigen. *J. Exp. Med.*, **121,** 671

Rowley, D. A. and Fitch, F. W. (1965b). The mechanism of tolerance produced in rats to sheep erythrocytes. II. The plaque-forming cell and antibody response to multiple injections of antigen begun at birth. *J. Exp. Med.*, **121,** 683

Schlossman, S., Levin, H. A., Rocklin, R. E. and David, J. R. (1971). The compartmentalization of antigen-reactive lymphocytes in desensitized guinea pigs. *J. Exp. Med.*, **134,** 741

Silobrcic, V. (1971). Life long tolerance and chimerism in parental mice induced with F_1 hybrid cells. *Europ. J. Immunol.*, **1,** 313

Simonsen, M. (1962). Graft-versus-host reactions. Their natural history and applicability as tools of research. *Prog. Allergy*, **6,** 349

Simpson, E. (1973). In preparation

Sjöberg, O. (1971). Antigen binding cells in mice immune or tolerant to *Escherichia coli* polysaccharide. *J. Exp. Med.*, **133,** 1015

Stobo, J. D. and Paul, W. E. (1973). Functional heterogeneity of murine lymphoid cells. III. Differential responsiveness of T cells to PHA and Con A as a probe for T cell sub-sets. *J. Immunol.*, **110,** 362

Taylor, R. B. (1964). An effect of thymectomy on recovery from immunological paralysis. *Immunology*, **7,** 595

Taylor, R. B. (1968). Immune paralysis of thymus cells to bovine serum albumin. *Nature (London)*, **220,** 611

Taylor, R. B. (1971). Induction and recovery from paralysis in two lines of cells. In *Immunological Tolerance to Tissue Antigens*, p. 75 (N. W. Nisbet and M. W. Elves, editors). Orthopaedic Hospital, Oswestry, England

Tong, J. L. and Boose, D. (1970). Immunosuppressive effect of serum from CBA mice made tolerant by the supernatant from ultracentrifuged bovine γ-globulin. *J. Immunol.*, **105,** 426

Uhr, J. W. and Moller, G. (1968). Regulatory effect of antibody on the immune response. *Adv. Immunol.*, **8,** 81

Voisin, G. (1971). Immunity and tolerance: A unified concept. *Cellular Immunol.*, **2,** 670

Wagner, H., Harris, A. W. and Feldmann, M. (1972). Cell-mediated immune response *in vitro*. II. Role of thymus and thymus-derived lymphocytes. *Cellular Immunol.*, **4,** 39

Warner, N. L. (1967). The immunological role of the avian thymus and bursa of

Fabricius. *Folia Biol. (Prague)*, **13,** 1

Wegmann, T. G., Hellström, K. E. and Hellström, I. (1971). Immunological tolerance: 'Forbidden clones' allowed in tetraparental mice. *Proc. Nat. Acad. Sci.*, **68,** 1644

Weigle, W. O., Chiller, J. M. and Habicht, G. S. (1971). Immunological unresponsiveness: Cellular kinetics and interactions. In *Progress in Immunology*, p. 311 (B. Amos, editor). New York and London: Academic Press

Wilson, D. B., Silvers, W. K. and Nowell, P. (1967). Quantitative studies in the mixed lymphocyte interaction in rats. II. Relationship of the proliferative response to the immunologic status of the donors. *J. Exp. Med.*, **126,** 655

8
Immunological Enhancement of Transplanted Organs

Frank P. Stuart

THE CLINICAL PROBLEM

Much of the improvement in results of human kidney transplantation during the past decade is due to increased familiarity with the use of immunosuppressive agents such as azathioprine, cyclophosphamide, prednisone and antilymphocyte globulin. Unfortunately, these agents are all immunologically non-specific in the sense that they suppress the immune response to all antigens, not just those that are present in the new graft. Their use deprives the recipient of part of his normal defenses against bacterial, viral and fungal pathogens. If the clinician administers them in doses that are always or nearly always capable of preventing rejection, he inevitably encounters an unacceptable incidence of lethal pulmonary and systemic infections. Consequently, he is challenged to find the narrow therapeutic zone in which many and hopefully most rejections can be controlled without losing the recipient. Even in those patients who tolerate immunosuppression without incurring infection or other toxic side-effects, there is after 2 or 3 years of therapy a distressingly high incidence of spontaneous malignancy. Their risk of developing cancer is increased by ten- to twenty-fold (Penn and Starzl, 1972).

The most recent reports from the Kidney Transplant Registry, an international registry maintained by the American College of Surgeons, indicate a two-year graft survival of 80 per cent for kidneys from living related donors and about 50 per cent for kidneys from cadaveric donors (Barnes *et al.*, 1972). A few individual centers have reported figures as high as 90 per cent for live donors and 70 per cent for cadaver donors, but the experience of many other centers has been less satisfying than that reported by the registry. It now seems unlikely that the goal of uniform 100 per cent survival of kidney grafts can be achieved with immunosuppressive agents that are in current clinical use. Rather than stretching them to the limit, we need to reduce the dependence on immunologically non-specific agents and turn toward immunologically specific suppression through induction of tolerance or enhancement.

TOLERANCE *v.* ENHANCEMENT

Tolerance and enhancement have both allowed long term survival of organ allografts in a variety of species. Much has been written about the mechanism of action of each. For years they were thought to be distinctly different, but recently several investigators have suggested that they may be no more than quantitative differences of a single phenomenon. Since discussion of enhancement and tolerance as separate entities is becoming increasingly difficult, it is appropriate to begin this review of enhancement with an historical sketch of tolerance and a presentation of some of the current thinking about tolerance.

In a recent review, Brent chose 1951 as the year in which tolerance had its beginnings (Brent, 1971); it was in that year that Medawar, Billingham and Brent began their experiments on induction of tolerance based on their observation that dizygotic cattle twins usually accept skin grafts exchanged between them. Their first report on tolerance induction appeared in 1953 (Billingham *et al.*, 1953) and they subsequently defined tolerance as a 'specific weakening or suppression of reactivity caused by the exposure of animals to antigenic stimuli before the maturation of the faculty of immunological response' (Billingham *et al.*, 1956). Later, the definition was modified in keeping with the observation that tolerance could be induced in immunologically mature animals as well as neonates.

Whether or not a particular antigen can induce tolerance depends on its dose, frequency, duration and route of administration and its immunogenicity as well as the animal's age and degree of immunological competence (Brent and Gowland, 1961, 1962, 1963; Gowland, 1965; Dresser and Mitchison, 1968; Silvers and Billingham, 1969). The dose, frequency and duration of antigen required to induce tolerance all increase as the genetic disparity between antigen donor and recipient increases. The most efficient route for antigen administration is by vein. Decreased immunological competence due either to young age or depletion of lymphoid tissue by drugs, radiation or antilymphocyte serum and thymectomy facilitates the induction of tolerance (Schwartz and Damashek, 1959; Schwartz, 1968; Lance and Medawar, 1969; Brent and Kilshaw, 1970; Brent *et al.*, 1971; Monaco *et al.*, 1966). Failure to select the optimal condition for each variable can lead to cell-mediated and humoral immunity rather than tolerance.

It is of interest that controversy concerning whether tolerance and immunological enhancement were the same phenomenon existed in the early 1950s. Snell, an early investigator concerned with enhancement, suggested that tolerance and enhancement should be called by the same term. However, Billingham and his colleagues took pains to differentiate the two in 1956 as follows (Billingham *et al.*, 1956): 'The properties that tolerance and enhancement possess in common are those which follow from the fact that both represent the outcome of specific central failures of response. But the means by which they are achieved, and in all probability their mechanisms, are so different as to make one cautious of describing them, as Snell has proposed, by the same term. The stimulus which confers tolerance on embryos merely incites immunity in adults; the stimulus which enhances the growth of homografts in adults does not prejudice the normal differentiation of immature antibody-forming cells. The one represents the effect of a complete antigen on an immature subject; the other, the effect of a modified antigenic stimulus on a system which is fully capable of an immune response. For the time being, perhaps the distinction should be made by the use of different terms.' Throughout most of the past two decades the suppression referred to as enhancement has been thought to be mediated by antibody (either administered to the recipient passively, or generated in the recipient by prior exposure to antigen) and considered to be largely peripheral in mechanism whereas tolerance has been considered to be an antigen-mediated central failure of the immune response.

The specific unresponsiveness of tolerance has been attributed at various times to elimination of the clone of cells capable of responding to a specific antigen or to a direct antigen-mediated change in antigen recognition cells that leaves them alive and intact but unable to respond (Brent, 1971a). Recently the Hellströms have provided another alternative by suggesting that tolerance depends on circulating serum-blocking factors which are most likely antibody–hapten complexes (Hellström *et al.*, 1971; Sjögren *et al.*, 1971). Since the numerous examples of cancellation of tolerance weigh heavily against the theory of elimination of cell clones (Brent, 1971a), the central unresolved issue with respect to tolerance is whether the unresponsiveness depends on existence of 'tolerant' cells or whether, as the Hellströms and others maintain, lymphocyte reactivity is simply held in check by serum-blocking factors.

Brent has recently reconfirmed the existence of classic tolerance in mice and maintains that serum-blocking factors play no role in it (Brent, 1972; Brent *et al.*, 1972). To emphasize another distinction between tolerance and enhancement he points out that lymphoid cells from truly tolerant animals do not respond to donor antigens in either mixed leukocyte culture or graft-versus-host reactions whereas cells from enhanced animals react normally (Wilson *et al.*, 1967; French, Batchelor *et al.*, 1971). Medawar emphasizes that lymphoid cell chimerism is always present in true tolerance. He suggests that Hellström serum-blocking factors are found only in cases of incomplete tolerance and points out that the reports that claim to show the presence of blocking factors in tolerant animals have failed to establish that the 'tolerant' animals were, in fact, lymphoid chimeras (Medawar, 1972).

Even though cell-mediated immunity and antibody or serum-blocking factors are absent in true tolerance, the process of tolerance induction may be a more 'active' one than is generally realized. It is of particular interest that frequently a transient immune response can be detected during the process of tolerance induction in adult animals and occasionally in neonates as well. Moreover, splenectomy has recently been shown to interfere with induction of high levels of tolerance in rats (Levinson and Silvers, 1973). Finally, using an *in vitro* system Diener and Feldmann have shown that an appropriate amount of antibody in conjunction with antigen (polymerized flagellin) greatly reduces the amount of antigen required to induce tolerance in cultured mouse spleen cells (Feldmann and Diener, 1971). They speculated that antibody helped to construct the lattice work of antigen molecules on the cell surface that is required for tolerance induction.

If a transient immune response is always part of true tolerance induction it would be easier to accept tolerance and enhancement as part of a single spectrum; incomplete tolerance and high degrees of enhancement may be the same phenomenon, as Medawar has suggested.

What then is immunological enhancement? It is generally accepted as the prolonged survival of a graft that results from presence in the recipient of endogenous or passively administered antibody against donor histocompatibility antigens. The initial observations were made on rodent tumor systems in the early 1900s (Flexner and Jobling, 1907). Inoculation of non-viable tumor cells into animals several days or weeks prior to challenge with viable cells results in progressive tumor growth and death; tumor growth followed by regression had always been the case in animals that were not pretreated with non-viable tumor. Enhancement was shown by Casey to be an immunological phenomenon (Casey, 1934) and Kaliss demonstrated its dependence on the presence of antibody in the recipient in 1953 by achieving prolonged survival of tumor allografts after passive immunization alone (Kaliss *et al.*, 1953; Kaliss, 1958). During the past two decades many investigators have reported prolonged survival of tumor and normal tissue allografts as a result of passive immunization or pretreatment with donor-type histocompatibility antigens. Prolonged graft survival that follows passive immunization alone is frequently referred to as passive enhancement whereas prolonged graft survival after antigen pretreatment is known as active enhancement.

ANTIGEN MEDIATED (ACTIVE) ENHANCEMENT

It is likely that most if not all instances of prolonged graft survival after pretreatment of adult recipients with antigen alone are examples of enhancement rather than true tolerance. There are no reports wherein true tolerance to complex histocompatibility antigens was induced in adult animals by antigen treatment alone (i.e. without additional manipulation of the immune system by drugs, antilymphocyte serum, thymectomy, or radiation). Wood has found that tolerance induction to histocompatibility antigens in adult mice requires thymectomy and antilymphocyte serum (ALS) in addition to antigen treatment; moreover, it was important that antigen be presented to the recipient as intact cells (bone marrow), rather than in the form of a crude sub-cellular preparation, presumably so that leukocyte chimerism could be established (Wood *et al.*, 1972). Although they have achieved indefinite skin graft survival in mice that were treated with ALS and bone marrow cells they were never able to demonstrate chimerism unless the recipient had also undergone thymectomy.

Antigen treatment, with and without addition of non-specific immunosuppressive agents such as ALS, azathioprine and steroid hormones, has led to prolonged survival of renal allografts in the dog, rabbit and rat.

Antigen pretreatment in the dog

Prolonged survival of renal allografts after antigen pretreatment was first reported in 1963 (Halasz and Orloff, 1963). Nineteen dogs were injected subcutaneously with 2 ml of donor whole blood on the tenth and again on the fifth day before transplantation. Mean survival of pretreated dogs was 29 days compared to 9 days for untreated controls. The authors did not mention the presence or absence of circulating antibody against the donor at the time of transplantation. A subsequent report from the same laboratory cited a mean survival of 31 days in dog renal allograft recipients that were treated with intravenous injections of a crude semi-soluble donor spleen extract (Seifert *et al.*, 1966). The extract was injected during a 10 day period prior to transplantation. In addition, the recipients were treated with prednisone and azathioprine in doses which, when given alone, failed to prolong survival. Again, no mention was made of circulating antibody in the recipients.

In 1966 Calne reported no prolonged survival of renal allografts in the dog after extensive trials of pretreatment with a variety of donor antigen preparations (whole blood, spleen, bone marrow and lymph node cells, and a crude semi-soluble extract of spleen) even though azathioprine was added as a therapeutic adjunct (Calne *et al.*, 1966).

In 1968, prolonged survival was reported after intravenous injection of a crude extract of spleen cell nuclei during the 3 weeks before transplantation (Zimmerman *et al.*, 1968). Maximum survival was 87 days; the presence of antibody was not sought.

In 1969, Wilson reported mean survival of 144 days for a group of 11 dogs that were treated with a 'soluble' cytoplasmic extract of spleen cells and low doses of methylprednisolone and azathioprine (Wilson *et al.*, 1969; Holl-Allen *et al.*, 1969). Some of the dogs had circulating lymphocytotoxic antibody in low titer against the donor at the time of transplantation. It is of special interest that they reported no instance of 'hyperacute' rejection.

Antigen pretreatment in the rabbit

Owen has achieved remarkable prolongation of survival of renal allografts and xenografts (guinea pig) in the rabbit by pretreatment of the recipient with donor antigen in the absence of additional non-specific immunosuppression (Owen *et al.*, 1968; Owen, 1969). A crude sonicated homogenate of liver, equivalent to 1000–2000 hepatic cells, was injected intravenously daily for 5 weeks before transplantation. Mean survival of treated allograft recipients was 26 days compared to 14 days for controls. Increase in the amount of antigen administered to allograft recipients during the 5 week period before transplantation resulted at times in no effect and sometimes in accelerated rejection. Xenografts produced urine for an average of 14 days in pretreated recipients in contrast to no more than a few hours for untreated controls. Owen was unable to detect circulating hemagglutinins against either the allograft or xenograft donors at the time of transplantation.

Antigen pretreatment in the rat

Several teams of investigators have reported prolonged survival of renal allografts in the rat after antigen pretreatment alone. Stuart observed an increase in mean survival to 89 days (compared to 17 days for untreated controls) from treating the recipient with a single intravenous injection of 10^8 donor spleen cells 24 hours before transplantation (Stuart *et al.*, 1968).

Taguchi reported prolonged urine formation after pretreatment of recipients with a crude homogenate of donor kidney that was injected by intraperitoneal route five times weekly for 4 weeks before transplantation (Taguchi *et al.*, 1968). No mention was made of circulating antibody.

Ockner pretreated recipients with a wide range of donor bone marrow cells by a single intravenous injection from one to 36 days before transplantation and found that maximal suppression of graft rejection was achieved by injecting between 10^7 and 10^8 cells within 6 to 13 days before transplantation (Ockner *et al.*, 1970). Five out of nine rats that received optimal treatment had nearly normal blood urea nitrogen concentration after more than 4 months.

During the past few years many laboratories have confirmed the relative ease with which survival of renal allografts can be prolonged in the rat by antigen treatment alone (Zimmerman, 1971; Fabre and Morris, 1972; Wilson, 1972). In all cases the dose and timing of optimal antigen pretreatment was such that circulating hemagglutinins, leukoagglutinins and lymphocytotoxic antibodies were present in the recipients in high titer at the time of transplantation.

The dramatic ease with which antigen mediated suppression of kidney rejection has been demonstrated in the rat, in contrast to other species such as the dog and rabbit, is related primarily to the vulnerability of grafts to hyperacute rejection in the different species.

It is a fortuitous peculiarity of the rat that intact allo-antibody against donor histocompatibility antigens results in prolonged survival of a kidney graft rather than hyperacute rejection. In other species, such as man, monkey, dog and rabbit, presence of cytotoxic antibody in the recipient usually leads to complement-mediated hyperacute rejection of kidney grafts. French maintains that a deficiency in the rat's complement system accounts for its inability to reject allografts in hyperacute fashion in the presence of alloantibody; addition of xenogeneic complement (guinea pig serum) does indeed lead to hyperacute rejection of the kidney graft (French, 1972).

Antigen mediated suppression of renal allograft rejection in a species that is vulnerable to antibody-mediated hyperacute rejection is a risky and unpredictable affair. The usual response to antigen treatment is some degree of cellular and humoral immunity, both of which are potentially dangerous for allografts (Brent, 1971). When both cellular and humoral responses are already well developed in a potential recipient it is the antibody response that inflicts most of the damage on a new graft. The peripheral blocking effect of antibody probably prevents direct cell-mediated injury from occurring.

The goal of antigen-mediated enhancement appears to be stimulation of a minimal antibody response that is insufficient to cause hyperacute rejection, yet sufficient to block the cellular response and also retard sensitization to a subsequent graft by binding peripherally with donor histocompatibility antigens. The combination of a continued antibody response and antigenic haptens from the graft could then provide the serum blocking factors which may be the key to enhancement homeostasis. In the reports already referred to in which renal graft suppression was achieved in the dog and rabbit after antigen pretreatment, the amount of antigen given was small and spread over several weeks. The antibody response at the time of grafting was modest or not easily detectable.

ANTIBODY-MEDIATED (PASSIVE) ENHANCEMENT

Specific suppression of allograft rejection by means of passive immunization with alloimmune serum was first demonstrated by Kaliss (Kaliss *et al.*, 1953) in a mouse sarcoma system. Small amounts of serum given intravenously within 24 hours of tumor inoculation caused the tumors to grow and ultimately kill their hosts, whereas tumor cells inoculated into untreated hosts grew into palpable tumors within a week or so but were then rejected by the host. The antibody involved in enhancement is directed against major histocompatibility antigens (H-2 locus in the mouse and Ag-B locus in the rat). Early reports indicated that antibody activity must be present against all of the major histocompatibility antigens that are present in the graft but absent from the recipient (Möller, 1963). It has been suggested, however, that complete coverage of all specificities is not always necessary (Mauel *et al.*, 1970).

Most investigators have found that the enhancing activity resides within the IgG class (Kaliss and Kandutsch, 1956; Takasugi and Hildemann, 1969; Kinsky *et al.*, 1972). In the mouse, which is the species that has been studied most, there is general agreement (with the exception of Kinsky *et al.*, 1972) that enhancing activity is limited to the IgG_2 subclass; IgG_2 fixes complement and moves more slowly than IgG_1 in an electrophoretic field. Whether or not passive immunization leads to graft enhancement depends at the outset on the susceptibility of the graft to antibody–complement mediated injury. The major determinant for such injury is the density of the target histocompatibility antigens on the graft's cell surface membranes (Winn, 1962; Möller and Möller, 1962; Linscott, 1970). For example, in the mouse the density of cell surface histocompatibility antigens is much greater for lymphomas than it is for sarcomas; it is also much more difficult to enhance lymphomas because the putative enhancing serum is cytotoxic for the grafted cells.

Point of action of enhancing antibody

The point at which enhancing antibody acts to prevent sensitization and graft destruction is not yet clear. For purposes of simplifying discussion, the immune response is usually broken down into three parts: afferent, central, and efferent. The afferent arc provides for contact between the immunizing antigen and the host's mass of lymphoid tissue. The central part of the response relates to the amount of immunologically competent lymphoid tissue and the cellular interactions that are initiated by its exposure to antigen. The efferent arc refers to the link between sensitized lymphoid cells or circulating antibody and the actual target cells in the graft.

It is fairly easy to show that target cells that have been coated with antibody are usually spared from injury and death when exposed to sensitized lymphocytes;

consequently, there is a consensus that efferent blockade by antibody does exist. It is much more difficult to differentiate between afferent and central blockade. Antibody might complex with and mask antigen in and from the graft and thus prevent it from immunizing the host; or antibody might have a central suppressive effect either directly on the host's immunologically competent cells or by affecting the way in which antigen is processed by macrophages. Although afferent inhibition doubtless exists, the bulk of evidence is in favor of a central effect for passively administered antibody (Rowley and Fitch, 1964; Uhr and Möller, 1968; Ryder and Schwartz, 1969; Snell, 1970; French, 1973).

The nature of central inhibition of the immune response may involve two quite different mechanisms. The first would depend on antibody against histocompatibility antigens. The second would depend on antibody against the variable portion (combining site) of antibody directed against histocompatibility antigens; this anti-antibody has been referred to as anti-receptor antibody. The first mechanism, the one involving traditional antibody against histocompatibility antigens, probably depends on adherence of antibody through its Fc piece to antigen processing macrophages. Presence of specific antibody on the macrophage not only helps attract antigen to macrophages, but apparently leaves it in a state which is incapable cf stimulating antigen recognition lymphocytes (Cruse *et al.*, 1973).

The second potential mechanism for central suppression (anti-receptor antibody) is based on the presence of lymphocyte cell surface immunoglobulins which serve as receptors to attract and bind the specific antigen (Rabellino *et al.*, 1971). If it were possible to prepare an antibody against just the combining site of the receptor antibody, one might achieve central suppression by preventing contact between antigen and antigen recognition lymphocytes. Indeed, recent reports from several laboratories indicate that antibody can be made against receptor IgG. Ramseier has prepared anti-antibody in F_1 hybrid rats by immunizing them with IgG obtained from serum of hyperimmune parents. His evidence for antibody (anti-receptor) activity is derived from a complex assay (Ramseier and Lindemann, 1971, 1973). McKearn has prepared antibody (anti-receptor) in $LBNF_1$ rats by injecting them repeatedly with glutaraldehyde crosslined L anti-BN IgG. His evidence for presence of anti-receptor activity comes from precipitin lines in appropriate gel diffusion assays and from ability to specifically suppress a GVH reaction in F_1 hosts (McKearn *et al.*, 1973) His preliminary studies indicate that survival of renal allografts in the rat is not prolonged by treatment with putative anti-receptor serum alone (McKearn and Stuart, 1973). Lucas, however, reports a modest prolongation of rat renal allograft survival after treatment with anti-receptor serum (Lucas and Enomoto, 1973).

Rowley, in an extensive review of specific suppression of the immune response, has suggested that what we usually consider to be purely anti-graft antibody may actually be a combination of anti-graft antibody (receptor antibody) and anti-receptor antibody (Rowley *et al.*, 1973). If he is correct, there would be additional support for the impression that passive enhancement works by suppression at all three levels, afferent, central and efferent.

Effectiveness of intact IgG v. antibody fragments

Limitation of enhancing activity to a single antibody class (IgG) suggests that the Fc portion of the molecule plays an important rôle in achieving enhancement. Indeed, removal of the Fc piece by pepsin digestion reduces the ability of passively administered antibody to suppress a variety of immune responses. IgG is 100–1000 times more effective than $F(ab')_2$ in suppressing the antibody response to sheep erythrocytes in intact mice and rats (Sinclair, 1969). The difference could be explained in part by differences in antibody concentration in tissue since $F(ab')_2$ is a smaller molecule and is lost readily into the urine. However, even when comparable antibody levels were maintained in the intact animal by repeated injections of $F(ab')_2$, the marked discrepancy in immunosuppressive ability remained (Sinclair *et al.*, 1970). Moreover, the immunosuppressive superiority of intact IgG over $F(ab')_2$ has been confirmed in an *in vitro* spleen cell culture system in which the question of increased catabolic rate of antibody fragments does not apply (Wason and Fitch, 1973). Intact IgG was at least ten times more effective in suppressing the response of cultured mouse spleen cells against sheep erythrocytes.

It is not known why IgG is more effective than $F(ab')_2$ in inhibiting antibody formation. Receptors for the Fc portion of the molecule have been demonstrated on the surfaces of lymphocytes (Basten *et al.*, 1972) and macrophages (Whitten *et al.*, 1973). Such receptors may play a rôle in the suppression of the immune response by antibody.

Passive enhancement of lymphomas

Lymphomas are particularly difficult to enhance with intact IgG because lymphoid cells which are rich in histocompatibility antigens can fix enough antibody and complement on the cell surface to cause cell death. By treating mice with Fab′, Chard was able to enhance the difficult E.L. 4 leukemia (Chard, 1967). Although enhancement was attributed to the digested antibody fragments, it may be that part of the effect was actually due to undigested IgG that might have been carried along with the fragments. The fragments may simply have acted as 'spacers' to separate the intact molecules far enough from each other so as to prevent antibody-complement mediated cell death. In any event, successful enhancement of the leukemia was an highly significant event in that it increased the likelihood that passive enhancement could be applied to transplanted organs in species that are subject to hyperacute rejection.

Enhancement of renal allografts in the rat by passive antibody

Despite the ease with which tumors were enhanced by antibody alone, many attempts at enhancement of skin allografts yielded only a day or so of extended survival. Although enhancement was an intriguing immunological phenomenon, there was doubt that it had much potential for prolonging the survival of normal tissues until passive enhancement of renal allografts was achieved in the rat (Stuart, 1968; French and Batchelor, 1969). In many instances rejection of rat renal allografts has been prevented completely by a single intravenous injection of antibody. Effective antisera have been raised in a wide variety of ways: with and without adjuvants such as Freund's complete adjuvant and *Bordatella pertussis* vaccine; against spleen cells, bone marrow cells and lymph node cells; and with single or multiple boosts over courses of three weeks to many months. Although almost all of the serum batches have high hemagglutinin and lymphocytotoxic titers, their enhancing ability varies greatly. With some batches as little as 1 ml given intravenously just before or after transplantation can prevent rejection indefinitely. Other batches may delay the onset of rejection and death by only a few days, even though multiple daily injections are continued for as long as 2 weeks. The effectiveness of a serum batch does not correlate well with hemagglutinin and lymphocytotoxic activity against donor strain cells; perhaps the effectiveness depends in part on presence or absence of anti-receptor antibody.

Enhancing activity resides in the IgG class of antibody which in the rat does not lead to hyperacute rejection. Experience with pepsin digest $F(ab')_2$ has been rather disappointing in that at least ten times as much antibody protein is required to achieve equivalent prolongation of graft survival (Shaipanich *et al.*, 1971; French, personal communication; Stuart, unpublished). It may be that the enhancing activity of $F(ab')_2$ preparations is due in part to undigested IgG that is carried along with the digest fragments.

Immunological status of long term rats with enhanced renal allografts

Survival for a normal life span with relatively normal renal function is a frequent occurrence after passive immunization. If rejection has not appeared within the first month after transplantation it is unlikely to do so later. Second kidney transplants from the original donor strain are readily accepted with no attempt at rejection even though the host receives no additional treatment. Yet, it is now quite clear that such long term recipients are not tolerant in the classic sense (Stuart *et al.*, 1970, 1971a; French *et al.*, 1971; Mullen *et al.*, 1973). They reject donor strain skin grafts in slightly delayed fashion (about 5 days later than controls) without concurrent injury to the well established renal graft; their spleen cells and peripheral blood leukocytes react normally with donor strain cells in MLC; their spleen cells mount vigorous graft-versus-host reactions in F_1 hybrid offspring; and they exhibit both cellular immunity and blocking serum factors in an *in vitro* microcytotoxicity assay. So, it appears that prolonged graft survival in passively immunized recipients depends on a continuing active response and perhaps some decrease in the immunogenicity of the well established graft.

Retransplantation of well established renal grafts to new hosts of the original recipient strain but without additional treatment leads to rejection in slightly delayed fashion. The onset of azotemia occurs 9 days after transplantation compared to 5 days for controls. Nevertheless, the rejection episode is vigorous and leads to death. The delayed onset of azotemia implies decreased immunogenicity that has been explained by loss of donor strain passenger leukocytes from the kidney during its residence in the first recipient. Rejection by the second recipient presumably depends on a response to vascular endothelial cells which remain donor in type (Stuart *et al.*, 1971b).

Paradoxically, presence of recipient type passenger leukocytes in the long term kidney leads to varying degrees of rejection if the kidney is transplanted back to a member of the original donor strain. A limited rejection episode is also observed frequently in the dog after retransplantation to the original donor (Murray *et al.*, 1962).

Adjuncts to passive enhancement in the rat

Prolonged survival of renal grafts has been achieved by a variety of approaches such as depletion of leukocytes in the donor prior to transplantation; splenectomy; treatment with heterologous antilymphocyte serum; and administration of some form of donor histocompatibility antigens. The enhancement effect of passive immunization is diminished by combining it with either depletion of donor passenger leukocytes or early recipient splenectomy. Both combinations cause delayed onset of rejection but they are inferior to antibody alone in producing long term stable kidney grafts. Perhaps an immunologic response to donor passenger leukocytes in the host's spleen leads to elaboration of antibody and blocking serum factors which may play a rôle in long term stability of the graft. However, late splenectomy (more than 2 months after transplant) is not deleterious to the enhanced graft (Lucas and Enomoto, 1973).

Both ALS and donor antigen treatment increase the immunosuppressive effect of passive immunization (Batchelor *et al.*, 1972). Since ALS acts by decreasing the number of immunologically competent lymphocytes, it is not surprising that its effect would be additive with that of passive antibody. Intravenous antigen pretreatment within 24 hours of transplantation is thought to act by deviation of the immune response toward antibody production which is readily suppressed by subsequent passive immunization. To the extent that intravenous antigen commits cells from a fixed population of antigen recognition cells toward a humoral response, there are fewer cells left to mount a cell mediated attack on the graft. Since it is generally agreed that it is the cell mediated response and not the humoral response that accounts for first set allograft rejection (Brent, 1971b), antigen pretreatment would presumably potentiate passive immunization simply by decreasing the potential magnitude of the cellular mediated response that needed to be controlled (Rowley *et al.*, 1973).

Enhancement of renal allografts in the rabbit

Passive immunization of rabbits with intact IgG against donor histocompatibility antigens leads to immediate destruction of renal allografts (Holter, 1972). $F(ab')_2$ fragments cause no injury to grafts. Moreover, when administered immediately prior to an infusion of intact IgG, the $F(ab')_2$ fragments prevent the hyperacute rejection that would otherwise occur (Holter *et al.*, 1972, 1973). Preliminary reports indicate that passive enhancement can be achieved in the rabbit either by repeated injections of $F(ab')_2$ or by infusions of $F(ab')_2$ followed by intact IgG (Sutherland *et al.*, 1973; Holter *et al.*, 1973). These are the first reports of successful passive enhancement of renal grafts in experimental animals that are susceptible to hyperacute rejection. They provide a model for the development of protocols for passive enhancement in man.

Enhancement of liver allografts in the baboon

Survival after orthotopic liver transplantation in the baboon has been prolonged from 13 days in controls to 27 days after passive immunization with polyspecific $F(ab')_2$ and 35 days after treatment with polyspecific whole serum (Myburgh and Smit, 1972). It is of particular interest that polyspecific whole serum did not lead to antibody mediated damage of the liver. Subhuman primate kidney grafts, in sharp contrast, are extremely susceptible to antibody mediated injury. Perhaps the liver with its sinusoidal blood supply is less vulnerable than the kidney.

ENHANCEMENT IN MAN

Intentional enhancement in man by means of antigen treatment or passive immunization has just barely begun. Clinical trials will be difficult and, initially at least, they will be confined to only a few transplantation centers. Yet, the 'antigen pretreatment' of natural pregnancy, blood transfusion, prior unsuccessful organ transplantation, and bacterial infection have at times inadvertently conditioned a potential host so as to allow enhancement of a subsequent graft. It is likely that much can be done with current clinical assays of cellular and humoral immunity to detect those patients who are already conditioned to enhance a subsequent graft.

Preconditioning for enhancement by blood transfusion, prior graft rejection, pregnancy and infection

Blood transfusion, an unsuccessful organ graft, pregnancy, and some bacterial infections present the individual with foreign histocompatibility antigens or cross-reacting antigens. In the case of blood transfusion it is the leukocytes and platelets, not the red cells, that are rich in histocompatibility antigens. Following a single transfusion of whole blood, an increased MLC response against the blood donor can be detected in virtually all patients, and an antibody response can be detected by microlymphocytotoxic assay in as many as 85 per cent (Caseley *et al.*, 1971; Oh *et al.*, 1972; Schechter *et al.*, 1972). The circulating antibody response is usually transient and weak but occasionally it persists for months. Presence of sufficient circulating antibody in a potential transplant recipient to kill donor lymphocytes (positive crossmatch) leads to hyperacute rejection of the kidney graft at least 80 per cent of the time (Patel and Terasaki, 1969). Even in the presence of a negative crossmatch with the actual donor, the risk of hyperacute rejection is higher in those individuals who have circulating cytotoxic antibody activity against lymphocytes from a high proportion of a panel of random cell donors (Patel *et al.*, 1971). If, however, an individual maintains negative crossmatches against such a cell panel, despite multiple transfusions, the likelihood of hyperacute rejection is virtually eliminated. Furthermore, his chance of maintaining good renal function in a transplant for more than a year is 85 per cent compared to approximately 50 per cent for the larger general experience reported to the Kidney Transplant Registry (Opelz *et al.*, 1972).

It is not yet clear whether patients who maintain negative crossmatches against a random panel, despite multiple transfusions, have failed to mount an antibody response at all. It is more likely that they have mounted a very modest antibody response which is insufficient to kill lymphocytes *in vitro*. Low levels of antidonor antibody can block the MLC response if recipient serum is added to the culture. Preliminary information indicates that many patients in the multiple transfusion category do have serum blocking activity in MLC (Terasaki *et al.*, 1973). One would expect such a limited antibody response to be ideal for enhancement of a subsequent organ graft.

The positive correlation between lymphocytotoxic antibody and hyperacute rejection and the realization that transfusions of whole blood can stimulate such antibodies has led to changes in the attitudes toward transfusion of patients on hemodialysis. Not only are fewer transfusions administered, but when a blood transfusion is needed, efforts are made to eliminate leukocytes and platelets by multiple washings with saline or by temporary freezing in glycerol. If, however, the antibody response to whole blood is beneficial (as long as one delays transplantation until the crossmatch is negative), then, perhaps the expense of eliminating leukocytes and platelets from whole blood is unnecessary and even unwise.

Paternal histocompatibility antigens expressed in the fetus during pregnancy stimulate a maternal lymphocytotoxic antibody response against paternal cells approximately 25 per cent of the time after a single pregnancy. Multiple pregnancies lead to cytotoxic antibody responses more often than not. Yet the clinical results of cadaver kidney transplantation for men and women are identical as long as positive crossmatches are avoided (Beleil *et al.*, 1972). In the case of living related donor transplants, women who have cytotoxins against a random panel (but not against the actual donor) fare slightly better than men.

The apparent enhancement effect of prior exposure to antigen may also apply to second kidney transplants. Recipients who rejected their first kidney had a 64 per cent incidence of good function for at least a year in the second transplant (compared to 58 per cent for first transplant controls) provided that lymphocytotoxic antibody failed to appear after rejection of the initial transplant (Opelz *et al.*, 1972).

Second transplants can also fare better in the dog, even when both are from the same donor, but the timing of the second transplant is critical (Miller *et al.*, 1971; Hattler and Miller, 1973). Hattler and Miller used a combination of lymphocytotoxic and MLC assays to determine the optimal timing for the second kidney. The first step was to wait until the lymphocytotoxic crossmatch became negative. There was then a period when the MLC reaction was blocked if it was performed in the presence of recipient plasma; furthermore, blocking persisted even after replacing recipient plasma with normal plasma. They called this the period of irreversible blocking and it was associated with accelerated rejection. Their explanation for irreversibility of the MLC reaction was that the recipient's serum was still toxic enough to kill the donor leukocytes even though killing had not occurred in the microlymphocytotoxicity assay. Approximately two months following transplantation, however, the culture assay became reversible; MLC of donor and recipient cells showed no stimulation when set in recipient plasma, but responded if the recipient plasma was removed and the culture period was resumed in normal plasma.

Although much less is known about bacterial antigens as a potential conditioning agent for enhancement, it appears that some do cross react with human histocompatibility antigens and lead to positive lymphocytotoxic crossmatches (McDonald,

1972). Conceivably, they could also lead to levels of antibody that are blocking rather than cytotoxic.

Clinical passive enhancement

Clinical trials of passive enhancement in man have been initiated at Guy's Hospital, London (Batchelor *et al.*, 1970). In the first clinical trial, the recipient's kidney was provided by his mother. The father was immunized with maternal leukocytes to prepare antiserum which was then digested to $F(ab')_2$ fragments with pepsin. The transplant was viable but did not function well during the first week after transplantation. It is not clear whether the impaired function was due to an ischemic injury or to antibody mediated injury. In any event, the kidney regained normal function and it was the author's impression that the recipient required less azathioprine and prednisone than do most recipients of living donor transplants.

The complexity of preparing serum with the appropriate specificities is certainly much simpler in the living related donor situation, but the serious clinical need is in the treatment of cadaver kidney recipients. No doubt additional clinical trials of passive enhancement will be forthcoming. Major questions to be answered before initiating such trials are: should antisera be raised in volunteers or obtained by plasmaphoresing postpartum women who exhibit antibody against paternal cells? Should the recipient be treated with a high polyvalent preparation or should HL-A typing be used to select a few 'appropriate' specificities? Should the patient receive intact IgG or should he receive antibody treated by enzyme digestion or some other means such as succinylation to remove or alter the Fc piece, or should he receive a combination of intact and modified antibody? Should the preparation used for treatment be free from antibody specificities that might combine with antigens that are present in the recipient but missing from the donor (anti-recipient alloantibody causes shock-like injury in the rat and mouse)? What should determine the dose and timing of treatment? Obviously, there is room for much more study in an animal model which, unlike the rat, is subject to antibody-mediated hyperacute rejection of organ grafts.

Clinical active enhancement

So far there have been no reports of successful prolongation of graft survival after intentional antigen pretreatment in man. In many ways active enhancement presents even greater problems and questions than does passive enhancement. One must determine for each antigen the form, route, dose and timing that will stimulate minimal cellular immunity, yet an amount and class of humoral immunity that will provide blocking activity but not cytotoxicity and hyperacute rejection. Much will depend on the recipient's pre-existing state of immunity. If he has already been exposed to the donor antigen in question, the dose and timing of antigen pretreatment required may be quite different. The hazards of active immunization are perhaps less predictable than for passive immunization; the possibility of inflicting damage on a graft may be greater for active immunization because of the variability with respect to primed cellular immunity. Optimal pretreatment may require several weeks. In that case, the limits imposed by current organ preservation techniques would eliminate active enhancement for recipients of cadaver kidneys. One could, however, re-examine the possibility of living unrelated or distantly related donors which have in recent years been excluded in most clinical transplant centers.

Less risky and less complicated logistically than extended antigen pretreatment may be the use of antigen within 24 hours before transplantation or during the first two weeks after transplantation as an adjunct to ALS, standard drug therapy, and even specific passive immunization.

Since its beginning in the late 1950s, clinical kidney transplantation has progressed stepwise through a series of plateaus. It has been stalled for several years, but the prospects are bright that immunologically specific suppression of allograft rejection can be achieved within this decade. The door will then be wide open for transplantation of any organ or tissue for which surgical techniques are available.

References

Barnes, B. A., and the Advisory Committee to the Renal Transplant Retistry (1972). The Tenth Report of the Human Renal Transplant Registry. *J. Amer. Med. Ass.*, **221,** 1495

Basten, A.. Miller, J. F. A. P., Sprent, J. and Pye, J. (1972). A receptor for antibody on B lymphocytes. I. Method of detection and functional significance. *J. Exp. Med.*, **135,** 610

Batchelor, J. R., French, M. E., Cameron, J. S., Ellis, F., Bewick, M. and Ogg, C. S. (1970). Immunological enhancement of human kidney graft. *Lancet*, **2,** 1007

Batchelor, J. R., Fabre, J. and Morris, P. J. (1972). Passive enhancement of kidney allografts, potentiation with antithymocyte serum. *Transplantation*, **13,** 610

Beleil, O. M., Mickey, M. R. and Terasaki, P. I. (1972). Comparison of male and female kidney transplant survival rates. *Transplantation*, **13,** 493

Billingham, R. E., Brent, L. and Medawar, P. B. (1953). 'Actively acquired tolerance' of foreign cells. *Nature* (*London*), **172,** 603

Billingham, R. E., Brent, L. and Medawar, P. B. (1956). Quantitative studies on tissue transplantation immunity. III. Actively acquired tolerance. *Phil. Trans. Roy. Soc. B*, **239,** 357

Brent, L. (1971a). Immunological Tolerance 1951–1971. In *Immunological tolerance to Tissue Antigens* (N. W. Nisbet and M. W. Elves, editors). Orthopaedic Hospital, Oswestry, England

Brent, L. (1971b). Pathogenic role of delayed hypersensitivity and antibody in allograft reactions. In *Cellular Interactions in the Immune Response*, pp. 250–263. Basel: S. Karger

Brent, L. (1972). Tolerance and enhancement in organ transplantation. *Transplant. Proc.*, **4**, 363

Brent, L. and Gowland, G. (1961). Cellular dose and age of host in the induction of tolerance. *Nature (London)*, **192**, 1265

Brent, L. and Gowland, G. (1962). Induction of tolerance of skin homografts in immunologically competent mice. *Nature (London)*, **196**, 1298

Brent, L. and Gowland, G. (1963). In *Conceptual Advances in Immunology and Oncology*, p. 335. New York: Harper and Row

Brent, L. and Kilshaw, P. J. (1970). Prolongation of skin allograft survival with spleen extracts and antilymphocyte serum. *Nature (London)*, **227**, 898

Brent, L., Hansen, J. A. and Kilshaw, P. J. (1971). Unresponsiveness to skin allografts induced by tissue extracts and anti-lymphocyte serum. *Transplant. Proc.*, **3**, 684

Brent, L., Books, C., Lubling, N. and Thomas, A. V. (1972). Attempts to demonstrate an in vivo rôle for serum blocking factors in tolerant mice. *Transplantation*, **14**, 382

Calne, R. Y., Davis, D. R., Medawar, P. B. and Wheeler, J. R. (1966). Effect of donor antigen on dogs with renal homotransplants. *Transplantation*, **4**, 742

Caseley, J., Moses, V. K., Lichter, E. A. and Jonasson, O. (1971). Isoimmunization of hemodialysis patients: 'Leukocyte-poor v. whole blood transfusions'. *Transplant. Proc.*, **3**, 365

Casey, A. E. (1934). Specificity of enhancing materials from mammalian tumors. *Proc. Soc. Exp. Biol. Med.*, **31**, 663

Chard, T., French, M. E. and Batchelor, J. R. (1967). Enhancement of the C57BL leukemia E.L. 4 by Fab fragments of isoantibody. *Transplantation*, **5**, 1266

Cruse, J. M., Whitten, H. D., Lewis, G. K. and Watson, E. S. (1973). Facilitation of macrophage mediated destruction of allogeneic fibrosarcoma cells by tumor enhancing IgG_2 *in vitro*. *Transplant. Proc.*, **5**, 961

Dresser, D. W. and Mitchison, N. A. (1968). The mechanism of immunological paralysis. *Adv. Immunol.*, **8**, 129

Fabre, J. W. and Morris, P. J. (1972). The effect of donor strain blood pretreatment on renal allograft rejection in rats. *Transplantation*, **14**, 608

Feldmann, M. and Diener, E. (1970). Antibody mediated suppression of the immune response in vitro. I. Evidence for a central effect. *J. Exp. Med.*, **131**, 247

Flexner, S. and Jobling, J. W. (1907). On the promoting influence of heated tumor emulsions on tumor growth. *Proc. Soc. Exp. Biol. Med.*, **4**, 156

French, M. E. (1972). The early effects of alloantibody and complement on rat kidney allografts. *Transplantation*, **13**, 447

French, M. E. (1973). Mechanism of the enhancement of rat kidney allografts. *Transplant. Proc.*, **5**, 1001

French, M. E., Batchelor, J. R., Watts, H. G. (1971). The capacity of lymphocytes from rats bearing enhanced kidney allografts to mount graft-versus-host reactions. *Transplantation*, **12**, 45

French, M. E. and Batchelor, J. R. (1969). Immunological enhancement of rat kidney grafts. *Lancet*, **2**, 1103

Gowland, G. (1965). Induction of transplantation tolerance in adult animals. *Brit. Med. Bull.*, **21**, 123

Halasz, N. A. and Orloff, M. J. (1963). Enhancement of kidney homografts. *Surg. Forum*, **14**, 206

Hattler, B. G. and Miller, J. (1973). Prospective in vitro prediction of enhancement of canine renal allografts. *Surgery* (in press)

Hellström, I., Hellström, K. E. and Allison, A. C. (1971). Neonatally induced allograft tolerance may be mediated by serum-borne factors. *Nature (London)*, **230**, 49

Holl-Allen, R. T., Scharli, A., Rippin, A., Busch, G. J., Simonian, S. J. and Wilson, R. E. (1969). Cytotoxic antibody after antigen pretreatment: Enhancement of renal allografts. *Surg. Forum*, **20**, 276

Holter, A., McKearn, T. J., Neu, M. R., Fitch, F. W. and Stuart, F. P. (1972). Renal transplantation in the rabbit. I. Development of a model for study of hyperacute rejection and immunological enhancement. *Transplantation*, **13**, 244

Holter, A. R., Neu, M. R., McKearn, T. J., Lynch, A. F. and Stuart, F. P. (1973). Abrogation of hyperacute rejection of renal allografts by pepsin digest fragments of antidonor antibody. *Transplant. Proc.*, **5**, 593

Kaliss, N. (1958). Immunological enhancement of tumor homografts in mice. A review. *Cancer Research*, **18**, 992

Kaliss, N., Molomut, N., Harriss, J. L. and Gault, S. D. (1953). Effect of previously injected immune serum and tissue on the survival of tumor grafts in mice. *J. Nat. Cancer Inst.*, **13**, 847

Kaliss, N. and Kandutsch, A. A. (1956). Acceptance of tumor homografts by mice injected with antiserum. I. Activity of serum fractions. *Proc. Soc. Exp. Biol. Med.*, **91**, 118

Kinsky, R. G., Voisin, G. A., Duc, H. T. (1972). Biological properties of transplantation immune sera. III. Relationship between transplantation (facilitation or inhibition) and serological (anaphylaxis and cytolysis) activities. *Trantplantation*, **13,** 452

Lance, E. M. and Medawar, P. (1969). Quantitative studies on tissue transplantation immunity. IX. Induction of tolerance with antilymphocyte serum. *Proc. Roy. Soc. B*, **173,** 447

Levinson, A. I. and Silvers, W. K. (1973). Effect of splenectomy on the induction of high degrees of tolerance to skin allografts in rats. *Cellular Immunol.*, **6,** 149

Linscott, W. D. (1970). Effect of cell surface antigen density on immunological enhancement. *Nature (London)*, **228,** 824

Lucas, Z. J. and Enomoto, K. (1973). Immunological enhancement of renal allografts in the rat. III. Role of the spleen. *Transplantation*, **15,** 8

Lucas, Z. J. and Enomoto, K. (1973). Enhancement of renal grafts by anti-receptor site serum. *Fed. Proc.*, **32,** 971

Mauel, J., Rudolf, H., Chapuis, B. and Brunner, K. T. (1970). Studies of allograft immunity in mice. II. Mechanism of target cell inactivation in vitro by sensitized lymphocytes. *Immunology*, **18,** 517

McDonald, J. C. (1973). A heterophile system in human renal transplantation. I. Distribution of antigens and reactivity of the antibodies. II. Relationship to clinical renal transplantation and the HL-A system. *Transplantation*, **15,** 116 and **15,** 123

McKearn, T. J., Fitch, F. W. and Stuart, F. P. (1973). Inhibition of reactivity to transplantation antigens by antibody against alloantibody. *Fed. Proc.*, **32,** 971 Abs.

McKearn, T. J. and Stuart, F. P. (1973). Unpublished observations

Medawar, P. B. (1972). Comments at ALG workshop. *Behring Institute Research Communication*, NO. 51, p. 219. Behringwerke A.G., Marburg, Germany

Miller, J., Hattler, B., Davis, M. and Johnson, M. C. (1971). Cellular and humoral factors governing canine mixed lymphocyte cultures after renal transplantation. I. Antibody. *Transplantation*, **12,** 65

Möller, G. (1963). Studies on the mechanism of immunological enhancement of tumor homografts. I. Specificity of immunological enhancement. *J. Nat. Canc. Inst.*, **30,** 1153

Möller, E. and Möller, G. (1962). Quantitative studies of the sensitivity of normal and neoplastic mouse cells to the cytotoxic action of isoantibodies. *J. Exp. Med.*, **115,** 527

Monaco, A. P., Wood, M. L. and Russell, P. S. (1966). Studies on heterologous anti-lymphocyte serum in mice. III. Immunologic tolerance and chimerism produced across the H-2 locus with adult thymectomy and anti-lymphocyte serum. *Ann. N.Y. Acad. Sci.*, **129,** 190

Mullen, Y., Takasugi, M. and Hildemann, W. H. (1973). The immunological status of rats with long surviving (enhanced) kidney allografts. *Transplantation*, **15,** 238

Murray, J. E., Balankura, O., Greenberg, J. B., and Dammin, G. J. (1962). Reversibility of the kidney homograft reaction by retransplantation and drug therapy. *Ann. N.Y. Acad. Sci.*, **99,** 768

Myburgh, J. A. and Smit, J. A. (1972). Passive and active enhancement in baboon liver allografting. *Transplantation*, **14,** 227

Ockner, S. A., Guttmann, R. D. and Lindquist, R. R. (1970). Renal transplantation in the inbred rat. XIII. Modification of rejection by active immunization with bone marrow cells. *Transplantation*, **9,** 30

Oh, J. H., Gault, M. H., Helle, S. J. and Dossetor, J. B. (1972). Development of lymphocytotoxic antibodies in hemodialysis patients. *Vox Sang.*, **22,** 208

Opelz, G., Mickey, M. R. and Terasaki, P. I. (1972). Identification of unresponsive kidney-transplant recipients. *Lancet*, 22 April, 1972, p. 868

Opelz, G., Mickey, M. R. and Terasaki, P. I. (1972). Prolonged survival of second human kidney transplants. *Science*, **178,** 617

Opelz, G., Sengar, D. P. S., Mickey, M. R. and Terasaki, P. I. (1973). Effect of blood transfusion on subsequent kidney transplants. *Transplant. Proc.*, **5,** 253

Owen, E. R. (1969). Preventing the rejection of transplanted organs. *Ann. Roy. Coll. Surg. Eng.*, **45,** 63

Owen, E. R., Slome, D. and Waterston, D. J. (1968). Prolongation of rabbit kidney allograft survival by desensitization. In *Advances in Transplantation*, p. 385. Baltimore: Williams and Wilkins

Patel, R. and Terasaki, P. I. (1969). Significance of the positive crossmatch test in kidney transplantation. *New Engl. J. Med.*, **280,** 735

Patel, R., Merrill, J. P. and Briggs, W. A. (1971). Analysis of results of kidney transplantation. Comparison in recipients with and without preformed antileukocyte antibodies. *New Engl. J. Med.*, **285,** 274

Penn, I. and Starzl, T. E. (1972). Malignant tumors arising de novo in immunosuppressed organ transplant recipients. *Transplantation*, **14,** 407

Rabellino, E., Colon, S., Grey, H. M. and Unanue, E. R. (1971). Immunoglobulins on the surface of lymphocytes. I. Distribution and quantitation. *J. Exp. Med.*, **133,** 156

Ramseier, H. and Lindenmann, J. (1971). Cellular receptors. Effect of anti-allo-antiserum on the recognition of transplantation antigens. *J. Exp. Med.*, **134,** 1083

Ramseier, H. and Lindenmann, J. (1972). Alliotypic antibodies. *Transplant. Rev.*, **10,** 57

Rowley, D. A. and Fitch, F. W. (1964). Homeostasis of antibody formation in the adult rat. *J. Exp. Med.*, **120,** 987

Rowley, D. A., Fitch, F. W., Stuart, F. P., Köhler, H. and Cosenza, H. (1973). Specific suppression of immune responses. *Science* (in press)

Ryder, R. J. W. and Schwartz, R. S. (1969). Immunosuppression by antibody; localization and site of action. *J. Immunol.*, **103,** 970

Schechter, G. P., Soehnlen, F. and McFarland, W. (1972). Lymphocyte response to blood transfusion in man. *New Engl. J. Med.*, **287,** 1169

Schwartz, R. S. (1968). In *Human Transplantation*, p. 440 (F. T. Rapaport and J. Dausset, editors). New York and London: Grune & Stratton

Schwartz, R. and Damashek, W. (1959). Drug-induced immunological tolerance. *Nature (London)*, **183,** 1682

Seifert, L. N., Halasz, N. A., Orloff, M. J. and Rosenfield, H. A. (1966). Antigen-induced prolongation of whole organ allograft survival. *Surg. Forum*, **17,** 278

Shaipanich, T., Vanwijck, R. R., Kim, J., Lukl, P., Busch, G. and Wilson, R. (1971). Enhancement of rat renal allografts with $F(ab')_2$ fragment of donor specific antikidney serum. *Surgery*, **70,** 113

Silvers, W. K. and Billingham, R. E. (1969). Influence of the Ag-B locus on reactivity to skin homografts and tolerance responsiveness in rats. *Transplantation*, **8,** 167

Sinclair, N. R. St. C. (1969). Regulation of the immune response. I. Reduction in ability of specific antibody to inhibit long-lasting IgG immunological priming after removal of the Fc fragment. *J. Exp. Med.*, **129,** 1183

Sinclair, N. R. St. C., Lees, R. K., Chan, P. L. and Khan, R. H. (1970). Regulation of the immune response. II. Further studies on differences in ability of $F(ab')_2$ and 7S antibodies to inhibit an antibody response. *Immunology*, **19,** 105

Sjögren, H. O., Hellström, I., Bansal, S. C. and Hellström, K. E. (1971). Suggestive evidence that the 'blocking antibodies' of tumor-bearing individuals may be antigen–antibody complexes. *Proc. Nat. Acad. Sci.*, **68,** 1372

Snell, G. D. (1970). Immunological enhancement. *Surg. Gynecol. Obstet.*, **130,** 1109

Stuart, F. P., Saitoh, T. and Fitch, F. W. (1968). Rejection of renal allografts: Specific immunologic suppression. *Science*, **160,** 1463

Stuart, F. P., Fitch, F. W. and Rowley, D. A. (1970). Specific suppression of renal allograft rejection by treatment with antigen and antibody. *Transplant. Proc.*, **2,** 483

Stuart, F. P., Fitch, F. W., Rowley, D. A., Biesecker, J. L., Hellström, K. E. and Hellström, I. (1971a). Presence of both cell-mediated immunity and serum blocking factors in rat renal allografts enhanced by passive immunization. *Transplantation*, **12,** 331

Stuart, F. P., Bastien, E., Holter, A., Fitch, F. W. and Elkins, W. L. (1971b). Rôle of passenger leukocytes in the rejection of renal allografts. *Transplant. Proc.*, **3,** 461

Sutherland, D. E. R., Howard, R. J. and Najarian, J. S. (1973). Immunological enhancement of renal allografts in an outbred animal susceptible to hyperacute rejection. *Fed. Proc.*, **32,** 971 Abs.

Taguchi, Y., Mackinnon, K. J. and Dossetor, J. B. (1968). Renal allograft modification by donor antigen in the rat: Evidence for significance of this principle in man. In *Advances in Transplantation*, p. 363. Baltimore: Williams and Wilkins

Takasugi, M. and Hildemann, W. H. (1969). Lymphocyte-antibody interactions in immunological enhancement. *Transplant. Proc.*, **1,** 530

Terasaki, P. I., Sengar, D. P. and Opelz, G. (1973). Enhancement in human kidney allografts. *Transplant. Proc.*, **5,** 641

Uhr, J. W. and Möller, G. (1968). Regulatory effect of antibody on the immune response. *Adv. Immunol.*, **8,** 81

Wason, W. M. and Fitch, F. W. (1973). Suppression of the antibody response to SRBC with $F(ab')_2$ and IgG in vitro. *J. Immunol.*, **110,** 1427

Whitten, H. D., Cruse, J. M. and Sprunt, D. H. (1973). Kinetics of the Fc receptors for tumor enhancing IgG_2 on the macrophage membrane. *Fed. Proc.*, **32,** 978 Abs.

Wilson, D. B., Silvers, W. K. and Nowell, P. C. (1967). Quantitative studies on the mixed lymphocyte interaction in rats. II. Relationship of the proliferative response to the immunologic status of the donors. *J. Exp. Med.*, **126,** 655

Wilson, R. E., Rippin, A., Dagher, R. K., Kinreart, P. and Busch, G. J. (1969). Prolonged canine renal allograft survival after pretreatment with solubilized antigen. *Transplantation*, **7,** 360

Wilson, R. E., Kim, J., Shaipanich, T., Sells, R. A., Maggs, P. and Lukl, P. (1972). Active enhancement of rat renal allografts with soluble splenic antigen. *Transplantation*, **13,** 322

Winn, H. J. (1962). The participation of complement in isoimmune reactions. *Ann. N.Y. Acad. Sci.*, **101,** 23

Wood, M. L., Gozzo, J. J. and Monaco, A. P. (1972). Use of antilymphocyte serum and bone marrow for production of immunological tolerance and enhancement Review and recent experiments. *Transplant. Proc.*, **4,** 523

Zimmermann, C. E., Busch, G. J., Stuart, F. P. and Wilson, R. E. (1968). Canine renal homografts after pretreatment with subcellular splenic antigens. *Surgery*, **63,** 437

Zimmermann, C. E. (1971). Active enhancement of renal allografts. *Transplant. Proc.*, **3,** 701

9
Immunological Engineering and Experimental Transplantation

Dennis W. Jirsch and Erwin Diener

INTRODUCTION

Clinical organ transplantation has achieved remarkable success in recent years. Transfer of a kidney from either a living related donor or a cadaver to a patient with end-stage renal disease has now become an accepted therapeutic measure. Technical problems inherent in transplantation surgery become ever less burdensome as clinical experience accumulates. Clearly the immune response of a patient to a foreign graft persists as the major obstacle preventing widespread allotransplantation therapy of a variety of diseases. Immunological factors centering around allograft acceptance are threefold and include proper donor selection, effective immunosuppression and the induction of immunological tolerance. Analyses of the results of tissue typing in renal allografting indicate the benefit of histocompatibility between recipient and donor (Patel *et al.*, 1968; Festenstein *et al.*, 1971). As more antigenic groups and immune response genetic loci are identified, however, the probability of finding a fully compatible donor recipient pair will diminish. In the unrelated cadaver donor situation, we are left with a residue of histoincompatibility which must be neutralized by either immunosuppression or the induction of tolerance. The immunosuppressive agents now in use, however, are non-selective and seriously impair host resistance to

---

From the MRC Transplantation Unit, the Departments of Surgery and Pathology and the Surgical-Medical Research Institute, The University of Alberta, Edmonton, Alberta, Canada.

the microbial environment, suppress vigilant immunologic surveillance mechanisms and are associated with toxicity.

The induction of specific graft-directed tolerance is thus the ultimate goal of the transplantation biologist. In the laboratory, this can be approached in a variety of ways. We will briefly survey significant work in this regard, describe in some detail laboratory systems which permit the induction of specific unresponsiveness both *in vivo* and *in vitro*, and speculate concerning possible clinical applications.

ANTIGEN RECOGNITION AND THE ORIGIN OF IMMUNOCOMPETENT CELLS

The lymphocyte, the spearhead of immune defence

The lymphoid system constitutes a specific adaptive mechanism whereby confrontation with an extrinsic antigenic molecule provokes lymphocytes to discriminate between 'self' and 'foreign' and leads to the production of antibody forming cells or specific 'killer' cells capable of destroying foreign tissue on direct contact. Only a small proportion of lymphoid cells are genetically committed to react against a given antigenic specificity (Burnet, 1959), and Medawar (1960) has defined an immunocompetent cell as one capable of recognizing antigen. Once activated by antigen, these cells enlarge, divide and differentiate into a population of pyronin positive cells which eventually give rise to further small lymphocytes (Gowans *et al.*, 1962). In the case of foreign graft tissue, these progeny of specifically sensitized lymphocytes are concerned with the actual destruction of the transplant (cell-mediated immunity). Other responses are expressed through circulating antibodies derived from descendants of another class of lymphocytes which have, through differentiation and multiplication, developed the intracellular machinery necessary for antibody production (humoral immunity). The end point of this process is the antibody secreting plasma cell.

Certain lymphocytes develop within the thymus and are termed T cells, while others differentiate within bone marrow, independent of thymic influence, and are designated as B cells. For most but not all antigens, the co-operation of these two cell types is necessary for an antibody response (Miller and Mitchell, 1969; Davies, 1969; Claman and Chaperon, 1969; Taylor, 1969). T cells evidently serve in a helper capacity in presenting antigen to relevant B cells, which are the immediate precursors of antibody forming cells (Nossal *et al.*, 1968). Other T cells become specifically activated upon contact with antigen and are the effector cells in cell-mediated immunity (Cerottini *et al.*, 1970; Miller *et al.*, 1971). Neonatal thymectomy thus greatly depresses both cell mediated immunity and humoral immunity to those antigens which require T–B cell co-operation (Miller, 1961; Miller and Osoba, 1967). Certain antigens do not require T cell help (Diener *et al.*, 1971) and humoral immunity in these instances remains intact following thymectomy (Miller and Osoba, 1967). These considerations are schematically represented in Figure 9.1.

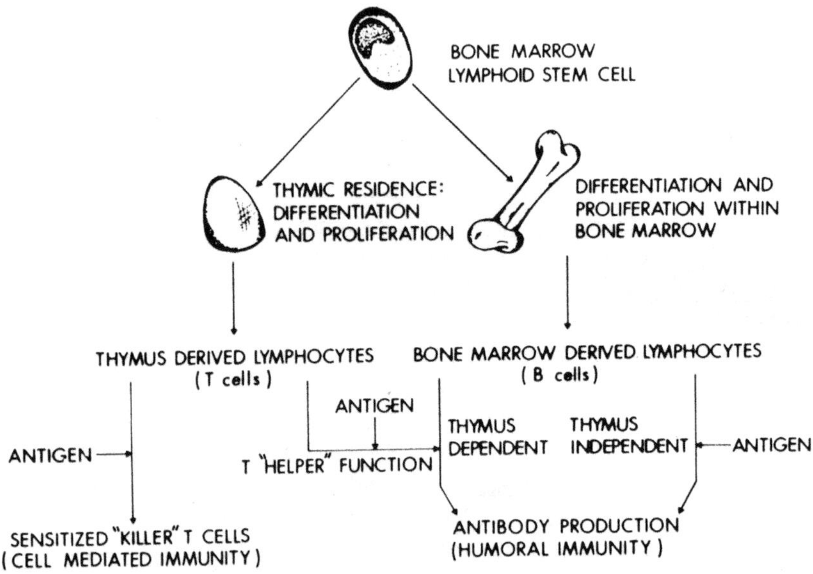

Figure 9.1 *Development of specialized T (thymus derived) and B (bone marrow derived) lymphocytes and their relationship to cellular and humoral immunity*

To initiate the events leading to either humoral antibody production or specifically sensitized 'killer' cells, immunocompetent cells must be triggered by foreign molecular structures, either soluble antigens or antigenic determinants on cell surfaces. What are the entities on lymphoid cells capable of discriminating between 'self' and 'non-self', and how does this recognition operate? The lymphocyte surface can be regarded as a switchboard from which signals are transmitted into the cell interior. Signals originate from molecular structures termed antigen recognition sites, which are sterically complementary to the structure of antigen molecules. In the case of B cells, these recognition sites are immunoglobulin IgM in character and are probably identical in basic structure with antibody. Helper T cells also appear to have specific surface receptors for antigen but T cell surface antibody is not readily demonstrable and differs from that found on B cells both qualitatively and quantitatively (Greaves and Hogg, 1971).

Origin of the immunocompetent cell

What is the origin of the lymphoid cells capable of recognizing a particular antigen, and how is this potential generated? All cells of the hematopoietic and lymphoid systems are derived from self-perpetuating bone marrow stem cells. Grafting of bone marrow into an animal which has received lethal X-irradiation (with consequent destruction of its own hematopoietic tissue) is a life saving procedure. Indeed, re-

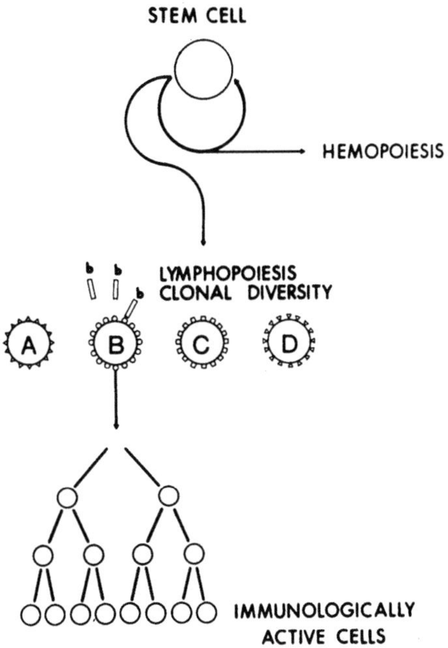

Figure 9.2 *The origin of immunocompetent cells. A, B, C and D are immunocompetent cells belonging to different cell clones. Each clone possesses recognition sites specific for only one antigen. b = specific antigen interacting with an immunocompetent cell.*
[*Reprinted with permission from* Medical Clinics of North America (*Diener and Jirsch, 1972*)]

population studies of Ford (1966), Micklem *et al.*, (1966) and Globerson and Auerbach (1967) showed that bone marrow has the capacity to recolonize not only bone marrow but also the thymus and peripheral lymphoid tissues. Further studies by Wu *et al.* (1968) demonstrated that single stem cells were capable of differentiation along lymphoid, erythroid, granulocytic or megakaryocytic lines.

It is evident that somewhere along the developmental pathway, from a few precursor cells (Figure 9.2) to the immensely large pool of specific immunocompetent cells in the lymphoid system, there occurs a critical phase during which the lymphocyte acquires the capacity to recognize a particular antigen and becomes immunocompetent. Since there are at the very least several thousand antigenic structures, and each lymphocyte recognizes only one antigenic specificity, we are faced with the problem that a single lymphocyte precursor must bear genetic information for the synthesis of several thousand different recognition sites. The hypothesis of Burnet (1959) has provided an answer to the dilemma. A limited number of genes undergo random somatic mutation during lymphopoiesis. The large number of mutant lymphocytes produced in this way are each genetically capable of recognizing a specific antigen. The potential for synthesis of recognition sites complementary to a given antigen then becomes the property of a single clone of cells. (This theory is known as the 'clonal selection theory of immunity'.) A single lymphoid precursor cell should thus generate a population of cells with gradually diversifying antigen recognition specificities. Yung *et al.* (1973) have, in fact, monitored the ontogenic development of immunocompetent cells in the mouse, and have found that a full antigen recognition spectrum is expressed within 20 days of clonal expansion from a single embryonic stem cell.

SPECIFIC SUPPRESSION OF THE IMMUNE RESPONSE

Immunological tolerance

Self tolerance

Immunological tolerance has been defined by Dresser and Mitchison (1968) as a state of partial or complete incapacity to respond to an immunogenic stimulus brought about by prior contact with antigen. The best example of this immunological unresponsiveness is the tolerant state we maintain toward our own body constituents. Attention was first directed to this phenomenon by Owen in 1945, who observed that dizygotic cattle twins are generally chimeric with respect to their red blood cell types due to synchorial placental anastomosis, which would permit free exchange of fetal blood *in utero*. Burnet and Fenner (1949) postulated shortly thereafter that a function of the lymphoreticuloendothelial system during embryonic life was to distinguish self from non-self constituents. Consequently, the presentation of foreign material to the developing embryo before it has learned to make this distinction would engender a specific lack of reactivity to this antigen. Experiments of Billingham *et al.* (1954) confirmed this interpretation. Skin grafts were permanently accepted between different inbred strains of mice if graft recipients were inoculated *in utero* with living donor spleen or kidney cells. The period during which tolerance may be induced during ontogeny of the immune system varies according to species, the tolerance responsive period extending several weeks after birth in rats (Woodruff and Simpson, 1955), while sheep embryos become immunocompetent well before parturition (Schinkell and Ferguson, 1953).

The rôle of the thymus in the induction and maintenance of the tolerant state has not yet been unequivocally established, but it is clearly important. Burnet (1962) suggested that one of the thymic functions was either the elimination or inactivation of self reactive clones. Antigens presented to the thymus would, therefore, be recognized as 'self' and not subject to immune attack. In accord with this concept, a number of investigators (Staples *et al.*, 1966; Isakovic *et al.*, 1965; Taylor, 1969) have been able to produce tolerance by direct intrathymic injection of antigens. The importance of this data is not clear since antigen specific tolerance can be induced in adult thymectomized animals (Mitchison, 1967) and the thymus does contain small numbers of lymphocytes capable of initiating an immune response (Mitchell and Miller, 1968). The suggestion is, therefore, that mature immunocompetent lymphocytes may be target cells in tolerance induction and that the thymus is not the only site available for this interaction. Since lymphocytes capable of reacting to alloantigens develop within the thymus, tolerance to self antigens may indeed occur within the thymus during ontogeny.

Methods of inducing tolerance in vivo

In experiments involving extrinsic antigens, several factors have been found important for tolerance induction. The route of antigen administration is important, for example, and tolerance is induced more easily following intravenous administration rather than subcutaneous, intradermal or intraperitoneal injection. The experiments of Triplett (1962) have suggested, moreover, that the permanent presence of antigen is necessary for the maintenance of tolerance. This is true probably because immunocompetent cells are generated throughout life and may replace tolerant cells unless they are rendered unresponsive themselves. Ever since the experiments of Smith and Bridges (1958), two factors have been found critically important in tolerance induction:

concentration and the molecular structure of the antigen used. For many antigens, there exist two distinct zones of concentration which can induce tolerance, a high and a low dosage zone, while intermediate concentrations provoke an immune response. This phenomenon has been characterized in experiments done with bovine serum albumen in adult mice and rabbits (Mitchison, 1964; Thorbecke and Benacerraf, 1967) and with the *Salmonella* flagellar antigens in rats (Shellam and Nossal, 1968; Ada and Parish, 1968). Immunological tolerance corresponding to these two zones has been defined as high zone and low zone tolerance.

The molecular state of most antigens is of paramount importance in determining the capacity to induce tolerance. Dresser (1962), for example, showed that monomeric (deaggregated) human gamma globulin, when injected into certain strains of mice rendered them unresponsive to subsequent injections of the aggregated human gamma globulin, a potent immunogen. Parish *et al.* (1969) have reported the isolation of fragments of cyanogen bromide treated flagellin (mol. wt. 40 000) of *Salmonella adelaide*. One of the fragments (Fragment 'A', mol. wt. 18 000) retains the main antigenic activity of flagellin and causes induction of tolerance but no immunity to flagellin when injected repeatedly at a particular dose level. Antigens may, therefore, exhibit tolerogenic or immunogenic qualities when administered *in vivo*. Since tolerogens can be converted into immunogens by nonspecific means such as by mixing them with adjuvants, Dresser (1963) has suggested that immunogenic antigens have properties called 'adjuvanticity', which, in the case of the bovine gamma globulin system, could be separated as aggregated material.

Tolerance to normally immunogenic substances can be induced in adult animals by administration of the antigen along with X-irradiation, immunosuppressive treatment (including antilymphocyte globulin) and by mechanical lymphocyte depletion (thoracic duct cannulation). Tolerance induction and immunity, though alternative effects at the single cell level, often coincide in adult animals. A balance between the two phenomena can apparently swing toward tolerance induction by non-specific removal of immunocompetent cells. This situation is most akin to that of the fetus: a stage of immunoincompetence most susceptible for tolerance induction during which stem cells proliferate and differentiate into mature lymphoid elements. Mitchison 1967) has shown that the threshold of antigen concentration for induction of tolerance under such conditions was 10^{-8} M for several different antigens. It has been calculated, moreover, that the dose of antigen per kilogram of body weight necessary to induce tolerance in an adult irradiated animal is comparable to that required in the neonate Smith, 1961).

As for potential clinical use, antilymphocyte serum as a means of immunosuppression during tolerance induction has been favored over X-irradiation for obvious reasons. For instance, rabbit anti-mouse ALS produces prolonged and profound lymphopenia and grossly deficient immune reactivity when injected into mice. Animals treated in this manner can be rendered tolerant to transplantation antigens of another mouse strain by injecting them with allogeneic spleen cells, similar to the phenomenon described in the neonate (Billingham and Brent, 1957). Recipients will then specifically retain skin grafts of the donor spleen cell strain. Since, as discussed earlier, thymectomy results in immunologic deficiency, tolerance is most easily induced by treatment of adult thymectomized mice with ALS prior to the administration of the tolerance inducing spleen cells (Monaco *et al.*, 1965). Adult thymectomized ALS-treated mice rendered tolerant by large doses of allogeneic lymphoid cells exhibit stable lymphoid chimerism (Monaco *et al.*, 1966) and a long-standing tolerance. In contrast, non-thymectomized mice rendered tolerant by ALS treatment accompanied with donor marrow infusion do not demonstrate long-standing lymphoid cell chimerism and the tolerant state is of short duration (Wood *et al.*, 1972).

Are both B and T cells involved in tolerance?

From the studies of Chiller *et al.* (1970), it appears that both B and T cells can be rendered tolerant. Neither thymus nor bone marrow cells from A/J mice injected 3 weeks previously with tolerogenic human gamma globulin could, with their normal counterpart, reconstitute secondary irradiated syngeneic recipients. With extrinsic proteins, both Mitchison (1971) and Rajevsky (1971) have found that the response of mice which exhibited low zone tolerance could be restored with the transfer of activated T cells but that high zone induced tolerance was unaffected. High zone tolerance may thus be due to specific inactivation of both T and B cells with low zone tolerance induction dependent only on T cell inactivation. In agreement with this, Chiller *et al.* (1971) have found that T cells could be rendered tolerant *in vivo* to human gamma globulin with concentrations of antigen far too low to specifically inactivate B cells.

Studies on tolerance induction *in vivo* have not answered the fundamental question as to the fate of the tolerant cell. Irreversible inactivation or cell death has been regarded as most consistent with current immunological data but there is recent alternative evidence which, in fact, considers at least certain types of immunological tolerance as an active state of cell repression rather than elimination (McCullagh, 1970a, b; 1972). Normal syngeneic lymphocytes could not restore immune reactivity when transferred to hosts tolerant to sheep erythrocytes and were, indeed, rendered unresponsive themselves. Allogeneic lymphocytes exposed to tolerant lymphocytes could, however, restore the immune response suggesting an 'unmasking' of immunocompetent cells. Nisbet (1971) has transferred tolerance to sheep erythrocytes in normal mice parabiosed to tolerant animals, and has been able to selectively transfer tolerance by injecting large numbers of tolerant thoracic duct lymphocytes or spleen cells into normal recipients.

Antibody-mediated enhancement and the immune response

The presence of humoral antibodies directed toward graft antigens can sometimes facilitate the growth of foreign tumor cells which would normally be rejected (Kaliss, 1956; 1958). Enhancing antibodies can be raised in response to normal immunization procedures (active enhancement) or the sera of animals previously exposed to tumor antigens may be passively administered to second graft recipients (passive enhancement). Kaliss (1956), for example, showed that serum from tumor bearing mice would promote tumor growth in secondary hosts if administered up to one week before or after the tumor inoculum. Although initial work on enhancement involved allografted tumors in rodents, the phenomenon has become relevant as a means of specifically facilitating the survival of allografted organs. Three main possibilities have been proposed as mechanisms by which enhancement may work:

Afferent blockage

Graft directed antibodies may cover antigenic determinants on foreign cells, thereby preventing activation of relevant immunocompetent cells (Uhr and Möller, 1968). For example, Snell *et al.* (1960) studied the lymph nodes draining the site of an allogeneic tumor. If mice were injected with hyperimmune antitumor antiserum before the tumor was transplanted, the lymph nodes were less reactive to the tumor thereafter, suggesting that the antiserum had covered tumor cell antigens. On the other hand, several workers (Terres and Wolins, 1961; Segre and Kaeberle, 1962) have demonstrated that specific antibody administered together with antigen may increase rather than diminish antigen immunogenicity. Similarly, Diener and Feldmann (1970) showed that polymerized flagellin from the bacterium *Salmonella adelaide* in the presence of antibody excess displayed an *in vitro* immune response comparable to controls stimulated with antigen alone. Uhr and Baumann (1961) in work with the tetanus toxoid antigen, could inhibit an antitetanus response with antibody with a quantity of antitoxin sufficient to cover only a small fraction of antigenic sites on the administered toxoid. Haughton and Nash (1969) provided further evidence against peripheral enhancement. The number of antibody molecules necessary to cover the antigenic sites of 5×10^8 sheep erythrocytes was 100-fold greater than that needed to suppress the immune response. Tumor allografts, moreover, can be enhanced by administration of antiserum at the time of peak rejection response (Kaliss, 1958) and, as shown by Möller (1965), smaller doses of antiserum were generally more effective than large doses in promoting tumor growth. Enhancing antiserum, moreover, suppressed the lymphocytosis accompanying allograft tumor immunity in cases where surgical excision of tumor was ineffective (Takasugi and Hildemann, 1969).

Central immunosuppression

Humoral antibodies may act directly on immunocompetent cells to specifically decrease immunological reactivity. This has been demonstrated convincingly by Amos *et al.* (1970) using a transplantable mouse tumor. Tumor cells were incubated with antiserum, washed free of excess serum, and then mixed with lymphoid cells from mice sensitized against the tumor. When these lymphoid cells were added to fresh tumor cells and injected into recipient mice, tumor growth was enhanced. Control experiments with lymphoid cells exposed to tumor and nonimmune serum failed to facilitate tumor growth. The work of Rowley *et al.* (1969a, b) is confirmatory and suggests that antibody may directly reduce the number of immunocompetent cells initially responsive to antigen.

Efferent enhancement

Humoral antibodies bound to the surface antigens of foreign cells considered as targets, conceivably protect such cells from the killing activity of sensitized lymphocytes. The first clear demonstration of efferent enhancement was given by Möller (1963) who grafted two identical homologous tumors simultaneously into the same non-sensitized mouse. One graft had been exposed *in vitro* to specific antiserum and this showed enhanced growth; the second, untreated graft was rejected in normal fashion. Further support for efferent blockage was given by recent work of the Hellströms. In tumor systems, sera of animals (Hellström and Hellström, 1969; Hellström, Evans and Hellström, 1969; Hellström, Hellström *et al.*, 1970a) or patients (Hellström, Hellström *et al.*, 1970b) bearing antigenically distinct tumors were shown to contain a factor that specifically inhibited the *in vitro* antitumor activity of lymphocytes from the tumor bearer or lymphocytes from specifically sensitized animals. Similarly, the sera from female mice mated with allogeneic males inhibited the *in vitro* activity of lymphocytes sensitized to paternal strain tissue (Hellström, Hellström *et al.*, 1969). A serum factor that abrogated the activity of sensitized lymphocytes has been demonstrated in chimeric dogs and mice (Hellström, Hellström *et al.*, 1970c; Hellström, Hellström *et al.*, 1971) and renal allografted humans (Quadracci, Hellström *et al.*, 1971; Hellström and Hellström, 1972a).

Although the initial proposal (Hellström and Hellström, 1970) was that the serum factor inhibiting the *in vitro* activity of sensitized lymphocytes was an antibody which combined with antigens on the target cell surface (efferent enhancement), a central form of immunosuppression was later postulated (Hellström and Hellström, 1971) for the so-called 'blocking antibody'. Ingenious experiments of Sjögren *et al.* (1971) indicated that blocking antibody might, in fact, be a complex of antigen and antibody.

Enhancing sera from mouse sarcomas were absorbed by tumor cells, which were spun down and resuspended in buffer. After mixing in buffer for one hour, tumor cells were discarded and the supernatant was passed through an ultrafilter which would retain molecules of molecular weight greater than 100 000. The filtrate was then passed through a second filter capable of retaining molecules of molecular weight greater than 10 000. Only a 1:1 combination of the material retained by the two filters optimally prevented lymphocyte mediated lysis of target cells, and neither of the two fractions alone were fully immunosuppressive. It was suggested that the two components separated by the molecular filters may have represented antigen and antibody and that uniting these two had led to blocking antigen–antibody complexes. This interpretation is supported by other experiments, in particular the work of Stuart and colleagues (Stuart *et al.*, 1968; Stuart *et al.*, 1970). Rat F_1 hybrid kidneys were grafted to parental strain animals. Graft recipients were inoculated with spleen cells of graft donor type in combination with homologous antiserum directed against graft alloantigens. Maximal allograft enhancement was achieved only when antiserum treatment was combined with the administration of donor spleen cells and, with this regimen, permanent survival of the transplanted kidneys was obtained in many recipients.

French and Batchelor (1969) transplanted allogeneic (F_1 to parent) rat kidneys in similar manner, but could enhance graft survival with passive administration of graft directed antiserum alone. It is possible however, that graft derived antigen itself may have permitted antigen–antibody complex formation. Enhanced graft survival has been obtained, moreover, in transplantation of skin, kidney or cardiac allografts in several laboratory species by injection of donor blood or blood elements at different intervals before and after grafting (Halasz, 1963; Marino and Benaim, 1958; Halasz *et al.*, 1964; Marquet *et al.*, 1971). Since the antibody response to rat renal allografts is not abrogated by passive administration of graft directed antisera (Lucas *et al.*, 1970), donor blood may indeed provide a ready source of antigen for complex formation with antibody. In the tumor cell system of Amos *et al.* (1970), described above, a similar combination of tumor cell antigen and specific antibody exposed to lymphocytes suppressed their ability to kill new cells. The combination of tumor plus antibody was more effective than exposure to either tumor or antibody alone. These studies were facilitated by a tissue culture system which allowed the maintenance of dispersed mouse lymphoid cells *in vitro*.

The concept of serum mediated blocking factors preventing the expression of cell mediated immunity is now firmly established in tumor and graft systems. The relationship of this phenomenon to the induction of neonatal tolerance or to normal self tolerance is not clear. There is, however, recent evidence that mice may react against antigens present on their normal (brain) cells *in vitro*, and expression of such induced cell mediated immunity is prevented by blocking factors present in normal sera (Hellström and Hellström, 1972b). This evidently contradicts the classic explanation for both neonatally induced tolerance and normal tolerance to self antigens, whereby lymphoid clones genetically capable of immune reactivity are eliminated during embryonic development.

A new concept in specific immunosuppression emanates from the work of Ramseier and Lindenmann (1972). Their work in the field of acquired tolerance may be relevant to self tolerance between lymphocytes. Antibodies can be raised against specific antigen receptors present on lymphoid cells, in their notation termed anti-RS, where RS signifies recognition structure. The specificity of these antibodies has been demonstrated in the following way. F_1 hybrid mice were immunized with repeated small doses of parental lymphoid cells, testing the subsequent serum for antibodies to histocompatibility antigens. They reasoned that F_1 cells would not bear receptors for either parental cell types but that parental cells themselves would bear receptors for the other parent. This parental recognition site directed toward the other parental lymphocyte would be the only unique structure that F_1 progeny could recognize and produce antibody against. The presence of these anti-RS antibodies has been demonstrated in several situations. The most convincing finding was the ability of anti-RS sera to inhibit graft-versus-host reactions (Joller, 1972). These anti-RS sera did not, however, inhibit MLC reactions. The relation of anti-RS sera to blocking factor is not yet clear but could be important, especially in transplantation of lymphoid tissues.

IN VITRO MANIPULATION OF THE IMMUNE RESPONSE

Tolerance induction *in vitro*

The abundant *in vivo* data relative to immunoregulative mechanisms have led to a number of interpretations which are conceptually disturbing. This has prompted experimentation by Diener and colleagues in an attempt to clarify the rôle, at the cellular level, of free antibody and of antigen–antibody complexes in immune suppression. Experiments were done on dispersed lymphocytes from mouse spleen which were kept alive using a tissue culture system devised by Marbrook (1967) (Figure 9.3). Spleen cells in an adequate medium were placed in a cylindrical tube closed off at the bottom by a dialysis membrane. This tube was then placed in an

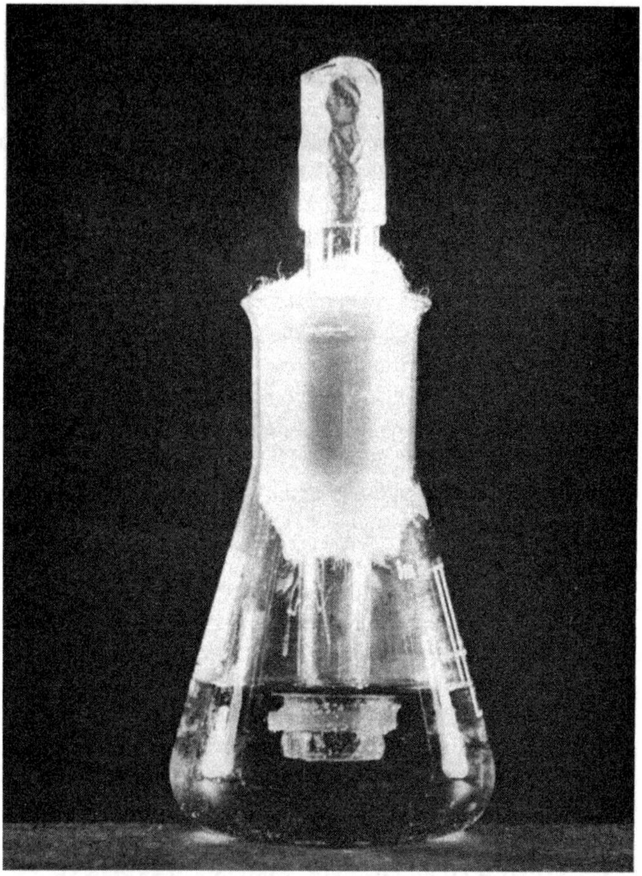

Figure 9.3 *Tissue Culture Flask: Dispersed mouse spleen cells are suspended in tissue culture medium inside an internal tube. The bottom end of the tube is closed off by a dialysis membrane and permits passage of nutrients from the reservoir across the membrane.*

Erlenmeyer-type flask containing sufficient tissue culture medium to equal the fluid level of the cell suspension in the inner cylinder. Cultures were maintained in a humidified incubator at 37 °C with a constant flow of a gas mixture consisting of CO_2, O_2 and N_2 (Mishell and Dutton, 1967). Direct interaction of splenic lymphocytes with antigen and/or antibody was thus permitted. Use was made of the H (flagellar) antigens of *Salmonella adelaide* (Ada *et al.*, 1964) which may be obtained in three different forms: polymerized flagellin (POL; mol. wt. $n \times 40\,000$), monomeric flagellin (MON; mol. wt. 40 000) and Fragment 'A' (mol. wt. 18 000), isolated from the cyanogen bromide digest of flagellin (Parish *et al.*, 1969). All three forms of the flagellar antigen share antigenic specificities but they express different degrees of immunogenicity and tolerogenicity *in vivo* and even more so *in vitro*.

In initial experiments, CBA mouse spleen cell suspensions were cultured *in vitro* for 4 days in the presence of polymerized flagellin (POL), monomeric flagellin (MON) and Fragment 'A'. Following the culture period, cells were harvested and the number of antibody forming cells (AFC) was determined (Diener, 1968). The degree of immunogenicity correlated with the molecular weight of the antigen: POL was the strongest immunogen, MON was intermediate in effect, and Fragment 'A' was virtually non-immunogenic (Diener and Feldmann, 1970). The effect of increasing concentrations of POL on the primary *in vitro* response was studied (Diener and Armstrong, 1967; 1969). CBA mouse spleen cells were cultured for 4 days in the presence of varying concentrations of POL. To control for antigen specificity, immunogenic concentrations of antigens different from *Salmonella adelaide* were added to the same cultures. It was found that a mere tenfold increase in POL concentration would convert an optimal *in vitro* immune response to virtually complete unresponsiveness (Figure 9.4). This effect was time dependent. If cells were exposed to supraimmunogenic levels of POL for intervals ranging from 15 minutes to 6 hours and were further incubated with immunogenic POL for 4 days, suppression was complete only after a 3-hour incubation with the high dose polymer. This phenomenon of antigen induced unresponsiveness *in vitro* fulfilled the criterion of tolerance since it was antigen specific as indicated by the normal response to unrelated antigens and furthermore, could be transferred to lethally X-irradiated recipients (Armstrong and Diener, 1969).

Antigen binding by relevant immunocompetent cells is evidently the first step in tolerance induction. If cells were exposed to a tolerance inducing concentration of POL for less than 3 days, and subsequently treated with trypsin, the tolerant state proved to be reversible. However, reversibility was abrogated when cells were exposed to a tolerance inducing concentration of the antigen longer than three days (Diener and Feldmann, 1972a). This may be interpreted as (1) initial attachment of tolerogenic antigen to immunocompetent cells, (2) proteolytic removal of cell surface antigen and possibly of recognition sites by trypsin, (3) regeneration of receptor sites after trypsinization and response to an immunogenic concentration of POL. In accord with this interpretation, pretreatment of dispersed mouse spleen cell suspensions with antimouse immunoglobulin serum (antibodies directed against the receptor

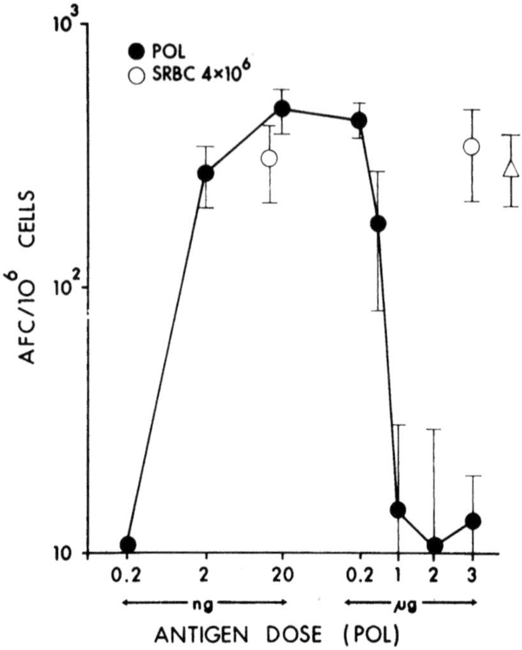

Figure 9.4 *Effect of increasing concentrations of antigen, polymer of* S. adelaide *flagellin (POL), on* in vitro *immune response. The number of antibody-forming cells (AFC) was estimated at 4 days of culture. Cultures had sheep erythrocytes (SRC) added along with POL. Each point and circle represents the mean of 8 to 12 cultures ± S.D.*
●*Immune response to POL of* S. adelaide. ○*Immune response to SRC.* △*Immune response to POL of* S. waycross.
[*Reprinted with permission from* J. Exp. Med. (*Diener and Armstrong, 1969*)]

site antibodies on mouse lymphocytes) could reversibly block the *in vitro* induction of both immunity and tolerance (Feldmann and Diener, 1971a).

The unresponsiveness induced *in vitro* with supraimmunogenic concentrations of POL may be considered analogous to the phenomenon of *in vivo* high zone tolerance referred to earlier. As determined *in vitro*, the mechanism of this tolerance involves first the attachment of antigen molecules to the surface of relevant immunocompetent cells. Because of the antigen dose relationship for tolerance induction, it has been suggested that the direct interaction of immunocompetent cells with more than

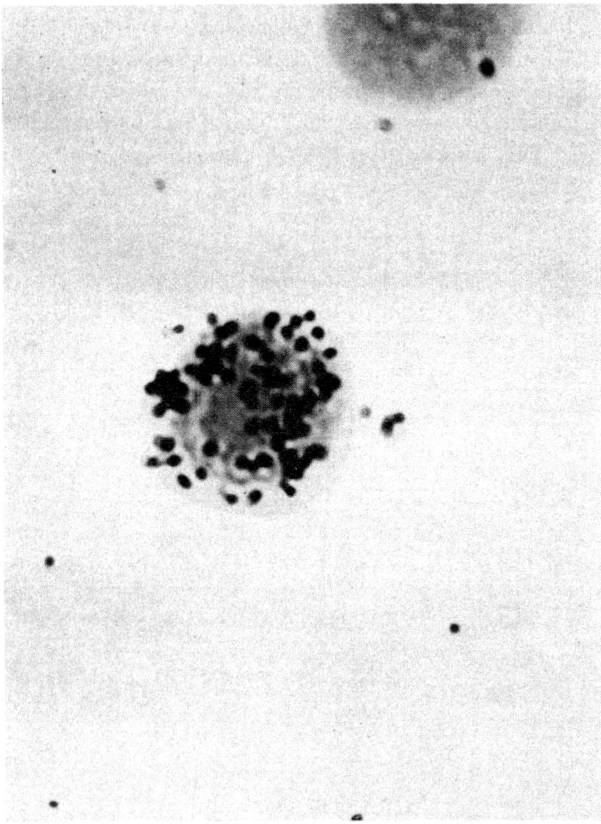

Figure 9.5 *Autoradiograph of mouse lymph node cell exposed to the antigen (POL) of polymerized flagellin, biosynthetically labeled with tritium. Antigen has attached to receptor sites randomly arrayed over the lymphocyte surface. Magnification × 2400*

a critical number of antigen molecules results in tolerance.The quality of the antigen POL, with available smaller antigenic units (MON and Fragment 'A') prompted investigation of this hypothesis. CBA spleen cells were incubated in tissue culture with MON or with Fragment 'A' for a period of 6 hours and were subsequently challenged with an immunogenic concentration of POL (20 ng) over a 4-day culture period. MON proved to be significantly less effective in its tolerance inducing capacity than POL, while Fragment 'A', an excellent tolerogen *in vivo* entirely failed to induce tolerance within the wide concentration range tested *in vitro* (Table 9.1). These results (Diener and Feldmann, 1970) conflict with the supposition of Dresser and Mitchison (1968) that the *in vivo* tolerance inducing capacity of an antigen is inversely related to its immunogenicity. The conclusion was that the induction of tolerance *in vivo* to a non-polymeric antigen such as Fragment 'A' must require a mediating mechanism not present in tissue culture.

Table 9.1 *Tolerance-inducing capacity* in vitro *of polymerized flagellin (POL), monomeric flagellin (MON), and fragment 'A'*

	Preincubation for 6 hours in vitro *with*	*AFC/culture S. adelaide*	*AFC/culture S. waycross*	*AFC/culture sheep erythrocytes*
POL	20 ng	4800 ± 215	1620 ± 93	2150 ± 78
	30 μg	115 ± 33*	1250 ± 115	2700 ± 185
MON	200 pg	4450 ± 105		
	2 ng	4425 ± 158		
	20 ng	3575 ± 314		
	30 μg	1350 ± 695†		
'A'	20 pg	4195 ± 459		
	200 pg	3850 ± 290		
	2 ng	3850 ± 312		
	20 ng	4700 ± 270		
	300 ng	3275 ± 536		
	30 μg	3750 ± 550		

*$P < 0.001$ compared with 20 ng POL
†$P < 0.02$ compared with 30 μg POL
'A': fragment 'A' of the cyanogen-bromide digest of flagellin. Each value represents the geometric mean of 8–10 cultures ± standard deviation. All cultures were challenged with 20 μg POL following preincubation
[Reprinted with permission from *J. Exp. Med.* (Diener and Feldmann, 1970).]

With this in mind, it was possible to construct an experimental model *in vitro* which could provide a hypothetical explanation for mechanisms of tolerance induction *in vivo*. Cell culture studies suggest that antigen (POL) becomes attached securely to the cell surface by virtue of the serial combination of repeated, identical antigenic determinants with a large number of recognition sites randomly arrayed over the cell surface (Figure 9.5; Diener and Paetkau, 1972). Indeed, the studies of Feldmann (1971) using the dinitrophenyl group (DNP) conjugated to *Salmonella* flagellin polymer, conclusively demonstrated that at least two groups per monomeric unit of flagellin were required for this hapten carrier unit to be tolerogenic. In other words, high hapten or ligand density permits closely spaced bonding to antigen sensitive receptors on the surface of the immunocompetent cell. The ease with which tolerance is established under tissue culture conditions is readily explained then for polymeric antigens or antigens which bear repeated antigenic determinants. Since, in contrast to the above *in vitro* studies, monomeric antigens most easily induce specific unresponsiveness *in vivo* (Ada and Parish, 1968), it was reasoned that (1) microanatomical or (2) humoral factors were operative in the intact animal but were absent under the conditions of cell culture.

The influence of humoral factors in tolerance induction is amenable to study *in vitro*. Studies of Dresser and Mitchison (1968) in adult animals, and Sterzl and Trnka (1957), and Sterzl (1966) in newborns had detected transient antibody production *in vivo* followed by an unresponsive state. This work suggested that the relevant humoral factor might indeed be antibody which could facilitate the mechanism proposed for POL by interlinking MON antigenic units. Given that the recognition antibody structures on the cell participate in this framework, the analogy becomes complete since cell surface recognition sites could become interlinked to the extent required for tolerance induction. Thus a lattice of antigen and antibody could build up at the surface of immunocompetent cells. The degree of linearity of such a complex would be determined by the molar ratio of antigen to antibody. The conditions for the formation of linear antigen–antibody complexes (simulating the linear structure of POL) occur most readily under conditions of slight antigen excess (Pauling, 1940). These hypothetical considerations are illustrated schematically in Figure 9.6. It was indeed possible to verify this concept experimentally: CBA spleen cells were cultured with MON or Fragment 'A' and various dilutions of specific hyperimmune antiserum for 6 hours. They were then washed and recultured in the presence of an immunogenic concentration of POL. As predicted (Figure 9.7), there was a distinct antigen–antibody concentration ratio which rendered immunocompetent lymphoid cells unresponsive (Diener and Feldmann, 1970). The hypothesis provides, moreover, that 'antibody mediated tolerance' should be inducible with bivalent $F(ab')_2$ fragments of antibody but

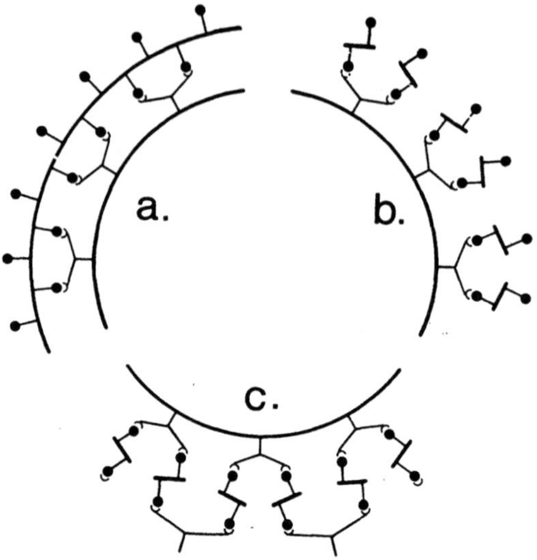

Figure 9.6 *Schematic drawing illustrating different ways of interaction on the cell surface between antigen or antigen and antibody, with antigen recognition sites.*
(a) Attachment to the recognition sites of a polymeric antigen.
(b) Attachment to the recognition sites of a monomeric antigen.
(c) Attachment to the recognition sites of a monomeric antigen in the presence of specific antibody.
Note: *In situation (a) and (c) antigen-recognition sites become interlinked by the antigen alone or by antigen–antibody complexes, respectively.*
[*Reprinted with permission from* Transplant. Rev. (*Diener and Feldmann, 1972b*)]

not with monovalent Fab. This requirement was met (Feldmann and Diener, 1972): antibody-mediated tolerance could be produced in the presence of bivalent, but not univalent, anti-POL antibody fragments.

Two different antigens were used in tissue culture to confirm the validity of tolerance obtained with flagellar antigens. CBA spleen cells exposed to ultrasonically fragmented sheep erythrocytes and antisheep erythrocyte antiserum were rendered tolerant at a defined ration of antigen–antibody *in vitro*. Similarly, mouse spleen cells could be rendered tolerant *in vitro* to chicken gamma globulin in the presence of antibody (Diener and Feldmann, 1972b).

Immunologic tolerance requires that cells rendered specifically unresponsive *in vitro*

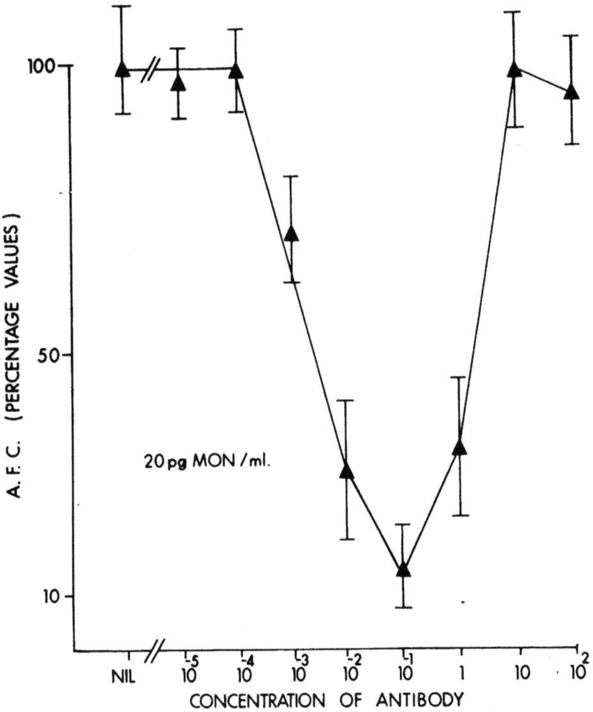

Figure 9.7 *Induction of tolerance to subimmunogenic concentration (200 pg/ml) of monomeric flagellin (MON). Spleen cells were incubated* in vitro *for 6 hours at 37 °C with various concentrations of MON and anti-POL before challenge with POL* in vitro. *Each value represents the arithmetic mean of 8–20 cultures ± standard error of the mean. Concentrations of antibody are expressed in immobilization titration units.*
[*Reprinted with permission from* Immunology (*Feldmann and Diener, 1971b*)]

may be transferred into lethally irradiated recipients without loss of tolerance. Accordingly, 3–5 million spleen cells, subjected to either high zone tolerance induction or antibody-mediated tolerance *in vitro*, were transferred into lethally irradiated syngeneic mice, which were then challenged with an immunogenic injection of POL. The animals were killed 7 or 8 days later and their spleens were tested for antibody forming cells with concomitant measurement of serum anti-POL activity. Both high zone and antibody-mediated tolerance could be transferred to an *in vivo* environment with maintained unresponsiveness (Armstrong and Diener, 1969; Feldmann and Diener, 1971b).

The main points emerging from this work are summarized in Table 9.2. Tolerance induction *in vitro* results from the direct interaction of immunocompetent cells with antigen at the level of surface recognition sites. The conditions which determine tolerance or immunity depend on the degree of interlinking of recognition sites by antigen. Interlinking beyond a certain level results not in immunity but tolerance. The conditions of tolerance induction are most easily achieved with polymeric antigens because they bear repeating antigenic units which can attach to large numbers of specific recognition sites. Monomeric antigens may be rendered 'polymeric' by interlinking them with bivalent antibody. With initial attachment of monomeric antigen to recognition sites, antigen and antibody at defined concentration ratios will readily form a lattice or complex on the surface of the lymphocyte. This focusing mechanism permits interlinking of receptors sufficient for tolerance induction. The following section will interpret these phenomena with speculations as to clinical relevance.

Interpretation and speculation

Low zone tolerance in vivo

The tolerance model provided by *in vitro* experimentation permits interpretation of the previously inexplicable phenomenon of low zone tolerance *in vivo*. The presence of antigen and antibody may provide a focusing mechanism at the level of the lymphoid cell with antigen–antibody complex formation and sufficient linkage of receptors as to induce tolerance. The experiments performed *in vitro* are convincing in this regard, since tolerance due to exposure of immunocompetent cells to sub-immunogenic levels of antigen alone is not possible. With addition of appropriate concentrations of antibody, as described above for MON and Fragment 'A', complex formation is again facilitated. Exposure of relevant lymphoid cells to this complex will interlink receptor sites and render cells tolerant. That this mechanism may operate *in vivo* is suggested by the fact that the antigen levels used for the induction of low zone tolerance *in vitro* are of the same order of magnitude as those used *in vivo* (Ada and Parish, 1968). *In vivo* the antibody required in this mechanism may be naturally occurring, or derived from stimulated lymphocytes and concomitant immunity (Dresser and Mitchison, 1968; Parish, 1969). Since antibody mediated tolerance *in vitro* could be induced with antibody concentrations as low as 10^{-14} M (Feldmann and Diener, 1971 (see discussion); Diener *et al.*, 1971), it may be suggested that a pertinent cell's own recognition antibody, when produced and secreted as part

Table 9.2 *Smmary of different methods of inducing immunological tolerance* in vitro

Antigen				*Treatment*			*Tolerance* in vitro	*Reversibility of tolerance*
Type	*Quality*	*Immunogenicity*		*Antigen*	*Antibody*	*Duration*		
		in vivo	in vitro					
S. adelaide	POL	+	+	supraimmunogenic		6 h	+	reversible
	POL	+	+	supraimmunogenic		3 days	+	not reversible
	POL	+	+	subimmunogenic		6 h	−	
	POL	+	+	immunogenic	+	6 h	+	
	MON	+	±	supraimmunogenic		6 h	±	
	MON	+	±	subimmunogenic		6 h	−	
	MON	+	±	immunogenic	+	6 h	+	
	MON	+	±	subimmunogenic	+	6 h	+	
	Fragment 'A'	±	−	various concentrations		6 h	−	
				various concentrations	+	6 h	+	
S.R.C.	Soluble	?	+	supraimmunogenic		6 h	−	
	Soluble	?	+	immunogenic	+	6 h	+	
Chicken								
gamma		±	−	various concentrations		16 h	−	
globulin		±	−	various concentrations		16 h	+	

POL: polymerized flagellin
MON: flagellin monomer
S.R.C.: sheep erythrocytes
Fragment 'A': cyanogen-bromide digest of flagellin (Parish *et al.*, 1969)
[Reprinted with permission from *Transplantation Review* (Diener and Feldmann, 1972]

of receptor turnover, may accumulate in the cells' microenvironment and suffice. Indeed, this situation may occur most reasonably in newborn animals, which are incapable of a measurable immune response despite demonstrable antigen recognition by immunocompetent cells (Dwyer and Warner, 1971). If antibody mediated tolerance applies both *in vitro* and *in vivo*, the phenomenon may explain immune homeostasis with regard to self antigens.This suggestion has been reinforced by the recent studies of Hellström and Hellström (1972) demonstrating that normal human serum can block cell mediated immunity to self-antigens.

Manipulation of the immune system

The ultimate goal in clinical transplantation is the induction of specific tolerance in a patient requiring an allograft. Selective production of blocking factors *in vivo* has not yet been possible and may indeed be a formidable task, due to our inability to control antigen and antibody dispersal and localization in the adult immunocompetent animal. Once the kinetics of blocking factors are known, administration to a relevant transplant recipient would ideally obviate the need for classical immunosuppressive treatment.

Recent developments in human bone marrow transplantation suggest an immediate approach in cases when the recipient is immunologically deficient. Here graft tissue is available for *in vitro* treatment similar to that previously described for mouse spleen cells. A forbidding difficulty with marrow allograft, however, has been the common occurrence of graft-versus-host disease in which the marrow cell inoculum or allograft recognizes the foreign antigens in its new host and proceeds to mount an immune response (Speck *et al.*, 1971). If, for example, bone marrow cells could be rendered tolerant *in vitro* to the antigens of the anticipated host, graft-versus-host disease would not occur. Transplantation antigens, the genetically determined tissue proteins important in provoking allograft responses, would be seemingly ideal for the induction of antibody-mediated tolerance *in vitro*. An attractive prediction involving antigen–antibody complexes as a tolerogen provides that an antiserum directed toward only one of the antigenic specificities of a transplantation antigen with multiple determinants, will mediate tolerance induction to the entire antigen (Diener and Feldmann, 1972b). This is illustrated in Figure 9.8. A molecule with three different antigenic determinants Q, Y and Z is capable of stimulating immunocompetent cells reactive to any of the three components. If antibody to determinant Z is present in a concentration favoring tolerance induction, interaction between Z and anti Z will not only render the lymphocyte reactive to determinant Z tolerant, but also cells reactive to Q and Y. Tolerance may thus be induced to any array of antigenic determinants that share the same 'backbone' provided antibody is present to any one such

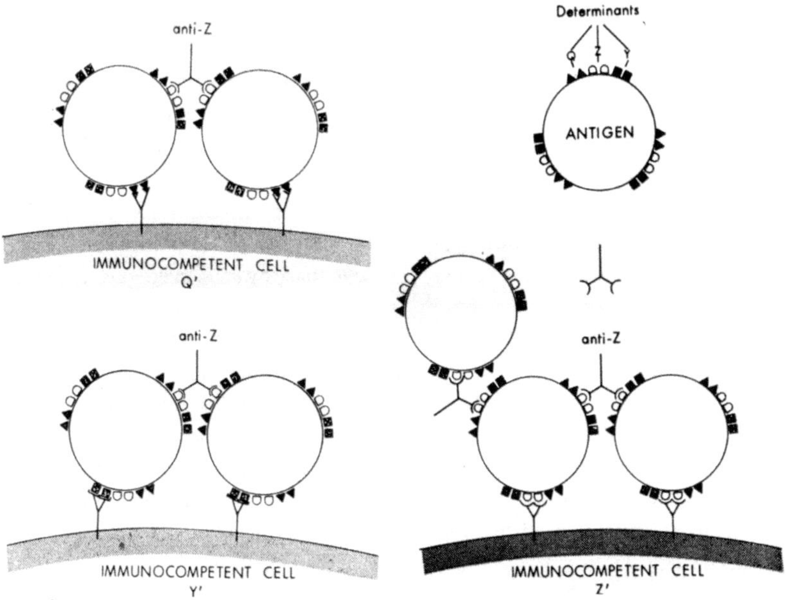

Figure 9.8 *Molecular model illustrating a possible mechanism of the cellular level that mediates tolerance by the interaction of cell-recognition sites, antigen, and antibody. For explanation, see text.*
[*Reprinted with permission from* Annals N.Y. Acad. Sci. (*Diener, Feldmann and Armstrong, 1971*)]

determinant. In the case of human transplantation antigens, antisera to only one of the HL-A antigens could elicit tolerance to all others carried on the same molecule, or conceivably on the same cell surface.

There have been technical difficulties with the isolation and characterization of histocompatibility antigens. The solubilization of these antigens from cell membranes yields materials with mosaics of antigenic determinants reflecting the genetic constitution of the donor. Glycoprotein moieties isolated have not had sufficient homogeneity or have carried indeterminate antigenic specificities, rendering *in vitro* studies unsuccessful thus far. As immunochemical isolation and purification of these substances become possible, however, *in vitro* tolerance induction in the presence of specific antisera may be realized. This approach can be regarded as *in vitro* production of blocking factors. If lymphocytes can be rendered tolerant *in vitro* in this manner, obviating the problem of graft-versus-host disease, direct infusion of blocking factors into recipients of other allografts may preclude cell mediated rejection. Baldwin *et al.* (1973) have achieved preliminary results in this regard. Tumor antigen derived from hepatoma cells was added to cytotoxic sera obtained from animals following tumor excision. A combination of tumor derived antigen and antiserum displayed *in vitro* blocking activity, preventing the cytotoxic activity of sensitized lymphocytes on cultured hepatoma cells.

Further immunochemical modification of transplantation antigens is conceivable. Polymerization of purified histocompatibility antigens would permit the induction of high zone tolerance *in vitro* to dispersed bone marrow cells analogous to the situation with polymerized antigens. A further use of transplantation antigen may be derived from the studies of Borel (1971) in which animals treated with the hapten DNP attached to a non-immunogenic carrier protein do not subsequently respond to DNP attached to an immunogenic carrier protein (carrier determined hapten specific tolerance). Further studies of Borel and Kilham (1973) have demonstrated that tolerance to DNP can be produced most effectively when DNP is attached to the isogeneic carrier IgG. If transplantation antigens, considered as haptenic molecules, can be conjugated similarly to an autologous protein, transplantation tolerance may be obtained clinically.

Experimental allograft tolerance *in vivo*

The permanent survival of allografts has been extraordinarily difficult to achieve across a major histocompatibility barrier in adult experimental animals. There are, of course, the already described experiments of Stuart *et al.* (1968) and French and Batchelor (1969) involving rat renal allografts enhanced with specific alloantiserum, and tolerance to rat and mouse skin allografts induced by Monaco and co-workers with ALG treatment and establishment of lymphoid chimerism. Notably absent, however, are reports dealing with transplantation tolerance to other organs and in other species. Renal allografts, for example, cannot be enhanced permanently in an outbred species such as the dog (Williams, 1973) and this may reflect only the inadequacy of current knowledge. A singular exception exists in the case of porcine liver allografts, dealt with separately in this volume. It has been suggested, in this regard, that allografts of pig liver survive well because the liver provides a good source of tolerogenic transplantation antigens and, possibly, that the normally reversed architecture of the pig lymph node, reminiscent of the early stages of development in the mouse lymph node (Williams, 1966), may facilitate tolerance induction.

Since tolerance may be induced with ease in the immunologically immature animal, temporary abolition of immunocompetence in the adult could conceivably mimic ontogenic mechanisms of the developing immune system and permit induction of allograft tolerance. 'Chimeric' animals with a functioning permanent allograft would provide a convenient means of determining whether adult allograft tolerance implies the presence or absence of graft directed cell mediated immunity and blocking factors.

The initial difficulty in developing such a model was the choice of an allograft. The two most common graft systems are skin grafts in laboratory rodents and renal allografts in rats and dogs. Each have particular disadvantages. Skin grafting, while technically easy, does not permit accurate evaluation of graft function and does not have a precise rejection end point. Renal allografts, on the other hand, can be followed functionally, but are tedious to implement, involving microvascular anastomoses, and are thus fraught with technical difficulties. There is an obvious need for an allograft model in small animals which is both technically simple and rapid and which permits functional evaluation. Because electrocardiographic evaluation of the heart is a convenient and precise measurement of the persistance of functioning graft tissue, we have turned to cardiac allografts as a transplantation model.

Free grafting techniques have been used to study transplanted whole hearts in the hamster (Poor, 1957), chick embryo (Katzberg, 1959), platyfish (Weinstein, 1960) and mouse (Conway *et al.*, 1958; Fulmer *et al.*, 1963). Only recently, however, has the model received attention as a means of monitoring transplantation immunity (Judd *et al.*, 1969).

Technique of cardiac allografting and subsequent evaluation

The original technique of neonatal or fetal heart transplantation in the mouse, as described by Fulmer *et al.* (1963) has been modified (Jirsch *et al.*, 1973a). As shown in Figure 9.9, hearts are removed from fetal mice *in utero* after 16–18 days gestation, by gentle blunt dissection under a stereomicroscope. The beating hearts, which measure approximately 1 mm diameter are placed in cold (4 °C) tissue culture medium. Using a tuberculin syringe with attached 26 gauge needle, 0.1 ml of saline is injected subcutaneously into the anterior aspect of the mouse ear, raising a small fluid filled bleb. This bleb is opened along its outer margin and the fetal heart is introduced into the subcutaneous space. Here the small graft is nourished by surrounding tissue fluid and serum until capillaries begin to grow into marginal myocardial tissue some days later.

Allograft cardiac function following transplantation is evaluated primarily by electrocardiography (Diener and Jirsch, 1972), with visual confirmation of graft pulsation through the thin overlying skin of the external ear. The limb leads of a standard ECG machine are attached to animals momentarily anesthetized with methoxyflurane (Figure 9.10). A smaller clip is attached to the periphery of the mouse ear containing the fetal heart graft and is connected proximally to the V-lead of the

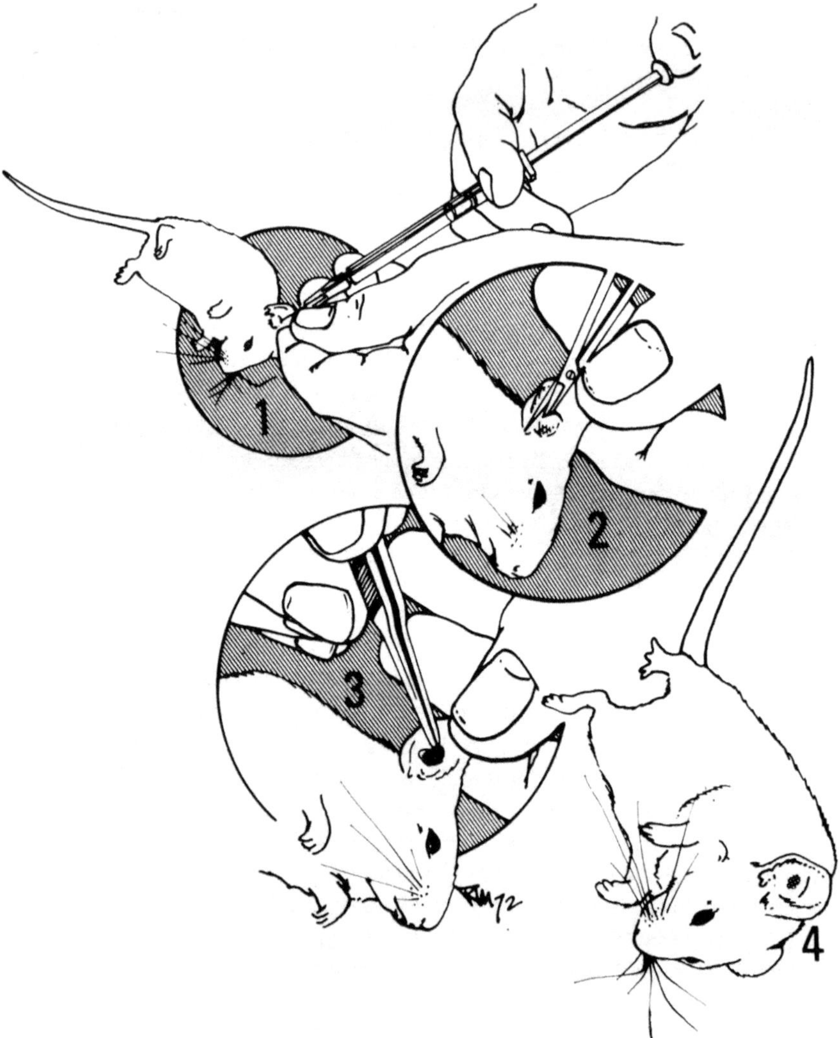

Figure 9.9 *Technique of cardiac allografting in the mouse.*
1, subcutaneous ear pocket formed by injecting a small amount of saline
2, bleb thus formed is opened along outer margin
3, insertion of 18–day gestation fetal mouse heart
4, graft in place.
[*Reprinted with permission from* Cardiovascular Research (*Jirsch* et al., *1973a*)]

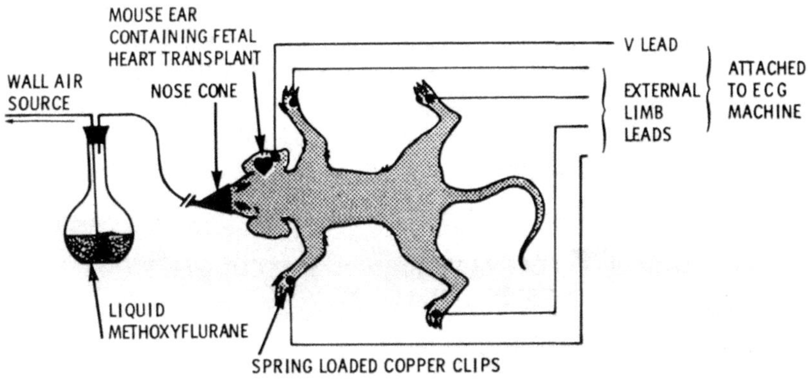

Figure 9.10 *Schematic representation of method of anesthesia and electrocardiography permitting evaluation of cardiac graft activity*

search electrode. In this manner, the electrical activity generated by both the adult host heart and that of the heterotopic fetal graft are recorded simultaneously as two distinct sets of independent rhythmical electrical activity (Figure 9.11). Whether or not allograft electrical activity is present provides a stringent and precise index of graft survival. The fetal heart bears transplantation antigens (Simmons and Russell, 1966), is tolerant to hypoxia and conveniently small to work with.

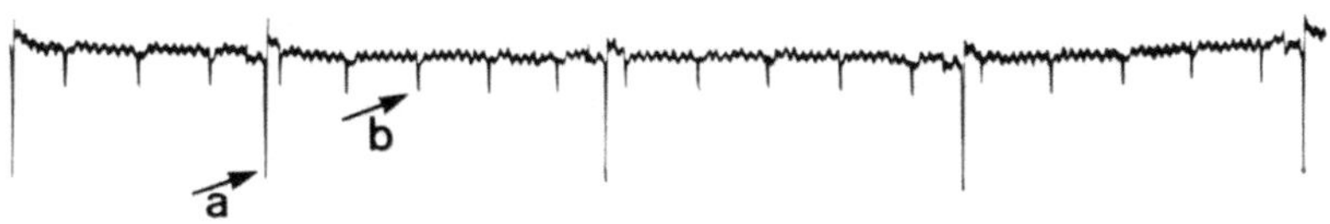

Figure 9.11 *Typical electrocardiogram obtained from a cardiac allografted mouse.*
a, electrical activity generated by the heterotopic graft
b, adult heart electrical activity

Syngeneic and allogeneic heart grafts

In a series of 20 adult CBA mice which received Balb/c fetal heart allografts (Jirsch *et al.*, 1973a), 19 of 20 mice began to show graft electrical activity on the fourth day following transplantation. This activity fell precipitously on the seventh day after allografting due to immune destruction of the heart, reflected histologically as a mononuclear cell infiltrate and beginning disruption of myocardial fibers. Second Balb/c grafts inserted in either the same or opposite ear of these mice reflected an anamnestic or memory response (Figure 9.12). Thus, only 50% of second grafts ever established electrical activity and, in these, rejection was more rapid with major loss of electrical activity on the fifth day post allografting. Fetal hearts transplanted between identical

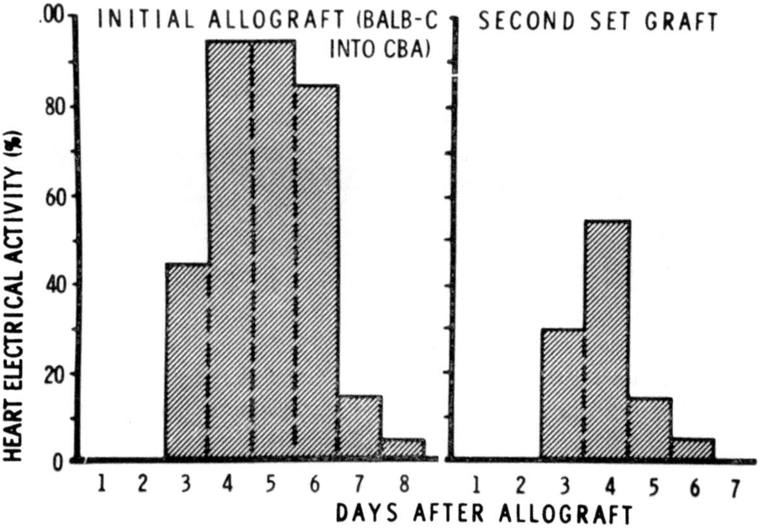

Figure 9.12 *Primary and secondary cardiac allograft survival and rejection. See text.* [*Reprinted with permission from* Cardiovascular Research (*Jirsch* et al., *1973a*)]

strain mice developed visible pulsation and detectable electrical activity in 95% of cases; these, however, did not reject and survived indefinitely. Visible monitoring of graft electrical activity was most rewarding in these cases for postoperative tissue swelling and bruising made direct observation of cardiac activity difficult in the first week after surgery. Syngeneic grafts did not grow to any significant extent, most probably due to the absence of a work load, but pulsation and electrical activity persisted indefinitely.

The apparent sensitivity of the fetal heart graft model prompted Jirsch and Kraft (1972) to test CBA recipients of Balb/c fetal hearts for evidence of cellular immunity at varying intervals following allograft insertion. The test system used was that described by Brunner *et al.* (1968). ^{51}Cr-labeled to Balb/c tumor target cells is released when such cells are attacked *in vitro* by allogeneic CBA spleen cells with killer activity. Spleen cells from CBA mice which received intravenous injections of 20×10^6 Balb/c spleen cells were quite capable of cell mediated immunity in the described system. Spleen cells from animals which had received single, multiple, repeated or even intraperitoneal Balb/c heart allografts were, however, not sensitized when tested from 5–14 days after transplantation. In contrast, flank skin allografts (Balb/c onto CBA; approximately 0.5 cm^2 area) demonstrated consistent sensitization within 10 days of transplantation. Evaluation of the allografted fetal heart was evidently superior to either an *in vitro* assay for cellular immunity or to skin allografting as a sensitive model of transplantation immunity.

Induction of tolerance was attempted without immunosuppressive treatment following the rationale depicted in Figure 9.13. Lethally irradiated CBA mice will die within a few days from hematopoietic failure if they are not reconstituted with syngeneic bone marrow. Two groups of animals are transplanted with Balb/c fetal hearts immediately after irradiation, at a time when they are immunologically incompetent. If the first group of mice are reconstituted with whole bone marrow, which includes both stem cells and immunocompetent cells, and the second group receives stem cells alone, the fate of the allografts in each case will, theoretically, differ. CBA recipients given syngeneic whole marrow should reject a Balb/c heart due to the presence of immunocompetent lymphocytes in the reconstituting marrow. However, Balb/c hearts placed in CBA recipients injected with hematopoietic stem cells alone should survive indefinitely, becoming permanently accepted as self as proliferation and differentiation of stem cells in the presence of antigens determines tolerance.

The problem revolves then around the isolation of the primordial stem cell, excluding it from the immunocompetent cell progeny. The immediate applicability of this approach to graft-versus-host disease is evident. In clinical bone marrow transplantation, one is aware of the fact that whole marrow or other lymphoid tissues contain immunocompetent cells which recognize alloantigens and mount an immune response against them. Immunocompetent cell deletion has, therefore, become one of the more promising experimental developments attempting to circumvent this problem. Pharmacological agents may be useful in this regard. Immunocompetent cells can be stimulated by nonspecific mitogens such as phytohemagglutinin (Nowell, 1960) or concanavalin A (Knight and Thorbecke, 1971), or by specific transplantation antigens (Reisfeld and Kahan, 1971; Viza *et al.*, 1968). Consequent proliferation of cells renders them susceptible to pharmacological attack by agents which interfere

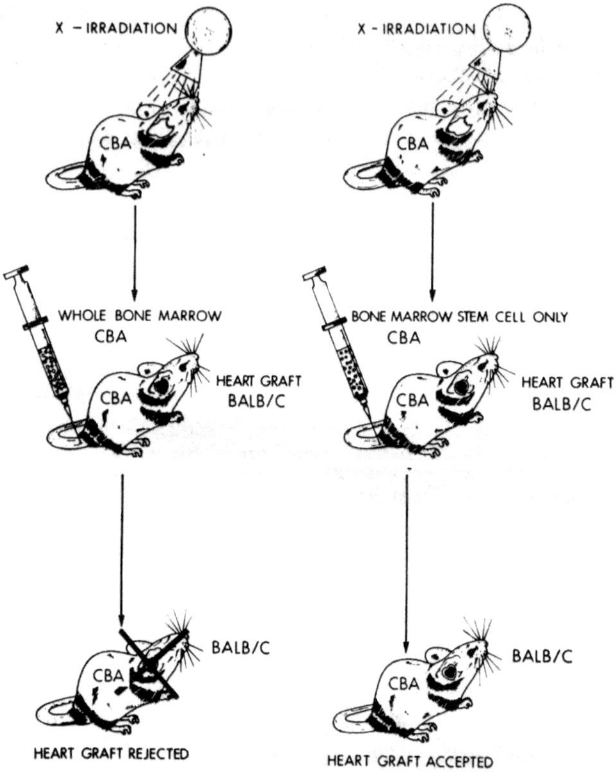

Figure 9.13 *Repopulation of an irradiated heart allografted animal with syngeneic bone marrow eventuates in allograft rejection. Repopulation with purified hematopoietic stem cells should induce tolerance in stem cell progeny with cardiac allograft survival.*
[*Reprinted with permission from* Medical Clinics of North America (*Diener and Jirsch, 1972*)]

with normal nucleic acid synthesis and results in the selective elimination of responsive cells. In recent experiments, both radioactive tritiated thymidine (Salmon *et al.*, 1971) and 5-bromodeoxyuridine (BUdR) (Zoschke and Bach, 1971) have been used to selectively remove stimulated (immunocompetent) lymphocytes from cell cultures. Cell cultures treated with cytotoxic agents active during cell division will, at an appropriate dosage level, retain stem cell activity because stem cells normally divide rather slowly and remain virtually unaffected (Bruce *et al.*, 1966; Lajtha, 1967). More extensive, however, have been experiments designed to purify bone marrow stem cells by physical methods. These have been based on differences between lymphoid cells with respect to size (Miller and Phillips, 1969) and density (Turner *et al.*, 1967; Dicke *et al.*, 1968; Phillips and Miller, 1970; Worton, McCullough *et al.*, 1969). The experiments of Phillips and Miller (1970) demonstrated that cells in mouse bone marrow and spleen which were capable of graft-versus-host activity could be defined as a population of small, slowly sedimenting cells which fell through a fetal calf serum gradient with a rate of modal distribution of about 3 mm/h. Stem cells, or cells defined by their ability to form hematopoietic colonies in the spleens of irradiated mice (Till and McCullough, 1961), tended to be larger in size and sedimented more quickly (Figure 9.14). Since clinical trials with hematopoietic tissue subjected to cell separation procedures have enjoyed only limited success (Speck *et al.*, 1971; Amato

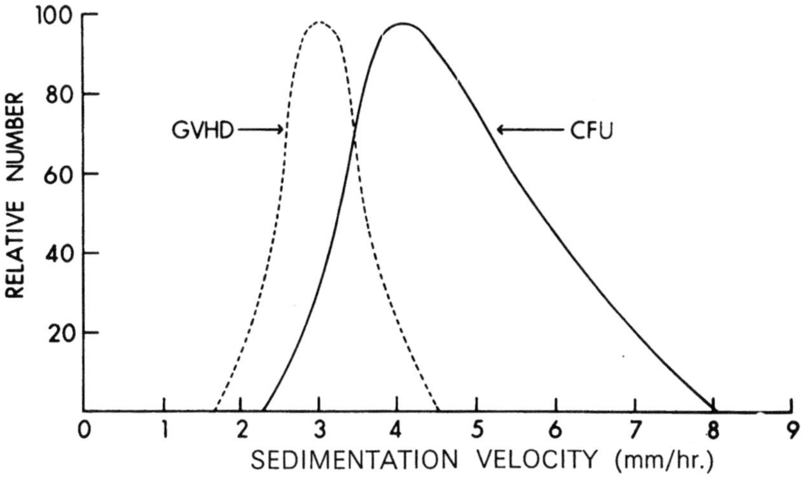

Figure 9.14 *Velocity sedimentation cell separation of mouse bone marrow and spleen: the modal distribution of immunocompetent (GVHD) and stem (CFU) cells. Purified stem cells sediment most rapidly and may be separable from immunocompetent cell fractions.* [*Adapted from Miller and Phillips (1970)*]

et al., 1971; Levey *et al.*, 1971) with evidence of delayed graft-versus-host disease, it became relevant to determine whether stem cells could be isolated from immunocompetent cells in an animal model.

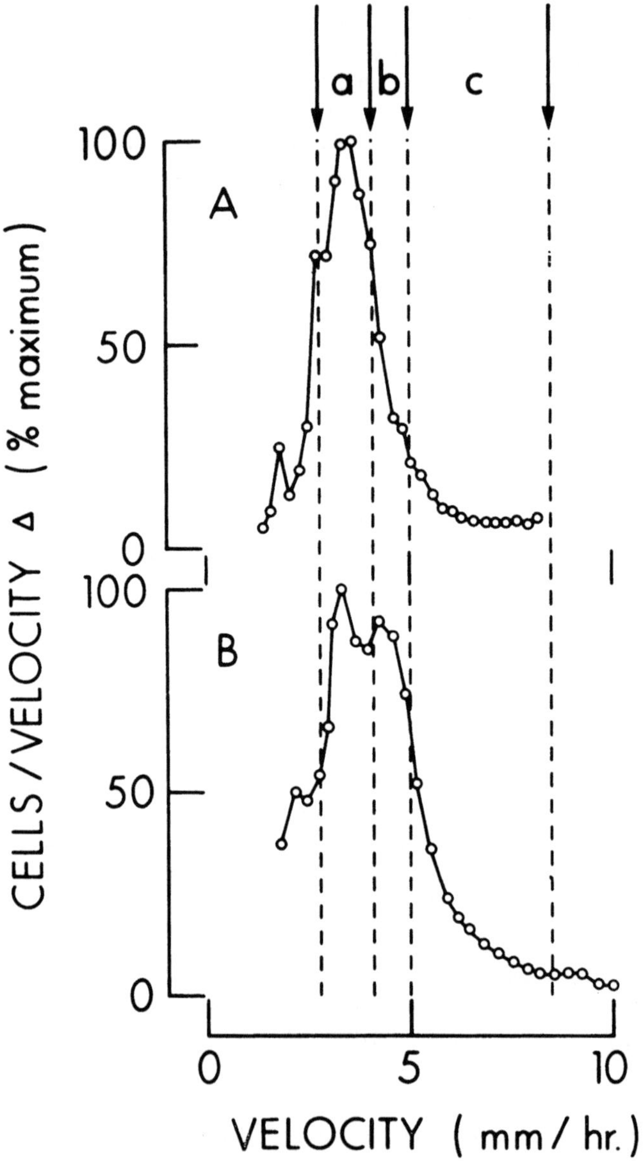

Figure 9.15 *A typical velocity sedimentation profile of A, normal spleen nucleated cells and B, normal bone marrow nucleated cells. Fraction a contains the majority of immunocompetent cells; fractions b and c are stem cell rich.* [*From Kraft* et al., *1973*]

Kraft *et al.* (1973) subjected mouse marrow and spleen to cell separation on the basis of velocity sedimentation and then used this fractionated marrow to reconstitute lethally irradiated fetal heart allografted mice. Figure 9.15 shows a typical velocity sedimentation profile of normal spleen and bone marrow nucleated cells which were pooled, sedimenting through three velocity ranges (a) 3–4 mm/h, (b) 4–5 mm/h and (c) 5–8 mm/h corresponding in each case to small, medium and large lymphoid cells. From the experiments of Phillips and Miller (1970) fraction (a) contains immunocompetent cells; fraction (b) should contain very few immunocompetent cells with fraction (c) virtually devoid of immunocompetent cells but stem cell rich. In initial experiments (Figure 9.16, A), lethally irradiated CBA mice were reconstituted with 0.1×10^6 syngeneic whole bone marrow cells and mean allograft heart rejection occurred within 4–5 weeks. In a further group of animals 2×10^6 syngeneic spleen cells were added to the reconstituting inoculum of bone marrow to determine whether or not the presence of large numbers of mature immunocompetent cells would increase the rate of allograft rejection. Rejection was not accelerated: the number of immunocompetent cells in the inoculum apparently did not affect the rejection process. Using fractionated marrow, surprising but similar results were found in that 0.1×10^6 cells of the slowly sedimenting fraction (immunocompetent cells) were no more efficient in immune destruction of the allograft than fractions presumably devoid of these cells (Figure 9.16, B). In fact, the fraction of bone marrow sedimenting most quickly and known to be rich in stem cells, disposed of the allograft heart in equal time.

An immunocompetent cell precursor normally present in the stem cell rich fraction of bone marrow could well differentiate and proliferate after transfer and provide lymphocytes capable of reacting against the allograft. In agreement with this, Kraft and Diener (1973, unpublished results) have found antibody forming cell precursors responding to POL in this fraction of marrow. Significantly, however, such immunocompetent precursor cells could not be identified in mouse spleen. The spleen possibly contains a more clear cut delineation between immunocompetent cells and stem cells without the large number of immunocompetent precursors found in bone marrow. Recent studies of Mond and Thorbecke (1973) are consistent with this interpretation: the immune responsiveness of splenic lymphocytes can be inhibited by *in vitro* treatment with anti-immunoglobulin antisera which is ineffective in suppressing bone marrow lymphocytes.

Velocity sedimentation of mouse spleen cells was carried out to test this possibility (Figure 9.16, C and D) (Kraft and Jirsch, 1973). In irradiated mice which were reconstituted with only the large or rapidly sedimenting spleen cells, allografts survived significantly longer than in recipients of whole or fractionated marrow. In addition,

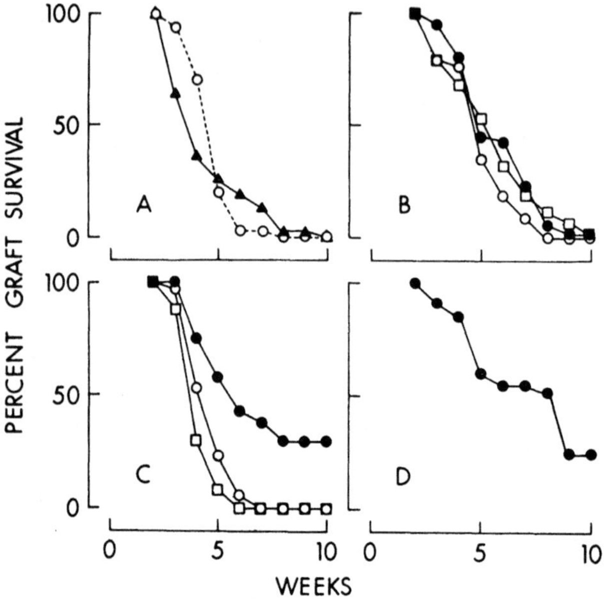

Figure 9.16 *Cardiac transplant survival in mice lethally irradiated, allografted and reconstituted with hematopoietic tissue:*

A △, *Unfractionated bone marrow*
(0.1 × 10^6 cells; 17 mice)
○, *Unfractionated bone marrow plus spleen*
(0.1 × 10^6 bone marrow cells; 2 × 10^6 spleen cells; 15 mice)
B □, *Fractionated bone marrow small cells*
(0.1 × 10^6 cells; 27 mice)
○, *Fractionated bone marrow, medium cells*
(0.1 × 10^6 cells; 20 mice)
●, *Fractionated bone marrow, large cells*
(0.1 × 10^6 cells; 36 mice)
C *Unfractionated bone marrow 0.1 × 10^6 cells plus*
□, *2 × 10^6 small spleen cells (17 mice)*
○, *2 × 10^6 medium sized spleen cells (14 mice)*
●, *2 × 10^6 large spleen cells (10 mice)*
D ●, *Large spleen cells alone (2 × 10^6 cells; 17 mice)*
[*From Kraft* et al., *1973*]

the high velocity spleen cell fraction gave evidence of inhibiting the rejection process, since a small number of animals carried functional allografts longer than 4 months following reconstitution with both large spleen cells and whole bone marrow. In contrast then, bone marrow cells permitting allograft rejection were spread over the entire range of velocity sedimentation values investigated but spleen cells differed, the large cell fraction thereof prolonging allograft function with permanent graft survival (>12 weeks) in a number of animals. The precursor cells present in bone marrow may thus be absent in spleen or alternatively, a class of large spleen cells which is absent in bone marrow may produce an inhibitor, such as blocking factor, causing allograft enhancement.

Twelve weeks after irradiation and reconstitution such immunocompetent chimeras, tolerant to a cardiac allograft following reconstitution with the large cell fraction of syngeneic spleen cells, were tested to determine whether they were still capable of recognizing the alloantigens of the foreign graft (Jirsch *et al.*, 1973b). Spleen cells from tolerant heart bearing animals could react *in vitro* to graft alloantigens with subsequent expression of cell mediated immunity using the assay of Brunner *et al.* (1970). More interestingly, perhaps, washed lymph node cells in small numbers ($2–10 \times 10^6$ cells) were transferred from graft tolerant animals to secondary allografted hosts which were irradiated and reconstituted with whole bone marrow. The addition of lymph node cells from such animals definitely prolonged cardiac allograft survival beyond that possible with bone marrow reconstitution alone, and permanent chimerism was produced in a number of instances.

Transfer of tolerance?

It is not known whether the specific immunosuppressive effect transferable with lymphocytes from tolerant animals is mediated via blocking factors, similar to those described earlier by the Hellströms, or by the direct suppressive effect of a thymus derived cell population, such as has been suggested by studies of Gershon *et al.* (1972). The phenomenon may be comparable to the transfer of sheep erythrocyte tolerance with tolerant lymphoid cells as described by McCullagh (1973). Whatever the mechanism, however, the ability to transfer a specific immunosuppressive agent opens exciting possibilities in the clinical arena.

SUMMARY AND CONCLUSIONS

Histocompatibility matching and the use of standard immunosuppressive agents remain the mainstay of clinical transplantation therapy. The recent discovery that humoral factors may prevent the effector phase of cell mediated immunity and permit allograft survival has renewed interest in the induction of specific tolerance. Experiments with bacterial antigens and antigen–antibody complexes have shown that tolerance can be induced *in vitro*; similar experiments with transplantation antigens may one day permit *in vitro* manipulation of lymphoid tissue with production of immunosuppressive blocking factors which can be administered to an allograft host *in vivo*. The precise nature of immunosuppressive serum factors and the characterization of cell populations responsible for their production await further experimental work. Future resolution of the lymphoid system's own immunosuppressive potential may enable the clinician to provide an optimal milieu for the induction of specific allograft tolerance.

References

Ada, G. L., Nossal, G. J. V., Pye, J. and Abbott, A. (1964). Antigens in immunity. I. Preparation and properties of flagellar antigen from *Salmonella adelaide*. *Aust. J. Exp. Biol. Med. Sci.*, **42,** 267

Ada, G. L. and Parish, C. R. (1968). Low zone tolerance to bacterial flagellin in adult rats. A possible role in antigen localized in lymphoid follicles. *Proc. Nat. Acad. Sci. (Washington)*, **61,** 556

Amato, D., Bergsagel, D. E., Clarysee, A. M., Cowan, D. H., Iscove, N. N., McCullough, E. A., Miller, R. G., Phillips, R. A., Ragab, A. H. and Senn, J. S. (1971). Review of bone marrow transplants at the Ontario Cancer Institute. *Transplant. Proc.*, **3,** 397

Amos, D. B., Cohen, I. and Klein, W. J. (1970). Mechanisms of immunologic enhancement. *Transplant. Proc.*, **2,** 68

Armstrong, W. D. and Diener, E. (1969). Immunological tolerance to a purified protein antigen *in vitro*. *Transplant. Proc.*, **1,** 619

Baldwin, R. W., Price, M. R. and Robins, R. A. (1973). Blocking of lymphocyte-mediated cytotoxicity for rat hepatoma cells by tumor specific antigen-antibody complexes. *Nature* (In press), 1973

Billingham, R. E. and Brent, L. (1957). A simple method for inducing tolerance of skin homografts in mice. *Transplant. Bull.*, **4,** 67

Billingham, R. E., Brent, L., Medawar, P. B. and Sparrow, F. M. (1954). Quantitative studies of tissue transplantation immunity. I. The survival times of skin homografts exchanged between members of different inbred strains of mice. *Proc. Roy. Soc. B*, **143,** 43

Borel, Y. (1971). Induction of immunological tolerance by a hapten (DNP) bound to a non-immunogenic protein carrier. *Nature New Biology*, **230,** 180

Borel, Y. and Kilham, L. (1973). Carrier determined tolerance in various strains of mice. (The role of isogeneic IgG in the induction of hapten specific tolerance.) (In press)

Bruce, W. R., Meeker, B. E. and Valeriote, F. A. (1966). Comparison of the sensitivity of normal hematopoietic and transplanted lymphoma colony-forming cells to chemotherapeutic agents administered *in vivo*. *J. Nat. Cancer Inst.*, **37,** 233

Brunner, K. T., Mauel, J., Cerottini, J. C. and Chapuis, B. (1968). Quantitative assay of the lytic action of immune lymphoid cells on ^{51}Cr-labeled allogeneic target cells *in vitro*: Inhibition by isoantibody and by drugs. *Immunology*, **14,** 181

Brunner, K. T., Mauel, J., Cerottini, J. C. and Chapuis, B. (1970). Studies on allograft immunity in mice. I. Induction, development and an *in vitro* assay of cellular immunity. *Immunology*, **18,** 501

Burnet, F. M. (1959). *The Clonal Selection Theory of Acquired Immunity*. Cambridge, Massachusetts: Vanderbilt University Press

Burnet, F. M. (1962). Role of the thymus and related organs in immunity. *Brit. Med. J.*, **2,** 807

Burnet, F. M. and Fenner, F. (1949). *The Production of Antibodies*. Melbourne: MacMillan

Cerottini, J. C., Nordin, A. A. and Brunner, K. T. (1970). Specific *in vitro* cytotoxicity of thymus-derived lymphocytes sensitized to alloantigens. *Nature*, **228,** 1308

Chiller, J. M., Habicht, G. S. and Weigle, W. O. (1970). Cellular site of immunologic unresponsiveness. *Proc. Nat. Acad. Sci.* (*Wash.*), **65,** 551

Chiller, J. M., Habicht, G. S. and Weigle, W. O. (1971). Kinetic differences in unresponsiveness of thymus and bone marrow cells. *Science*, **171,** 183

Claman, H. W. and Chaperon, E. A. (1969). Immunologic complementation between thymus and marrow cells—A model for the two cell theory of immunocompetence *Transplant. Rev.*, **1,** 92

Conway, H., Griffith, B. H., Shannon, J. E. and Findley, A. (1958). Survival of the transplanted fetal heart in the mouse, as determined by pulsatile activity. *Transplant. Bull.*, **5,** 121

Davies, A. J. S. (1969). The thymus and the cellular basis of immunity. *Transplant. Rev.*, **1,** 43

Dicke, K. A., van Hooft, J. I. M. and van Bekkum, D. W. (1968). The selective elimination of immunologically competent cells from bone marrow and lymphatic cell mixtures. II. Mouse spleen fractionation as a discontinuous albumin gradient. *Transplantation*, **6,** 571

Diener, E. (1968). A new method for the enumeration of single antibody-producing cells. *J. Immunol.*, **100,** 1062

Diener, E. and Armstrong, W. D. (1967). Induction of antibody formation and tolerance *in vitro* to a purified protein antigen. *Lancet*, **2,** 1281

Diener, E. and Armstrong, W. D. (1969). Immunological tolerance *in vitro*. Kinetic studies at the cellular level. *J. Exp. Med.*, **129,** 51

Diener, E. and Feldmann, M. (1970). Antibody mediated suppression of the immune response *in vitro*. II. A new approach to the phenomenon of immunological tolerance. *J. Exp. Med.*, **132,** 31

Diener, E. and Feldmann, M. (1972a). Mechanisms at the cellular level during induction of high zone tolerance *in vitro*. *Cell. Immunol.*, **5,** No. 1, 130

Diener, E. and Feldmann, M. (1972b). Relationship between antigen and antibody-induced suppression of immunity. *Transplant. Rev.*, **8,** 76

Diener, E., Feldmann, M. and Armstrong, W. D. (1971). Induction *in vitro* of immunological tolerance to the H-antigens of *Salmonella adelaide*. *Ann. N.Y. Acad. Sci.*, **181,** 119

Diener, E. and Jirsch, D. (1972). The future of transplantation immunology. *Med. Clin. N. Amer.*, **56,** 453

Diener, E., O'Callaghan, E. and Kraft, N. (1971). Immune response *in vitro* to *Salmonella* H-antigens, not affected by anti-Theta serum. *J. Immunol.*, **107,** 1775

Diener, E. and Paetkau, V. (1972). Antigen recognition: Early surface-receptor phenomena induced by binding of a tritium-labeled antigen. *Proc. Nat. Acad. Sci. (USA)*, **69,** 2364

Dresser, D. W. (1962). Paralysis induced in adult mice by small quantities of protein antigen. *Immunology*, **5,** 378

Dresser, D. W. (1963). Specific inhibition of antibody production. III. Apparent changes in the half-life of bovine gamma globulin in paralyzed mice. *Immunology*, **6,** 345

Dresser, D. W. and Mitchison, N. A. (1968). The mechanism of immunological paralysis. *Advances Immunol.*, **8,** 145

Dwyer, J. M. and Warner, N. L. (1971). Antigen binding cells in embryonic chicken bursa and thymus. *Nature New Biology*, **229,** 210

Feldmann, M. (1971). Induction of immunity and tolerance to the dinitrophenyl determinant *in vitro*. *Nature (London)*, **231,** 21

Feldmann, M. and Diener, E. (1971a). Reversible blocking effect of anti-mouse immunoglobulin serum on the induction of immunity and tolerance *in vitro*, *Nature (London)*, **231,** 183

Feldmann, M. and Diener, E. (1971b). Antibody mediated suppression of the immune response *in vitro*. III. Low zone tolerance *in vitro*. *Immunology*, **21,** 387

Feldmann, M. and Diener, E. (1972). Antibody-mediated suppression of the immune response. IV. Effect of antibody fragments *in vitro*. *Immunology*, **108,** 93

Festenstein, H., Sachs, J. A., Oliver, R. T. D., Burke, J. M., Adams, E., Divver, W., Hyams, A., Pegrum, G. D., Blafour, I. C. and Moorehead, J. F. (1971). Multi-centre collaboration in 162 tissue typed renal transplants. *Lancet*, **2,** 225

Ford, C. E. (1966). Traffic of lymphoid cells in the body. In *Ciba Foundation Symposium. Thymus: Experimental and Clinical Studies*, p. 131 (G. E. Wolstenholme and R. Porter, editors). London: Churchill

French, M. E. and Batchelor, J. R. (1969). Immunological enhancement of rat kidney grafts. *Lancet*, **2,** 1103

Fulmer, R. I., Cramer, A. T., Liebelt, R. A. and Liebelt, A. G. (1963). Transplantation of cardiac tissue into the mouse ear. *Amer. J. Anat.*, **113,** 273

Gershon, R. K., Cohen, P., Hencin, R. and Liebhaber, S. (1972). Suppressor T cells. *J. Immunol.*, **108,** 586

Globerson, A. and Auerbach, R. (1967). Reactivation *in vitro* of immunocompetence in irradiated mouse spleen. *J. Exp. Med.*, **126,** 223

Gowans, J. L., McGregor, D. D. and Vowen, D. M. (1962). Imitation of immune response by small lymphocytes. *Nature (London)*, **196,** 651

Greaves, M. F. and Hogg, N. M. (1971). Immunoglobulin determinants on the surface of antigen-binding T- and B-lymphocytes in mice. *Proceedings of the First International Congress of Immunology*, p. 111 (B. Amos, editor). New York and London: Academic Press

Halasz, N. A. (1963). Enhancement of skin homografts in dogs. *J. Surg. Res.*, **3,** 503

Halasz, N. A., Orloff, M. J. and Hirose, F. (1964). Increased survival of renal homografts in dogs after injection of graft donor blood. *Transplantation*, **2,** 453

Haughton, G. and Nash, D. R. (1969). Specific immunosuppression by minute doses of passive antibody. *Transplant. Proc.*, **1,** 616

Hellström, I., Evans, C. A. and Hellström, K. E. (1969). Cellular immunity and its serum mediated inhibition in shope-virus inducted rabbit papillomas. *Int. J. Cancer*, **4,** 601

Hellström, I. and Hellström, K. E. (1971). The rôle of immunological enhancement for the growth of autochthonous tumors. *Transplant. Proc.*, **3,** 721

Hellström, I. and Hellström, K. E. (1972a). Cell mediated immunity and blocking antibodies to renal allografts. *Transplant. Proc.*, **4,** 369

Hellström, I. and Hellström, K. E. (1972b). Can 'blocking' serum factors protect against autoimmunity? *Nature (London)*, **240,** 471

Hellström, I., Hellström, K. E. and Alluson, A. C. (1971). Neonatally induced allograft tolerance may be mediated by serum-borne factors. *Nature (London)*, **230,** 49

Hellström, I., Hellström, K. E. and Sjögren, H. O. (1970a). Serum mediated inhibition of cellular immunity to methylcholanthrene-induced murine sarcomas. *Cell Immunol.*, **1,** 18

Hellström, I., Hellström, K. E., Bill, A. H., Pierce, G. E. and Yang, J. P. S. (1970b). Studies on cellular immunity to human neuroblastoma cells. *Int. J. Cancer*, **6,** 172

Hellström, I., Hellström, K. E., Storb, R. and Thomas, E. D. (1970c). Colony inhibition of fibroblasts from chimeric dogs mediated by the dogs' own lymphocytes and specifically abrogated by their serum. *Proc. Nat. Acad. Sci. (USA)*, **66,** 65

Hellström, K. E. and Hellström, I. (1969). Cellular immunity against tumor antigens. *Adv. Cancer Res.*, **12,** 167

Hellström, K. E. and Hellström, I. (1970). Immunological enhancement as studied by cell culture techniques. *Ann. Rev. Microbiol.*, **24,** 373

Hellström, K. E., Hellström, I. and Brawn, J. (1969). Abrogation of cellular immunity to antigenically foreign mouse embryonic cells by a serum factor. *Nature (London)*, **224,** 914

Isakovic, K., Smith, S. B. and Waksman, B. H. (1965). Role of the thymus in tolerance. I. Tolerance to bovine gamma globulin in thymectomized, irradiated rats grafted with thymus from tolerant donors. *J. Exp. Med.*, **122,** 1103

Jirsch, D. W. and Kraft, N. (1972). Cellular immunity *in vitro* and heterotopic transplantation of the mouse heart. *Transplantation*, **14,** 396

Jirsch, D., Kraft, N. and Diener, E. (1973a). Transplantation of the mouse heart—A useful research model. *Cardiovasc. Res.* (In press)

Jirsch, D. W., Kraft, N. and Diener, E. (1973b). Tolerance induction and transplantation of the mouse heart. In preparation

Joller, P. W. (1972). Graft-versus-host reactivity of lymphoid cells inhibited by anti-recognition serum. *Nature, New Biology*, **240,** 214

Judd, K. P., Allen, C. R., Jr., Guiberteau, M. J. and Trentin, J. J. (1969). Prolongation of murine cardiac allografts with antilymphocyte serum. *Transplant. Proc.*, **1,** 470

Kaliss, N. (1956). Course of production of an isoantiserum affecting tumor homograft survival in mice. *Proc. Nat. Acad. Sci.*, **42,** 269

Kaliss, N. (1958). Immunological enhancement of tumor homografts in mice: A review. *Cancer Res.*, **18,** 992

Katzberg, A. A. (1959). Cardiac rhythm as a prerequisite for the survival of fetal heart transplants. *Plast. Reconstr. Surg. and Transplant. Bull.*, **23,** 113

Knight, S. G. and Thorbecke, G. J. (1971). Ontogeny of cellular immunity: Development in rat thymocytes of mixed lymphocyte reactivity to allogeneic and xenogeneic cells. *Cell. Immunol.*, **2,** 91

Kraft, N., Jirsch, D. W. and Diener, E. (1973). Heart allograft survival as an index of stem cell purification in the mouse. Submitted to *Transplantation*

Lajtha, L. G. (1967). Bone marrow stem cell kinetics. *Serum Hematol.*, **4,** 293

Levey, R. H., Klemperer, M. R., Gelfand, E. W., Sanderson, A. R., Batchelor, J. R., Berkel, A. I. and Rosen, F. S. (1971). Bone marrow transplantation in severe combined immunodeficiency syndrome. *Lancet*, **2,** 571

Lucas, Z. J., Markley, J. and Travis, M. (1970). Immunologic enhancement of renal allografts in the rat. I. Dissociation of graft survival and antibody response. *Fed. Proc.*, **29,** 2041

Marbrook, J. (1967). Primary immune response in cultures of spleen cells. *Lancet*, **2,** 1279

Marino, H. and Benaim, F. (1958). Experimental skin homografts: effect of homohemotherapy on their survival time. *Amer. J. Surg.*, **95,** 267

Marquet, R. L., Heystek, G. A. and Tinbergen, W. J. (1971). Specific inhibition of organ allograft rejection by donor blood. *Transplant. Proc.*, **3,** 708

McCullagh, P. (1970a). The immunological capacity of lymphocytes from normal donors after their transfer to rats tolerant of sheep erythrocytes. *Aust. J. Exp. Biol. Med. Sci.*, **48,** 369

McCullagh, P. (1970b). The abrogation of sheep erythrocyte tolerance in rats by means of the transfer of allogeneic lymphocytes. *J. Exp. Med.*, **132,** 916

McCullagh, P. (1972). The nature of the response of the cells of the sheep erythrocyte tolerant rat to transferred allogeneic lymphocytes. *Aust. J. Exp. Biol. Med. Sci.*, 50, 49

McCullagh, P. (1973). The transfer of immunological tolerance with tolerant lymphocytes. (In press)

Medawar, P. B. (1960). Theories of immunological tolerance. In *Ciba Foundation Symposium. Cellular Aspects of Immunology*, p. 134. London: Churchill

Micklem, H. S., Ford, C. E., Evans, E. P. and Gray, J. (1966). Inter-relationships of myeloid and lymphoid cells: Studies with chromosome marked cells transferred into lethally irradiated mice. *Proc. Roy. Soc., B.*, **165,** 78

Miller, J. F. A. P. (1961). Immunological function of the thymus. *Lancet*, **2,** 748

Miller, J. F. A. P., Brunner, K. T., Sprent, J., Russel, P. J. and Mitchell, G. F. (1971). Thymus derived cells as killer cells in cell-mediated immunity. *Transplant. Proc.*, **3,** 915

Miller, J. F. A. P. and Mitchell, G. F. (1969). Thymus and antigen reactive cells. *Transplant. Rev.*, **1,** 3

Miller, J. F. A. P. and Osoba, D. (1967). Current concepts of the immunological functions of the thymus. *Physiol. Rev.*, **47,** 437

Miller, R. G. and Phillips, R. A. (1969). Separation of cells by velocity sedimentation. *J. Cell Physiol.*, **73,** 191

Miller, R. G. and Phillips, R. A. (1970). Separation of cells by velocity sedimentation. In *The Separation of Hemopoietic Cell Suspension* (D. W. van Bekkum and K. A. Dicke, editors). Rijswijk: The Netherlands

Mishell, R. and Dutton, R. W. (1967). Immunization of dissociated spleen cell cultures from normal mice. *J. Exp. Med.*, **126,** 423

Mitchell, G. F. and Miller, J. F. A. P. (1968). Immunological activity of thymus and thoracic-duct lymphocytes. *Proc. Nat. Acad. Sci. (Wash.)*, **59,** 296

Mitchison, N. A. (1964). Induction of immunological paralysis in two zones of dosage. *Proc. Roy. Soc. Biol. Sci. B*, **161,** 275

Mitchison, N. A. (1967). Immunological paralysis as a dosage phenomenon. In *Regulation of the Antibody Response*, p. 54 (B. Anader, editor). Springfield: Thomas

Mitchison, N. A. (1971). The relative ability of T and B lymphocytes to see protein antigen. In *Cell Interactions in Immune Responses*, p. 249 (A. Cross, T. Kosuren and O. Mäkelä, editors). New York: Academic Press

Möller, G. (1963). I. Studies on the mechanism of immunological enhancement of tumor homografts. II. Specificity of immunological enhancement. *J. Nat. Cancer Inst.*, **30,** 1153

Möller, H. (1965). Antagonistic effects of humoral isoantibodies on the *in vitro* cytotoxicity of immune lymphoid cells. *J. Exp. Med.*, **122,** 11

Monaco, A. P., Wood, M. L. and Russell, P. S. (1965). Adult thymectomy: Effect on recovery from immunological depression in mice. *Science*, **149,** 432

Monaco, A. P., Wood, M. L. and Russell, P. S. (1966). Studies on heterologous antilymphocyte serum in mice. III. Immunological tolerance and chimerism produced across the H-2 locus with adult thymectomy and antilymphocyte serum. *Annals N.Y. Acad. Sci.*, **129,** (Article 1), 190

Mond, J. J. and Thorbecke, G. J. (1973). Greater sensitivity to inhibition by anti-immunoglobulin of splenic than of bone marrow B lymphocytes. *J. Immunol.*, **110,** 605

Nisbet, N. W. (1971). Some aspects of immunological tolerance investigated by parent to F_1 hybrid parabrosis in mice. *Transplantation*, **11,** 318

Nossal, G. J. V., Cunningham, A., Mitchell, G. F. and Miller, J. F. A. P. (1968). Cell to cell interaction in the immune response. III. Chromosomal marker analysis of single antibody forming cells in reconstituted, irradiated or thymectomized mice. *J. Exp. Med.*, **128,** 839

Nowell, P. C. (1960). Phytohemagglutinin: an initiator of mitosis in cultures of normal human lymphocytes. *Cancer Res.*, **20,** 462

Owen, R. D. (1945). Immunogenetic consequences of vascular anastomoses between

bovine twins. *Science*, **102,** 400
Parish, C. R. (1969). Immunochemical studies of bacterial flagellin. Ph.D. Thesis, University of Melbourne, Melbourne, Australia
Parish, C. R., Wistar, R. and Ada, G. L. (1969). Cleavage of bacterial flagellin by cyanogen bromide. Antigenic properties of the protein fragments. *Biochem. J.*, **113,** 501
Patel, R., Mickey, M. R. and Terasaki, P. I. (1968). Serotyping for homotransplantation. XVI. Analysis of kidney transplants from unrelated donors. *New Engl. J. Med.*, **279,** 501
Pauling, L. (1940). A theory of the structure and process of formation of antibodies. *J. Amer. Chem. Soc.*, **62,** 2643
Phillips, R. A. and Miller, R. G. (1970). Physical separation of hemopoietic stem cells from cells causing graft-versus-host disease. I. Sedimentation properties of cells causing graft-versus-host disease. *J. Immunol.*, **105,** 1168
Poor, E. (1957). Brephoplastic homotransplantation of hamster heart: A preliminary report. *Transplant. Bull.*, **4,** 143
Quadracci, L. J., Hellström, I., Striker, G. E., Marchioro, T. L. and Hellström, K. E. (1971). Immune mechanisms in human recipients of renal allografts. *Cell Immunol.*, **1,** 561
Rajewsky, K. (1971). The carrier effect and cellular co-operation in the induction of antibodies. *Proc. Roy. Soc. B*, **176,** 385
Ramseier, H. and Lindenmann, J. (1972). Aliotypic antibodies. *Transplant. Rev.*, **10,** 57
Reisfeld, R. A. and Kahan, B. D. (1971). Biological and chemical characterization of human histocompatibility antigens. *Fed. Proc.*, **172,** 1134
Rowley, D. A., Fitch, F. W., Axelrad, M. A. and Pierce, C. W. (1969a). The immune response suppressed by specific antibody. *Immunology*, **16,** 549
Rowley, D. A., Fitch, F. W., Saitoh, T. and Stuart, F. P. (1969b). Specific suppression of cell-mediated immune responses. *Transplant. Proc.*, **1,** 580
Salmon, S. E., Krakauer, R. S. and Whitmore, W. F. (1971). Lymphocyte stimulation: selective destruction of cells during blastogenic response to transplantation antigens. *Science*, **172,** 490
Schinkell, P. G. and Ferguson, K. A. (1953). Skin transplantation in the fetal lamb. *Aust. J. Exp. Biol.*, **6,** 533
Segre, D. and Kaeberle, M. L. (1962). The immunological behavior of baby pigs. *J. Immunol.*, **89,** 782
Shellam, G. R. and Nossal, G. J. V. (1968). Mechanism of induction of immunological tolerance. IV. The effects of ultra low doses of flagellin. *Immunology*, **14,** 273
Simmons, R. L. and Russell, P. S. (1966). The histocompatibility antigens of fertilized

mouse eggs and trophoblast. *Ann. N.Y. Acad. Sci.*, **129,** 35

Sjögren, H. O., Hellström, I., Bansal, S. C. and Hellström, K. E. (1971). Suggestive evidence that the 'blocking antibodies' of tumor bearing individuals may be antigen–antibody complexes. *Proc. Nat. Acad. Sci. (Wash.)*, **68,** 1372

Smith, R. J. and Bridges, R. A. (1958). Immunological unresponsiveness in rabbits produced by neonatal injection of defined antigens. *J. Exp. Med.*, **108,** 227

Smith, R. T. (1961). Immunological tolerance of non-living antigens. *Adv. Immunol.*, **1,** 67

Snell, G. D., Winn, H. J., Stimpfling, J. H. and Parker, S. J. (1960). Depression by antibody of the immune response to homografts and its role in immunological enhancement. *J. Exp. Med.*, **112,** 293

Speck, B., Pooren, L. J., de Koning, J., van Bekkum, D. W., Eernisse, J. G., Elkerbout, F., Vossen, J. M., and van Rood, J. J. (1971). Clinical experience with bone marrow transplantation: failure and success. *Transplant. Proc.*, **3,** 409

Staples, P. J., Gery, I. and Waksman, B. H. (1966). Role of the thymus in tolerance. III. Tolerance to bovine gamma globulin after direct injection of antigen into the shielded thymus of irradiated rats. *J. Exp. Med.*, **124,** 127

Sterzl, J. (1966). Immunological tolerance as the result of terminal differentiation of immunologically competent cells. *Nature (London)*, **209,** 416

Sterzl, J. and Trnka, Z. (1957). Effect of very large doses of bacterial antigen on antibody production in newborn rabbits. *Nature (London)*, **179,** 918

Stuart, F. P., Bastien, E., Fitch, F. W. and Rowley, A. (1970). Mechanisms of antigen and antibody induced suppression of renal allograft rejection in the rat. *Fed. Proc.*, **29,** 3052

Stuart, F. P., Saitoh, T. and Fitch, F. W. (1968). Rejection of renal allografts: Specific immunologic suppression. *Science*, **160,** 1463

Takasugi, M. and Hildemann, W. H. (1969). The regulation of immunity toward allogeneic factors in mice. II. Effect of antiserum and antiserum fractions on the cellular and humoral response. *J. Nat. Cancer Inst.*, **43,** 857

Taylor, R. B. (1969). Cellular co-operation in the antibody response of mice to two serum albumins: Specific function of thymus cells. *Transplant. Rev.*, **1,** 114

Terres, G. and Wolins, W. (1961). Enhanced immunological sensitization of mice by simultaneous injection of antigen and specific antiserum. *J. Immunol.*, **86,** 361

Thorbecke, G. J. and Benacerraf, B. (1967). Tolerance in adult rabbits by repeated non-immunogenic doses of bovine serum albumin. *Immunology*, **13,** 141

Till, J. E. and McCullough, E. A. (1961). A direct measurement of the radiation sentivity of normal mouse bone marrow. *Radiation Res.*, **14,** 213

Triplett, E. L. (1962). On the mechanism of immunologic self recognition. *J. Im-*

munol., **89**, 505

Turner, R. W. A., Siminovitch, L., McCullough, E. A. and Till, J. F. (1967). Density gradient separation of hemopoietic colony forming cells. *J. Cell Physiol.*, **69**, 73

Uhr, J. W. and Baumann, J. B. (1961). Antibody formation—the suppression of antibody formation by passively administered antibody. *J. Exp. Med.*, **113**, 935

Uhr, J. W. and Möller, G. (1968). Regulatory effect of antibody on the immune response. *Adv. Immunol.*, **8**, 801

Viza, D. C., Degani, O., Dausset, J. and Davies, D. A. L. (1968). Lymphocyte stimulation by soluble human HL-A transplantation antigens. *Nature (London)*, **219**, 704

Winstein, R. R. (1960). Behavior of transplanted hearts in platyfish. *Trans. N.Y. Acad. Sci.*, **22**, 647

Williams, G. M. (1966). Ontogeny of the immune response. II. Correlation between the development of the afferent and efferent limbs. *J. Exp. Med.*, **124**, 57

Williams, G. M. (1973). Transplantation. *Surg. Gynecol. Obstet.*, **136**, 212

Wood, M. L., Gozzo, J. J., Heppner, G. and Monaco, A. P. (1972). Cell-mediated immunity and serum blocking factor in tolerance produced in mice with anti-lymphocyte serum and bone marrow cell infusion. *Transplant. Proc.*, **4**, 383

Woodruff, M. F. and Simpson, L. W. (1955). Induction of tolerance to skin homografts in rats by injection of cells from the prospective donor soon after birth. *Brit. J. Exp. Path.*, **36**, 494

Worton, R. G., McCullough, E. A. and Till, J. E. (1969). Physical separation of hemopoietic stem cells from cells forming colonies in culture. *J. Cell Physiol.*, **74**, 171

Wu, A. M., Till, J. E., Siminovitch, L. and McCullough, E. A. (1968). Cytological evidence for a relationship between normal hematopoietic colony forming cells and cells of the lymphoid system. *J. Exp. Med.*, **127**, 455

Yung, Lilly L. L., Wyn-Evans, T. Cheryl and Diener, E. (1973). Ontogeny of the murine immune system: Development of antigen recognition and immune responsiveness. *European J. Immunol.* (In press)

Zoschke, D. C. and Bach, F. H. (1971). Specificity of allogeneic cell recognition by human lymphocytes *in vitro*. *Science*, **172**, 1380

10
Kidney and Skin Allografts in the Rat

E. White

INTRODUCTION

Until the late 1960s the results from organ grafting were usually predictable. The rules for survival of, or immunological rejection of, grafts were defined in the early 1940s. Human kidney isografts regularly survive and kidney allografts usually experience rejection episodes even with immunosuppressive therapy. Survival and normal function of canine kidney allografts were difficult to achieve even with immunosuppression. These observations conformed to and substantiated the immunological principles of transplantation. Simply stated, the principles are:

(1) A host does not normally respond immunologically to histocompatibility antigens that he possesses, and,
(2) A host may respond to foreign histocompatibility antigens that he does not possess.

Response, in this context, is generally considered to be immunological rejection of grafted tissues. Subsequent grafting from the original disparate donor would result in accelerated rejection. These principles were developed primarily from observations of skin and tumor grafts. For quite some time both cellular and humoral responses have been detected with rejection of grafts. Until recently the humoral response has been an enigma for the transplantation biologists because the resultant antibodies could not be convincingly related to graft destruction. It now appears that certain antibodies are destructive while others prolong survival of grafts (enhancement).

Results from enhancement of tumor grafts provided the basis for our initial interpretation of the unexpected, prolonged survival of disparate kidney grafts in rats (White and Hildemann, 1968). When indigenous and freely growing tumors from one strain of mice are injected or transplanted into another strain, the tumor is usually rejected and the animal survives. However, when the recipient animal is properly pretreated with donor histocompatibility antigens (active immunization) or alloantibodies specific against the donor antigens (passive immunization) the tumor may grow and result in the death of the animal. In this event immunization does not result in accelerated rejection but in enhanced growth of the tumor. Accelerated rejection of tumors may be achieved by varying the immunizing protocol, however. Emerging information from tumor immunology is critical to an explanation of the results from kidney and skin grafting in rats. Enhancement, mediated by alloantibody, is the keystone to current theories offered to explain many anomalous phenomena.

Throughout the recorded history of transplantation, sporadic aberrations of the rules of transplantation have been reported. Grafted tissues or organs are observed to survive when they should have been rejected. Prolonged survival of ovary, pituitary, and parathyroid glands occurred in antigenically disparate combinations (Linder, 1962; Gittes *et al.*, 1964). However, neither the site nor the method of grafting these organs were typical for vascular anastomosis of kidneys or graft-bed preparation for skin. The observations were early indicators that not all allografts would be subject to the same dismal prognosis as skin grafts. In many instances extended survival of kidney allografts in dogs could be achieved by utilizing immunosuppressive drugs. Surprisingly, many of these allografts would survive even when immunosuppressive therapy was curtailed or discontinued.

The prognosis of human kidney allografts prior to effective immunosuppression was generally unfavorable. However, the prolonged survival of some allografted individuals suggested that the rules of transplantation were not absolute (Hume *et al.*, 1955). The reported aberrations were disconcerting for the immunobiologists, but nurtured their research interest. The results also offered hope to clinicians whose patients require renal grafts. Many of the early anomalous results were totally unpredictable and not easily reproduced. Unpredictability resulted primarily from a lack of genetic definition and control in allografted populations.

Kidney grafting in the rat

Until 1965, microsurgical limitations of vascular anastomosis precluded utilization of highly inbred strains of laboratory animals for experimental renal grafting. Kidney transplants were generally limited to genetically and antigenically disparate random populations. Sun Lee made a most significant contribution to the field of immunological surgery (Fisher and Lee, 1965; Lee, 1967). His simple and routinely successful technique allowed for kidney grafting within genetically defined strains of rats and pointed the way to an ever increasing understanding of basic principles or organ graft survival and rejection. Highly inbred strains of rats have been available for some years. Fortunately, extensive genetic and histocompatibility characterization of established lines is documented. A resurgence of interest in rat immunogenetics has occurred because of the popularity of the rat for experimental organ transplantation. The enormous potential for advances in transplantation immunobiology through utilization of the rat model is just beginning to be tapped. This will surely sustain the impetus for further characterization of established lines and development of additional congenic strains, as has been developed with mice. Availability of more congenic strains of rats will help define the effects of discrete antigenic differences in grafts.

Immunogenic relationships—histocompatibility typing

A brief overview of the current status of histocompatibility typing in the rat should be helpful for subsequent discussion in this chapter. Similar to most species studied, the rat seems to have a major or 'strong' histocompatibility locus termed H-1 or Ag-B. Conceptually, this locus corresponds to the H-2 locus in mice or the HL-A locus in humans, and governs the expression of 'strong' histocompatibility antigens. An undetermined number of loci control the expression of minor or 'weak' histocompatability antigens. Classification of histocompatibility genes (and/or antigens as strong or weak) originally derived from observed rejection times for skin or tumor grafts. Antigenic disparities were characterized as strong when acute rejection occurred and weak when chronic rejection occurred. Allogeneic skin grafts between inbred strains of rats are rejected usually in an acute fashion regardless of compatibility or incompatibility at the major H-1 locus, however. Other adjunctive parameters have therefore been used to distinguish between strong and weak histocompatibility antigens. In the past it was presumed that strong histocompatibility antigens induced alloantibodies, graft-versus-host reactions (GVHR) and blastogenesis in mixed lymphocyte cultures (MLC), exclusively. Alloantibody is easily induced and detected by hemagglutination and/or cytoxicity tests. Classical GVHR presumably does not occur in weakly disparate combinations (those matched for major histocompatibility alleles), and only minimal to zero blastogenesis occurs in MLC between weakly disparate lymphoid cell populations.

In summary, strong antigenic disparities result in acute rejection of skin allografts, induction of alloantibody, GVHR, and blastogenesis in MLC. Weak antigens may induce acute rejection of skin and alloantibody formation (Thoenes *et al.*, 1969; Thoenes *et al.*, 1970; White *et al.*, 1969).

An example of the utilization of these factors for histocompatibility typing is the relationship between Lewis (Lew) and Fischer (Fi) rats. It is presumed that these two strains of rats share the same major histocompatibility allele, $H\text{-}1^l$ or $Ag\text{-}B^1$, because earlier investigators were unable to demonstrate alloantibody, GVHR, or positive MLC between these strains. Acute rejection of skin grafts occurs between Fi and Lew rats, but this is not surprising because the cumulative effect of weaker antigens also results in acute rejection in mice (Hildemann and Cohen, 1967). It would appear difficult, if not impossible, to demonstrate GVHR or positive MLC between these rat strains. Our subsequent findings, anti-Fi antibody from long surviving Lew recipients of Fi kidneys, illustrated that alloantibodies could be induced in weaker disparate combinations (Thoenes *et al.*, 1970; White *et al.*, 1969). This finding also provided further evidence that enhancement may contribute to the prolonged survival of these renal allografts, as discussed below. We may need to reassess the significance of alloantibody induction for rat histocompatibility typing to include facile detection in strongly disparate combinations as a factor rather than the mere presence or absence of antibodies. The same principle may be true for other factors, e.g. GVHR and MLC, because GVHR has been convincingly demonstrated between mice strain combinations disparate at non H-2 loci (Cantrell and Hildemann, 1972). A review of the above information is important because many of the anomalous events initially observed from experiences with skin and kidney grafting in rats were thought to be unique for weaker incompatibilities and not applicable for stronger differences. Table 10.1 summarizes the current classification of inbred strains of rats relative to their genetic

Table 10.1 *Histocompatibility type of rat strains**

	H-1 or *Ag-B Locus*	
Strain	*Allele*	*Allele*
Lewis (Lew)	$H\text{-}1^l$	$Ag\text{-}B^1$
Fischer (Fi)	$H\text{-}1^l$	$Ag\text{-}B^1$
AS	$H\text{-}1^l$	$Ag\text{-}B^1$
Brown Norway (BN)	$H\text{-}1^n$	$Ag\text{-}B^3$
Buffalo (Buf)	(H-1?)	$Ag\text{-}B^6$
AS2	$H\text{-}1^f$	Ag-B?
August	($H\text{-}1^c$?)	$Ag\text{-}B^5$

*Adapted from Štark *et al.*, 1971; Palm, 1971

and histocompatibility designations and should be helpful in following the grafting combinations to be discussed later.

Early observations from skin and kidney grafts

With the advent of a simple and adequate grafting method by Sun Lee (Fisher and Lee, 1965; Lee, 1967), several laboratories began transplanting kidneys in rats. Guttmann and his associates, the most productive group in this field, reported in 1967 that strongly disparate (BN × Lew)F_1 → Lew grafts resulted in early loss of renal function, usually within seven days (Guttmann *et al.*, 1967). These important results were not too surprising in view of the prevailing immunological rules for transplantation and more intriguing results awaited future developments, i.e. disparate survivals between organs and skin. Early reports whetted the investigative appetite of laboratories around the world. The commercial supply of BN rats was quickly utilized by a few laboratories. Because most investigators had to utilize different rat strains the resultant diversity of results was significant, and I believe was a fortuitous event. Animal availability dictated that we use Fischer, Buffalo and Lewis animals in early experiments because we simply could not get Brown Norway. Our interests in 1967 were initially focused on testing the effects of immunosuppressive drugs on weakly disparate kidney graft combinations (Fi and Lew). There was considerable interest in immunosuppression for weakly disparate grafts at this time because of the obvious similarity of these rat combinations to human renal allografts matched for HL-A antigens. Preliminary expectations were that non-related human kidney grafts, matched for major HL-A antigens, would have better survival and rejection would be more easily suppressed than mismatched kidney grafts. In retrospect, these assumptions were erroneous. The results of kidney grafting in weakly disparate rats proved to be distinctively different from similar human grafting combinations.

A protocol to test the effects of immunosuppression of Fi → Lew kidneys required that control allografts be done in the absence of any immunosuppressive drugs on normal recipients. We fully expected prompt rejection of control kidney grafts. Surprisingly, the animals had prolonged or indefinite survival with grafted kidney only, in spite of the fact that skin grafted between these strains was rejected within two weeks. This was one of the earliest reports of predictable, prolonged survival of vascular anastomosed organ allografts in otherwise normal inbred animals (White and Hildemann, 1968). Tolerance could not be considered seriously as a mechanism to explain this unexpected graft survival, because skin grafts from the original donor strain were rejected by long-surviving kidney allografted recipients (White and Hildemann, 1968; White *et al.*, 1969; White and Hildemann, 1969). Our initial expectations with skin grafting were that kidney allografted recipients would reject both kidney and skin, or reject neither. The confusing results observed raised more questions than answers.

An intriguing report regarding the ease of prolonging the survival of rat kidney allografts across major histocompatibility barriers appeared (Stuart *et al.*, 1968). These results were achieved in BN to Lew combinations by pretreatment of recipients with either antigen (active enhancement) or alloantibody (passive enhancement). Surprisingly prolonged kidney allograft survival in combinations of out-bred strains of rats were reported (Salaman, 1968). Skin grafts between these strains survived for eight to ten days. Skin grafts from the original donor strains subsequent to kidney allografting survived without apparent rejection. Tolerance was suggested as a mechanism to explain both kidney and skin graft survival in this situation. Our earliest attempts at skin and kidney grafting within an out-bred Sprague Dawley strain resulted in prolonged survival of kidney but early rejection of skin grafts (White, unpublished results). Survival of August or (August × AS) $F_1 \rightarrow$ AS kidney allografts, enhanced by treatment of recipients with alloantibody specific against donor August histocompatibility antigens, was reported (French and Batchelor, 1969). It was also evident that F_1 donor kidneys were more easily enhanced than parent strain kidneys. Sakai demonstrated that reciprocal grafting (reversal of donor and recipient strains) dramatically altered the rejection times for kidney grafts. Using AS and AS2 combinations he found that F_1 kidney grafts were rejected within fifteen days in AS recipients and survived longer than 30 days in AS2 recipients (Sakai, 1969). His findings of acute renal rejection for parent strain AS $\rightarrow$ AS2 were not in agreement with subsequent reports (Salaman *et al.*, 1971; Bildsoe *et al.*, 1971).

Further disparaties between survival of allografted tissues, e.g. skin, heart and kidney, were found (Freeman and Steinmuller, 1969; Bildsøe *et al.*,1970). Heart grafts in weak combinations (Lew × Fi) $F_1 \rightarrow$ Lew, were rejected in acute times approximating those of skin while kidneys survived for extended periods of time. Ease of enhancement in treated recipients, prolonged survival in normal recipients, and differential modes of rejection for skin, kidney and heart allografts were the highlights of the early efforts in allografting in the rat. Elucidation of mechanisms to explain these observations will be increasingly available as research continues in grafting in the rat.

FACTUAL CONSIDERATIONS — DESCRIPTION OF SKIN AND KIDNEY GRAFTING

The editor has suggested distinct separations between factual information and theoretical considerations. We have documented observations concerning grafting animals with skin and kidney, and will theorize on the mechanisms which dictate these events. It would seem appropriate to discuss the theories of the mechanisms in three general categories: (a) skin grafting, (b) kidney grafting, and (c) a combination of both.

Skin grafting across major and minor transplantation barriers

At present the results of skin grafting seem to be the most predictable. Skin grafting is usually accomplished by the preparation of a graft-bed on a recipient and application of the donor graft. Healing is by ingrowth of vessels and complete vascularization of the graft is achieved after several days post surgery. Initially it was felt by some investigators that the difference in healing and vascularization of kidney and skin contributed to their differential survival times. Modes and amounts of antigenic exposure may be different in these two situations and may have an effect on the immune status of a recipient. Several lines of investigation have made differences of grafting technique seem less important than previously projected. Pedicle skin grafts with direct vascular anastomosis give similar rejection times when compared with traditional methods (Cho *et al.*, 1972). Hearts with vascular anastomosis transplanted between Fischer and Lewis rats are rejected in an acute fashion similar to skin as compared to prolonged survival for kidneys in this combination (Freeman and Steinmuller, 1969). Therefore, it would appear that skin grafts between highly inbred strains of rats are regularly rejected by normal recipients within 2 weeks using either graft-bed or vascular techniques. Acute rejection of skin allografts occur whether the genetic or antigenic differences are strong or weak in the majority of rat strains studied. One interesting and curious aspect of interstrain skin graft survival is the constant, but minor, difference in rejection times dependent on the direction of grafting. These observations have been made in many grafting combinations. For example, AS → AS2 skin grafts had a median survival time of 10.1 days and AS2 → AS rejected in 8.3 days. This modest difference of approximately two days may be expanded dramatically with kidney grafting. Kidney graft survival in an AS → AS2 combinations may be indefinite while rejection occurred within two weeks in AS2 → AS direction (Salaman *et al.*, 1971; Bildsøe *et al.*, 1971).

Prolonged survival of skin grafts between rats can be achieved under a variety of conditions. One of the better examples of chronic rejection of skin in normal rat populations is seen between male and female intrastrain grafts. Chronic rejection running into the hundreds of days is the general rule in this instance (Mullen and Hildemann, 1972). Skin graft survival may also be prolonged by a variety of immunosuppressive regimes. The use of Imuran, cyclophosphamide, antilymphocyte globulin, etc. are moderately successful in prolonging the survival of skin grafts. Surprisingly, a few H-1 incompatible skin grafts showed extended survival in actively enhanced recipients (prior rejection of skin or injection of lymphocytes) (Heslop, 1971).

Grafting across major transplantation barriers (H-1 disparities)

Kidney—normal recipients

A whole spectrum of rejection patterns occur with kidney grafts. Rejection may range from acute (death of the animal within seven days) to a rejection reaction so chronic that the animal survives indefinitely. Both F_1 or parent strain donors to parent strain recipients have been used for kidney grafting. The more frequently used strain combinations are BN or Buf $\rightarrow$ Lew, August $\leftrightarrows$ AS and AS $\leftrightarrows$ AS2. To repeat, initial results indicated that grafting across major disparities resulted in acute rejection of kidneys within 7 to 10 days especially for the BN and Lewis. These conclusions were based on the observation that recipients became oliguric or anuric with markedly decreased renal plasma flow about day seven (Guttmann *et al.*, 1967). Many strongly disparate grafts between BN and Lewis undergo spontaneous reversal of rejection crisis and survive for surprisingly long times (White, unpublished results). This has been observed also with Buffalo to Lewis combination (Mullen *et al.*, 1973; Mullen and Hildemann, 1971; Ippolito *et al.*, 1972). As a generalization, F_1 to parent strain grafts survive much longer and are more easily enhanced by pretreatment of recipients than parent strain to parent strain grafts. This $F_1 \rightarrow$ parent kidney combination seems to present quantitatively less antigens to a recipient. The lowered antigenic density or dosage effect may contribute to prolonged survival as compared with parent $\rightarrow$ parent. Dramatic differences demonstrated in survival of kidneys are not seen with skin grafts.

Striking results have been reported in AS $\leftrightarrows$ AS2 kidney combinations. AS2 $\rightarrow$ AS grafts were all rejected within 18 days. In the opposite direction, AS $\rightarrow$ AS2, seven of ten animals survived beyond 50 days (Salaman *et al.*, 1971). AS $\rightarrow$ AS2 grafts were reported to survive for many months (Bildsøe *et al.*, 1971). Chronic rather than acute rejection occurred in spite of major H-1 disparities between donor and recipient animals.

Kidney—immunized recipients

Proper pretreatment of recipients with either histocompatibility antigens (injection of lymphoid cells or soluble antigenic preparations) or preformed alloantibodies directed against the donor strain may result in prolonged survival of kidney grafts. These animals are immunized, in a sense, by their treatment with lymphoid cells or allo-antibody, but are also specifically immunosuppressed because the kidney survives. Contrarily, *accelerated* rejection of kidney allografts can be achieved by somewhat similar methods.

With strongly disparate combinations one might expect that presensitization by rejection of a skin graft prior to kidney grafting would result in acute rejection of the kidney. Seven AS2 rats were preimmunized by rejection of a single AS skin graft and subsequently grafted with AS kidneys (Salaman *et al.*, 1971). Three of the seven rats survived beyond 80 days. Kidney grafting subsequent to rejection of two consecutive AS skin grafts precluded survival beyond 8 days in AS2 recipients. Injection of either whole alloantiserum with exogenous complement (French, 1972), or IgM fractions (Mullen *et al.*, 1973; Mullen and Hildemann, 1971) into kidney allografted recipients may cause accelerated rejection of the graft.

Kidney—nonspecific immunosuppressed recipients

Almost any of the contemporary immunosuppressive drugs or xenogeneic antilymphoid globulins may extend the viability of allografted kidneys in bilaterally nephrectomized rats. The ease of extending the function of these grafts is impressive compared to human and canine kidney grafts.

Skin and kidney grafting

In studies referred to earlier (Salaman *et al.*, 1971), AS2 rats that survived transplantation with AS kidneys retained subsequent AS skin grafts up to the time of their death. The time of skin grafting after kidney transplantation was not stated. By contrast, recipients that were preimmunized by rejecting an AS skin graft prior to renal grafting rejected AS skin grafts subsequent to renal grafting.

Other investigators reported that enhanced (alloantibody mediated) Lewis recipients of (Buf $\times$ Lew)F_1 renal grafts rejected subsequent Buffalo skin grafts at times dependent on the interval between kidney and skin grafts. Buffalo test skin grafts showed increasing median survival, up to 40 days, when placed at 0, 40 and 100 days post kidney grafting. Specific immunity for rejection of Buffalo skin grafts decreased in intensity but nonetheless persisted in successfully enhanced Lewis recipients (Mullen *et al.*, 1973).

Prolonged survival can be achieved in strongly disparate combinations by nonspecific immunosuppression. Sixty days after renal grafting Lewis recipients (treated with cyclophosphamide) of (BN $\times$ Lew)F_1 kidneys were grafted with F_1 skin. The skin grafts were rejected normally and renal function was not impaired during or after rejection (Kawabe *et al.*, 1972).

In the reports of concurrent kidney and skin graft studies discussed above third party control grafts were rejected in normal times. One may conclude that nonspecific immunosuppression of long-surviving kidney allografted recipients has minimal to zero effect on the animals' ability to reject third party grafts. Specific suppression allows for kidney survival but rarely extends to skin grafts in strongly disparate combinations. It would appear that the AS → AS2 situation is exceptional (Salaman *et al.*, 1971).

Grafting across minor transplantation barriers (H-1 compatible)

Kidney—normal recipients

Weakly disparate kidney allografts into otherwise normal recipients resulted in very prolonged survival or extremely chronic rejection in all strain combinations tested. Fischer to Lewis kidney allografts usually survive for many months and Lewis to Fischer seem to survive indefinitely (White *et al.*, 1969). Histologically the tempo of rejection is drastically different in these reverse combinations. Fischer to Lewis renal grafts exhibited minimal to moderate inflammatory infiltrations throughout their survival. By contrast, it was histologically difficult to distinguish between Lewis → Fischer allografts and isografts months after kidney grafting (White *et al.*, 1969). Using AS and Lewis combinations, other investigators also found consistent long survival in this H-1 compatible combination (Thoenes and White, 1973).

Kidney—immunized recipients

Preimmunization of Lewis recipients by rejection of a primary Fischer skin graft resulted in slightly curtailed Fischer kidney graft survival with subacute rejection times (2–5 weeks with maximal survival of 8 weeks). No Lewis animal which previously rejected two Fischer skin grafts lived beyond 17 days with a Fischer kidney graft. Preimmunized animals thus showed progressively worse clinical courses after renal transplantation than normal recipients. Other sensitization methods, e.g. injection of lymphoid cells or dispersed kidney tissue, resulted in accelerated rejection of subsequent Fischer skin. Transplantation of a Fischer kidney, leaving one host kidney *in situ*, resulted in accelerated rejection of subsequent skin grafts as well. Curiously, it was noted in other studies that Fischer kidney grafts were rapidly rejected if Lewis recipients were unilaterally nephrectomized (White *et al.*, 1969). Sex associated histocompatability antigens are generally considered to be weak disparities which can cause chronic rejection of skin grafts. Mullen and Hildemann found that kidney rejection could not be demonstrated between male and female intrastrain grafts with both parent strain and F_1 combinations. Rejection of kidneys did not occur even with preimmunization through rejection of skin, or injection of lymphoid cells (Mullen and Hildemann, 1971, 1972).

Skin and kidney grafting

Kidney allografted animals, subsequently skin grafted, survived as long as kidney grafted animals. Lewis recipients of Fischer kidney allografts rejected subsequent Fischer skin grafts in slightly extended times of 17 days for first-set grafts, but rejected second- and third-set grafts in an accelerated manner. In this series one rat exhibited prolonged survival of a second-set Fischer skin graft (80 days) and promptly rejected a third-set graft in an accelerated fashion (8 days), a curious occurrence (White *et al.*, 1969). It would appear from studies of Mahabir *et al.* that the longer one delays skin grafting after renal grafting the longer the median survival of the skin graft in this combination (Mahabir *et al.*, 1969). In another weakly disparate combination Thoenes, using AS, Lewis and F_1 found that skin grafts from the original donor strain had surprisingly prolonged, perhaps indefinite, survival times if the skin grafts were placed 5–8 months after kidney grafting (Thoenes and White, 1973).

THEORETICAL CONSIDERATION—MECHANISM FOR SURVIVAL

Enhancement versus tolerance

Differential vulnerability of skin and kidney allografts is evident from the above discussion. A kidney allografted rat will reject skin from the original donor strain and retain adequate to normal kidney function for reasons which remain obscure. Several mechanisms and reasons have been offered to explain this phenomenon. Originally tolerance and enhancement competed for pre-eminence as the most logical explanation since tolerance and enhancement were thought to be mutually exclusive, although we still understand very little about the underlying mechanisms. Classically, tolerance is induced by proper neonatal exposure to alloantigens (lymphoid cells). Animals which have been rendered tolerant are non-reactive to subsequent exposure to these specific histocompatibility antigens. Specific non-reactivity is critical to the concept of tolerance. Thus the inability of investigators to demonstrate immune reactivity against donor cells or grafts by long-surviving recipients of kidney allografts would be consistent with a tolerant state. Measurements of immunological reactivity may be achieved by several methods, including rejection of skin, detection of allo-antibody, cell mediated immunity (CMI), blastogenesis in mixed lymphocyte cultures (MLC), and graft-versus-host reaction (GVHR). In our earlier studies tolerance was excluded as an explanation for the survival of Fischer → Lewis kidneys because these long-surviving Lewis recipients rejected subsequent Fischer skin grafts with no detriment to renal function. Quite early we proposed that active enhancement could account for these observations (White and Hildemann, 1968). To implicate enhancement it was critical to demonstrate alloantibodies in long-surviving allograft recipients.

Alloantibody

Alloantibody induction after immunization between H-1 compatible rat or H-2 compatible mice strains has been difficult to demonstrate. Utilizing a sensitive ^{51}Cr cytotoxicity assay, Lewis recipients of Fischer kidney allografts were found to produce anti-Fischer antibodies which persisted for at least several months after grafting (Thoenes *et al.*, 1969, 1970; White *et al.*, 1969). Enhancement was a more justifiable assumption than tolerance. Thoenes has recently extended his findings by monitoring alloantibody levels of long-surviving AS and Lewis recipients of allografted kidneys (weakly disparate combination). Antibody levels fall to normal background values between 5 and 8 months after kidney grafting. Kidney donor strain skin grafts placed when alloantibody returns to control level display remarkable survival, perhaps indefinite for most grafts (Thoenes and White, 1973). In this instance enhancement (early reactivity evidenced by antibody) with a gradual shift to later tolerance (non-reactivity evidenced by fall of antibody and skin graft survival) could be operative. Thus enhancement and tolerance would not necessarily be mutually exclusive, but rather dependent on the temporal events. This is conjectural, however, because the assay used measured cytotoxic antibodies whereas immunoblocking antibodies are probably not cytotoxic in the presence of endogenous rat complement. Whether levels of lymphocytotoxic antibodies are related to efficacy of kidney enhancement remains unclear. Direct tests for enhancing antibody may be positive by passive transfer even though cytotoxic or hemagglutinating antibodies are undetectable *in vitro*. A recent report further amplifies the importance of active antibody production in survival of enhanced kidney allografted rats. Splenectomy around the time of renal grafting abolished the effects of enhancement in recipients pretreated with antigen or antibody. Too early splenectomy or delay had no effect on survival (Enomoto and Lucas, 1973). For passive enhancement the effectiveness of immunoblocking allo-antibodies is increased as histoincompatibility becomes weaker (Hildemann, 1973).

Cell mediated immunity (CMI)

Direct *in vitro* test of CMI with lymphocytes from long-surviving renal allografted rats have consistently revealed reactivities similar to control normal or preimmunized animals (Stuart *et al.*, 1971; Mullen *et al.*, 1973), but not tolerance of non-reactivity.

Mixed lymphocyte culture (MLC)

Lymphocytes from long-surviving AS2 recipients of AS kidneys showed decreased blastogenesis in MLC compared to normal controls and results generated speculation that tolerance was induced by kidney grafting (Salaman *et al.*, 1971). By contrast, hyporeactivity in MLC was demonstrated as a characteristic of immunized animals (Virolainen *et al.*, 1969). Lymphocytes from long-surviving Lewis recipients of (BN × Lew)F_1 responded in MLC similarly to cells from normal rats (Ippolito *et al.*, 1972).

Graft-versus-host reactions

GVHR results indicate that lymphoid cells from long-surviving kidney allografted rats have activity similar to normal animals (French *et al.*, 1971), hyperreactive (Mullen *et al.*, 1973) or slightly hyporeactive (Bildsøe *et al.*, 1971). The latter, using the same AS and AS2 combination as Salaman (Salaman *et al.*, 1971), showed that lymphocytes from long-term surviving allografted recipients had decreased GVHR compared to normal control animals. Hyporeactivity was typical for other animals which had been repeatedly immunized by rejection of skin and injection of allogeneic lymphoid cells. By contrast, animals made tolerant at birth by injection of bone marrow cells yielded no GVHR (Bildsøe *et al.*, 1971).

These evidences of alloantibody induction and lymphoid cell reactivity preclude tolerance as a mechanism in the classical sense.

Other factors

Several other factors may contribute to differential survival of kidney and skin.

Adaptation

Adaptation was postulated at an early date and implied that some donor tissues of a graft, primarily vascular endothelium, were replaced by host cells (Woodruff, 1952). Graft histocompatibility antigens would be, in effect, cloistered by host cells from the effector cells of rejection. Several recent reports have suggested that adaptation may occur but does not appear to be a significant factor in survival of grafts at this time (Nirmul *et al.*, 1972; de Bono, 1972; Williams *et al.*, 1971).

Differential antigenicity

It is becoming increasingly evident that specific tissues or cell types have different and distinct spectra and concentrations of antigens. Histocompatibility antigens seem to be expressed in maximal concentrations on lymphoid cells and skin. Histocompatibility antigens are expressed on renal tissues and probably exist in lower concentration than skin or lymphocytes (Jones *et al.*, 1972). Teleologically, high concentrations of histocompatability antigens on epithelia or immunocytes may be essential for maximal recognition, accounting for the differences. A number of studies have shown that F_1 kidneys are more easily enhanced than parent strain kidneys. Ease of enhancement may be related to allelic suppression in the hybrid with half the antigens of either parent strain represented (Batchelor *et al.*, 1973). Kidney tissue injected into normal recipients sensitized for accelerated rejection of subsequent skin grafts and transplantation of a kidney (removed prior to skin graft) also immunized recipients for accelerated rejection of skin (White *et al.*, 1969). Regardless of any quantitative differences, enough antigens are available on renal tissues to cause rejection of kidneys, even at an accelerated rate, and to immunize recipients under proper circumstances. The rôle of organ specific antigens in rejection is unknown at the present time. The author believes that quantitative and qualitative antigenic differences contribute substantially to the disparate survival times of kidney and skin, but little direct evidence exists to confirm or reject this hypothesis.

Quantity of tissue—Antigenic dosage

Kidney grafts provide more tissue to a recipient than most skin grafts. However, equivalent weights of skin are still rejected early while kidneys survive for prolonged periods in weakly disparate combinations (White *et al.*, 1969). Quantitative differences of tissue may have some significance related to the ability of a kidney grafted animal to survive with extensive destruction of renal tissue.

Phenotypic suppression

It has been proposed that alloantibody may suppress or inhibit expression of histocompatibility antigens on grafted tissues. One report showed modulation of HL-A phenotype in an immunodeficient child (Sanderson *et al.*, 1972). Although antigenic modulation frequently occurs in micro-organisms and tumor cells, the role of allotypic suppression in prolonged survival of allografts is still unclear.

Weak complement system of the rat

Rat complement seems to be inefficient in some cytotoxicity testing situations. Rat kidneys are susceptible to hyperacute rejection but rats, even strongly preimmunized, do not generally reject kidneys in a hyperacute manner (Chavez-Peon *et al.*, 1971). Exogenous xenogeneic complement may facilitate hyperacute rejection (French, 1972). These observations suggest that rat complement may be deficient in some manner. However, any deficiency that exists does not preclude rejection of skin, kidneys, and hearts even at an acute rate in some instances.

Effects of uremia

The immunosuppressive effects of uremia are difficult to analyze. For long-surviving rats grafted with kidney and skin, any immunosuppression that may exist does not protect skin from rejection. If a rat is kidney allografted and the removal of the contralateral kidney is delayed, rejection is vigorous for the grafted kidney. This occurs in situations where survival of the grafted kidney would occur if the recipient were bilaterally nephrectomized (Fi → Lew) (White *et al.*, 1969) or enhanced (BN × Lew) F_1 → Lew (Zimmerman, 1971). Mild uremia may be quite important for kidney allograft survival.

Bacterial effects

The consequences of bacterial infection may not be fully appreciated in the overall rejection response of allografted kidneys. Infectious disease may be a significant factor in the ultimate death of a kidney allografted rat. Critical experiments to evaluate the bacterial component need to be done under germ-free conditions, and are in progress in this laboratory. Skin allografts on germ-free mice rejected in times similar to conventional control animals (Smith *et al.*, 1972) and bacterial infection apparently has little effect in this instance.

COMMENTS ON MICROSURGICAL TECHNIQUE

The microsurgical technique of kidney grafting is quite simple for the experienced operator but extremely demanding for the novice. It would seem appropriate to share experiences in this area with those who may be planning to transplant rat kidneys. Rigorous repetition and practice are required to master the technique in dissection, suturing, etc. After observing several talented operators learn this technique it would appear one needs to accomplish approximately fifty successful operations before an ischemia time of 30 to 45 minutes is consistently achieved. This is important becasue of the obvious deleterious effects of poor technique on the kidney graft.

Most early investigators utilized a bladder-to-bladder anastomosis (Lee, 1967). After considerable experience with this technique and the ureter-to-ureter anastomosis (Daniller *et al.*, 1968; White *et al.*, 1969) we strongly favor the latter. The ureter-to-ureter anastomosis results in considerably less hydronephrosis and urinary calcification, and eliminates necrosis or rejection of transplanted bladder. In particular, necrosis or rejection of allografted bladder is a problem in strongly disparate combinations. Little information is available to adequately characterize the events relative to bladder rejection. It appears that bladder rejection is similar to skin rejection; a loss of epithelium with replacement by host cells and a gradual replacement or fibrosis of deeper stromal tissue (White, unpublished results).

For most studies bilateral nephrectomy at the time of allografting may be appropriate because of the rapid kidney rejection concomitant with leaving one of the host kidneys *in situ*. Finally, successful transplantation and accuracy of results are dependent on a healthy rat population. Most rat colonies are affected by chronic respiratory disease. Optimal vivarium conditions and diet are prerequisites for healthy rats and for successful kidney grafting.

SUMMARY

It would appear that enhancement, mediated by specific immunoblocking antibody, largely contributes to the prolonged survival of kidney grafts in rats. Incumbent on enhancement is specific immunologic reactivity to produce the essential immunoglobulins and specific inhibition to prevent rejection of the graft. Several hypotheses have been offered to explain the mechanism of enhancement, and are discussed elsewhere in this text. Central blocking probably occurs by curtailment of cell mediated immunity through T lymphocyte series and/or by inhibiting cytotoxic IgM antibody production through the B lymphocyte series. Peripheral blocking is equally plausible and may not necessarily be mutually exclusive with central blocking. Enhancing antibody may preferentially bind to antigenic sites and protect the graft from cell mediated immunity or cytotoxic antibody. None of these hypotheses adequately explain the disparate survival of kidney and skin allografts. Probably a combination of many factors, i.e. differential antigenicity, vulnerability, uremia, bacterial, account for these events. Some of these factors have been discussed; others are as yet unknown. Further characterization of immunoblocking antibodies will encourage their use in the clinical practice of kidney transplantation whether or not the mechanisms of action are completely understood.

References

Batchelor, J. R., Shumak, K. H. and Watts, H. G. (1973). ^{125}I-labeled rat transplantation alloantibody. II. Studies on antibody identity and comparative antigen site numbers per cell. *Transplantation*, **15,** 80

Bildsøe, P., Ford, W. L., Pettirossi, O. and Simonsen, M. (1971). GVH analysis of organ-grafted rats which defy the normal rules for rejection. *Transplantation*, **12,** 189

Bildsøe, P., Sorensen, S. F., Pettirossi, O. and Simonsen, M. (1970). Heart and kidney transplantation from segregating hybrid to parental rats. *Transplant. Rev.*, **3**, 36

Cantrell, J. L. and Hildemann, W. H. (1972). Characteristics of disparate histocompatibility barriers in congenic strains of mice. *Transplantation*, **14**, 761

Chavez-Peon, F., Monchik, G., Winn, H. J. and Russell, P. S. (1971). Humoral factors in experimental renal allograft and xenografts rejection. *Transplant. Proc.*, **3**, 573

Cho, S. I., Marcus, F. S. and Kountz, S. L. (1972). A model for study of allograft rejection in the rat: use of skin with an intact vascular pedicle. I. Effects of vascularity on allograft survival. *Transplantation*, **13**, 486

Daniller, A., Buchholz, R. and Chase, R. A. (1968). Renal transplantation in rats with the use of microsurgical techniques: A new method. *Surgery*, **64**, 956

de Bono, D. P. (1972). Host repopulation of endothelium in human kidney transplants. *Transplantation*, **14**, 438

Enomoto, K. and Lucas, Z. J. (1973). Immunological enhancement of renal allografts in the rat. III. Rôle of the spleen. *Transplantation*, **15**, 8

Fisher, B. and Lee, S. (1965). Microvascular surgical techniques in research, with special reference to renal transplantation in rats. *Surgery*, **58**, 904

Freeman, J. S. and Steinmuller, D. (1969). Acute rejection of skin and heart allografts in rats matched at the major rat histocompatibility locus. *Transplantation*, **8**, 530

French, M. E. and Batchelor, J. R. (1969). Immunological enhancement of rat kidney grafts. *Lancet*, **2**, 1103

French, M. E. (1972). The early effects of alloantibody and complement on rat kidney allografts. *Transplantation*, **13**, 447

French, M. E., Batchelor, J. R. and Watts, H. G. (1971). The capacity of lymphocytes from rats bearing enhanced kidney allografts to mount graft-versus-host reactions. *Transplantation*, **12**, 45

Gittes, R. F., Kastin, A. J., Groff, D. B. and Ketcham, A. S. (1964). Deficiency of effective histocompatibility antigens in pituitary and parathyroid tissue. *Surg. Forum*, **15**, 154

Guttmann, R. D., Lindquist, R. R., Parker, R. M., Carpenter, C. B. and Merrill, J. P. (1967). Renal transplantation in the inbred rat. I. Morphologic, immunologic, and functional alterations during acute rejection. *Transplantation*, **5**, 668

Heslop, B. F. (1971). Spontaneous deceleration of skin allograft rejection in the rat. *Transplantation*, **11**, 497

Hildemann, W. H. (1973). The weaker the histoincompatibility, the greater the effectiveness of specific immunoblocking antibodies. *Transplantation*, **15**, 221

Hildemann, W. H. and Cohen, N. (1967). *Histocompatibility Testing 1967*, p. 13

(E. S. Curtoni, P. L. Mattiuz and R. M. Tosi, editors). Copenhagen: Munksgaard

Hume, D. M., Merrill, J. P., Miller, B. F. and Thorn, G. W. (1955). Experiences with renal homotransplantation in the human: report of 9 cases. *J. Clin. Invest.*, **34,** 327

Ippolito, R. J., Mahoney, R. J. and Murray, I. M. (1972). Renal transplantation between histoincompatible rats. I. Acute rejection and prolonged survival of reciprocal renal allografts in immunocompetent rats. *Transplantation*, **14,** 183

Jones, J. V., Hamblin, T. J., Margree, G. and Moore, B. (1972). Leucocyte alloantigens in the kidney. *Transplantation*, **14,** 29

Kawabe, K., Guttmann, R. D., Levin, B., Merrill, J. P. and Lindquist, R. R. (1972). Renal transplantation in the inbred rat. XVIII. Effect of cyclophosphamide on acute rejection and long survival of recipients. *Transplantation*, **13,** 21

Lee, S. (1967). An improved technique of transplantation in the rat. *Surgery*, **61,** 771

Linder, D. E. A. (1962). Further studies on the state of unresponsiveness against skin homografts, induced in adult mice of certain genotypes by a previous ovarian homograft. *Immunology*, **5,** 195

Mahabir, R. N., Guttmann, R. D. and Lindquist, R. R. (1969). Renal transplantation in the inbred rat. X. A model of 'weak histocompatibility' by major locus matching. *Transplantation*, **8,** 369

Mullen, Y. and Hildemann, W. H. (1971). Kidney transplantation genetics and enhancement in rats. *Transplant. Proc.*, **3,** 669

Mullen, Y. and Hildemann, W. H. (1972). X- and Y-linked transplantation antigens in rats. *Transplantation*, **13,** 521

Mullen, Y., Takasugi, M. and Hildemann, W. H. (1973). The immunologic status of rats with long-surviving (enhanced) kidney allografts. *Transplantation*, **15,** 238

Nirmul, G., Severin, C. and Taub, R. N. (1972). Adaptation of skin allografts in mice treated with antilymphocyte serum. *Transplantation*, **13,** 27

Palm, J. (1971). Classification of inbred strains for Ag-B histocompatibility antigens. *Transplant. Proc.*, **3,** 1965

Sakai, A. (1969). Antigenicity of skin and kidney in the rat as studied in the transplantation model. *Transplantation*, **8,** 882

Salaman, J. R. (1968). Renal transplantation between two strains of rats. *Nature (London)*, **220,** 930

Salaman, J. R., Elves, M. W. and Festenstein, H. (1971). Factors contributing to survival of rats transplanted with kidneys mismatched at major locus. *Transplant. Proc.*, **3,** 577

Sanderson, A. R., Gelfand, E. W. and Rosen, F. S. (1972). A change in HL-A phenotype associated with a specific blocking factor in the serum of an infant with

severe combined immunodeficiency disease. *Transplantation*, **13,** 142
Smith, C. S., Pilgrim, H. I. and Steinmuller, D. (1972). The survival of skin allografts and xenografts in germ-free mice. *Transplantation*, **13,** 38
Štark, O., Kren, V. and Günther, E. (1971). RtH-1 antigens in 39 rat strains and six congenic lines. *Transplant. Proc.*, **3,** 165
Stuart, F. P., Saitoh, T. and Fitch, F. W. (1968). Rejection of renal allografts: specific immunologic suppression. *Science*, **160,** 1463
Stuart, F. P., Fitch, F. W., Rowley, D. A., Biesecker, J. L., Hellström, K. E. and Hellström, I. (1971). Presence of both cell-mediated immunity and serum-blocking factors in rat renal allografts 'enhanced' by passive immunization. *Transplantation*, **12,** 331
Thoenes, G. H., White, E. and Hildemann, W. H. (1969). Alloantibodies against weaker histocompatability antigens. *Fed. Proc.*, **28,** 379
Thoenes, G. H., White, E. and Hildemann, W. H. (1970). Alloantibodies induced by weaker histocompatability antigens in rats. *J. Immunol.*, **104,** 1447
Thoenes, G. H. and White, E. (1973). Enhancement induced specific non-reactivity in experimental kidney transplantation. *Transplantation*, **15,** 308
Virolainen, M., Hayry, P. and Defendi. V. Effect of presensitization on the mixed lymphocyte reaction of rat spleen cell cultures. *Transplantation*, **8,** 179
White, E. and Hildemann, W. H. (1968). Allografts in genetically defined rats: difference in survival between kidney and skin. *Science*, **162,** 1293
White, E. and Hildemann, W. H. (1969). Kidney versus skin allograft reactions in normal adult rats of inbred strains. *Transplant. Proc.*, **1,** 395
White, E., Hildemann, W. H. and Mullen, Y. (1969). Chronic kidney allograft reactions in rats. *Transplantation*, **8,** 602
White, E. (Unpublished results)
Williams, G. M., Krajewski, C. A., Dagher, F. J., ter Haar, A. M., Roth, J. A. and Santos, G. W. (1971). Host repopulation of endothelium. *Transplant. Proc.*, **3,** 869
Woodruff, M. F. A. (1952). The transplantation of homologous tissue and its surgical applications. *Ann. Royal Coll. Surg. Eng.*, **11,** 173
Zimmerman, E. (1971). Active enhancement of renal allografts. *Transplant. Proc.*, **3,** 701

11
New Possibilities for Organ Allografting in the Mouse

Robert J. Corry and Paul S. Russell

INTRODUCTION

It is now firmly established that the most important factor governing the long-term survival of living cells transferred from one mammal to another of the same species is the degree of immunogenetic disparity between donor and recipient. Thus, the existence of highly inbred strains, of which all of the members are isohistogenic with one another, has been a weapon of major proportions to the transplantation biologist. Only by the use of inbred strains of animals is it possible to construct experiments in which donors and recipients differ from one another by precisely the same degree in repeated experiments. Inbred strains of several species have now been developed, including the mouse, rat, hamster, guinea pig, and rabbit (Billingham and Silvers, 1959) and efforts are well advanced to produce increasingly inbred dogs. Nevertheless, the process or characterization of inbred strains is much more advanced in the mouse than in any other species as a consequence of much careful work by many investigators over the last four decades. For the work which we will report in brief in this chapter, we have depended most heavily upon the achievements of Dr. George Snell and his colleagues who have developed highly inbred strains of mice which differ from one another by no more than single antigenic specificities of varying strength, termed 'coisogenic' strains. These strains of mice, especially those which are coisogenic with one another, have therefore offered opportunities for designing experiments in transplantation which are not possible in any other species. It is not surprising that the mouse has been used very extensively as an experimental animal in cellular immunology, and many tissues of various types have been grafted between mice by

---

This work was supported by grants AI-06320 and AM-07055 from the United States Public Health Service.

free transfer of bits of tissue which must survive on the basis of establishing a blood supply from small vessels in the graft bed. This type of vascularization is commonly achieved by skin grafts placed onto an open wound prepared for them or by small pieces of endocrine or other tissue freely implanted into an appropriate site in the recipient (Russell, 1961). Thus, in the past, extensive experiments have been performed with mice in which all sorts of free grafts of cells and tissues have been employed including skin, bone, endocrines, and even fetal or newborn heart implants (Judd and Trentin, 1971a, b), as well as infusions of suspensions of living cells. Because of technical limitations on the construction of anastomoses of minute blood vessels, however, no systematic studies of *primarily vascularized* organ transplants have heretofore been reported in the mouse. The crucial step in the transfer of an organ which will depend upon primary vascular union with the recipient for its survival is the construction of vascular anastomoses which will remain patent in a high proportion of cases. Our techniques are simple and represent no more than a miniaturization of the methods of vascular suture used extensively by Carrel (1908) in the early years of this century. They have since been applied by many ingenious workers to progressively smaller vessels with much recent success in organ transplantation in the rat.

The purpose of this chapter will be to present brief descriptions of our techniques for the performance of primarily vascularized heart and kidney transplants in the

Table 11.1

Strains		*Organ transplanted*	*Incompatibilities involved*
Donor	*Recipient*		
B10.D2 →	B10.D2	Heart	0
$(C3 \times D2)F_1$ →	$(C3 \times D2)F_1$	Kidney	0
B10.D2 →	$(B6 \times A)F_1$	Heart and Kidney	H-2 K.31
B10.BR →	$(B6 \times A)F_1$	Heart and Kidney	H-2D.32
C57BL/10 →	$(C3 \times D2)F_1$	Kidney	H-2.2, 22, 33, 39 plus multiple non-H-2
A/J →	$(B10 \times 129)F_1$	Heart	H-2.1, 3, 4, 8, 13, 23, 25, 41, 43 plus multiple non-H-2
129 →	C57BL/10	Heart	Multiple non-H-2 only

mouse and some of the early results which have been achieved in these studies. Some of the data presented briefly in this chapter are taken from projects currently in progress, and will be presented more completely elsewhere.

The strains of mice utilized have been carefully selected for their immunogenetic relationships to one another and for their general hardiness. Most of them have already been used in a series of studies of immunological enhancement of skin graft survival in our laboratory (Jeekel *et al.*, 1971), so that much useful information, such as the duration of survival of skin grafts between normal members of the various strains, was already available. In Table 11.1 are set out the donor and recipient strains chosen for these experiments, and the incompatibilities involved in each combination.

TRANSPLANTATION OF THE MOUSE HEART

We have recently perfected a technique for the transplantation of the mouse heart to a heterotopic position in the recipient's abdomen by primary vascular anastomosis, in a fashion similar to that described by Ono and Lindsey (1969) in the rat. Mann *et al.* (1933) was the first to describe the circulation of such an auxiliary heart transplant in the neck of a dog. By union of the aorta of the transplant to a major artery of the host, oxygenated blood perfuses the coronary vessels and then drains into the right heart where it is then ejected into the host's venous circulation via the pulmonary artery. Barker *et al.* (1971) has transplanted the rat heart to its recipient's abdomen to study the ability of donor strain lymph node cells to induce tolerance to a primarily vascularized heart transplant. The cardiac impulse of the transplant can be palpated easily in its abdominal location and its intensity graded on a daily basis. The success of this operation depends upon the immediate return to a normal sinus rhythm of the transplanted heart (see below).

Technique of heterotopic heart transplantation in the mouse

Donor and recipient mice are anesthetized with a single intraperitoneal injection of chloral hydrate. The ventral surface of the abdomen and chest is shaved and then cleansed with 70% alcohol. Under × 16 magnification, a 2mm segment of recipient aorta and vena cava below the renal vessels is dissected free. Usually, ligation of a single lumbar artery and vein is necessary. Proximal and distal ligatures of 6-0 silk are then placed loosely around both the aorta and vena cava. These ties will be used later for temporary vascular occlusion.

A midline abdominal incision is then made in the donor mouse and heparin is injected through its inferior vena cava. The abdominal incision is extended cephalad through a median sternotomy, and the heart is expeditiously removed, usually in 3 or 4 minutes. The inferior and superior vena cavae are ligated and transected distal to the ligatures. The aorta and pulmonary artery are divided as far distally as the first branch in the former and the bifurcation in the latter. A mass ligature is placed around the pulmonary veins which are divided distal to the ligature. The excised heart is then transferred to a vessel containing Ringer's lactate solution at 0–4 °C.

The recipient animal is placed under the microscope and the ties around the aorta and vena cava are tightened with a single knot to temporarily occlude the aorta and vena cava for construction of the anastomoses. A venotomy in the vena cava and then an aortotomy are made adjacent to one another to correspond in size with the donor aorta and pulmonary artery. The donor heart is then removed from the chilled solution and its aorta is joined in end to side fashion to the recipient aorta. Next, the donor pulmonary artery is sutured to the inferior vena cava of the recipient. To accomplish the anastomoses, 9–0 nylon sutures (Ethicon) have been used in all cases. Careful everting anastomoses must be carried out to avoid platelet aggregation and subsequent clotting at the suture lines. At the completion of the anastomoses, the ties are gradually released and recipient blood is allowed to flow into the donor aorta, thus perfusing the coronary system. Following perfusion, fibrillation and then sinus rhythm ensue. With onset of sinus rhythm, the blood in the right atrium is ejected into the right ventricle where it is then forced by contraction of the right ventricle into the recipient's inferior vena cava. After resuscitation of the transplanted heart, the abdomen is then closed and the animal is placed in a constant temperature incubator during recovery from anesthesia.

Assessment of survival and rejection of the transplanted heart

During the early stages of perfecting the technique described above, it became clear that resuscitation of the heart to a normal sinus rhythm within minutes after perfusion of the coronary vessels with oxygenated blood was essential for the survival of the transplant. If the heart transplant could not be resuscitated as a result of a prolonged period of ischemia, the heart would simply dilate and the blood within it would clot. Frequently the recipient animal would survive this event, although postoperatively an abdominal heart beat could not be felt. On reopening the abdomen of several of these animals within 24 hours, a completely arrested and dilated heart with clotted chambers and anastomoses was found. Histological studies of such hearts have shown thrombi throughout the chambers and at the anastomoses associated with variable degrees of myocardial necrosis depending upon the time interval after transplantation which had elapsed before the heart had been removed. In short, if these very small heart transplants did not resume a normal rhythm, they did not survive.

As the microvascular technique improved with experience, the ischemia time was shortened, and resuscitation of the arrested heart to fibrillation and thence to normal sinus rhythm was possible in about 90 per cent of the cases. Ischemia times of less than half an hour usually resulted in almost immediate return to a sinus rhythm following external warming and perfusion of the coronary vessels with recipient oxygenated blood. Occasionally, gentle cardiac massage with cotton applicator sticks was required to revert ventricular fibrillation to a sinus rhythm.

Abdominal palpation of the heart beat proved to be the most reliable form of assessing the activity of the transplant. Palpation of the impulse was performed daily and its intensity graded on a scale of 4 to 0. Electrocardiograms can be readily recorded from these mice when they are lightly anesthetized with ether. Figure 11.1 shows such an electrocardiogram in which two separate QRS complexes can be seen. This method of assessment of function of the transplant proves to be no more reliable than careful abdominal palpation, however, in establishing the times at which a sharp change in

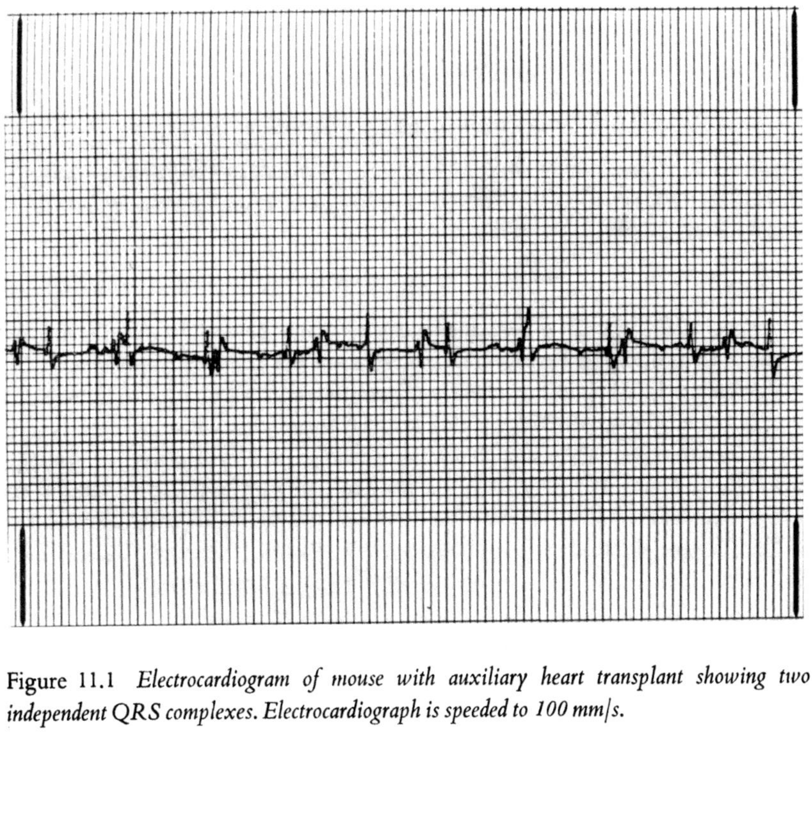

Figure 11.1 *Electrocardiogram of mouse with auxiliary heart transplant showing two independent QRS complexes. Electrocardiograph is speeded to 100 mm/s.*

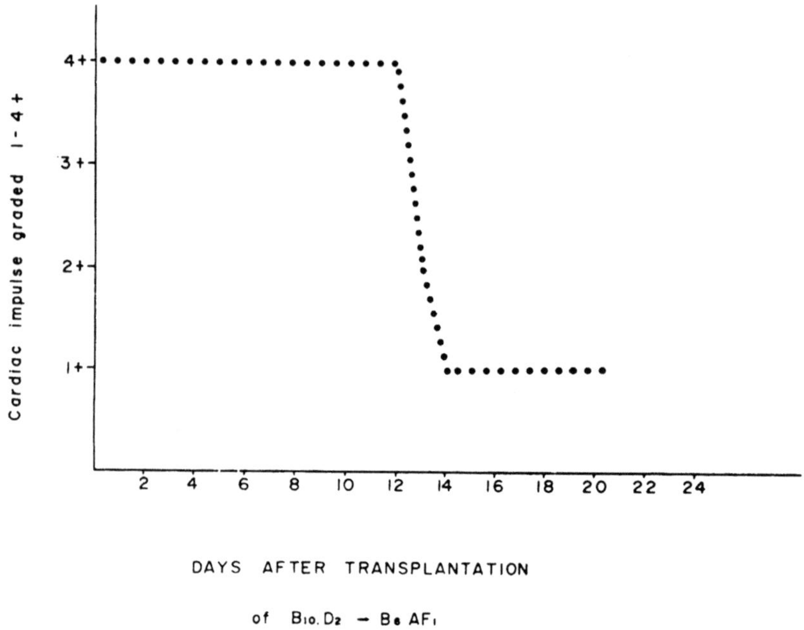

Figure 11.2 *Typical abrupt decline of intensity of cardiac impulse (rejection episode) of B10.D2 heart transplant in a B6AF1 recipient occurring over a two day period between 12 and 14 days after transplantation*

the vigor of the impulse occurs. Nevertheless, it may be useful in confirming the presence of cardiac activity when the impulse is so weak as not to be palpable.

A substantial decline in the intensity of the palpable cardiac impulse from 4 to 1 usually occurred over a 1–2 day period in an allografted heart that had been beating normally for at least a week. This abrupt decline of activity is illustrated diagrammatically in Figure 11.2. Decline of intensity of the heart beat was recorded as the initial rejection episode.

Since a precipitous alteration in the activity of cardiac allografts was regularly detectable, it is possible to compute a Median Time of Impulse Decline = (MTID) after the method of Litchfield (1949) for each group of animals studied. This MTID was thus arrived at in much the same way as the Median Survival Time of skin grafts, although we have guarded against using this same terminology for heart transplants as the observation of a decline in pulsatile activity cannot always be taken as being tantamount to the complete and irreversible death of the transplant. This point was emphasized in a particularly dramatic way in one group of animals described below in which a distinct recovery of heart transplant activity was observed after an initial period of marked reduction of the pulse.

Behavior of heart transplants between mice with well defined histoincompatibilities

The donor–recipient combinations are detailed in Table 11.1 which also includes the organ studied in each case.

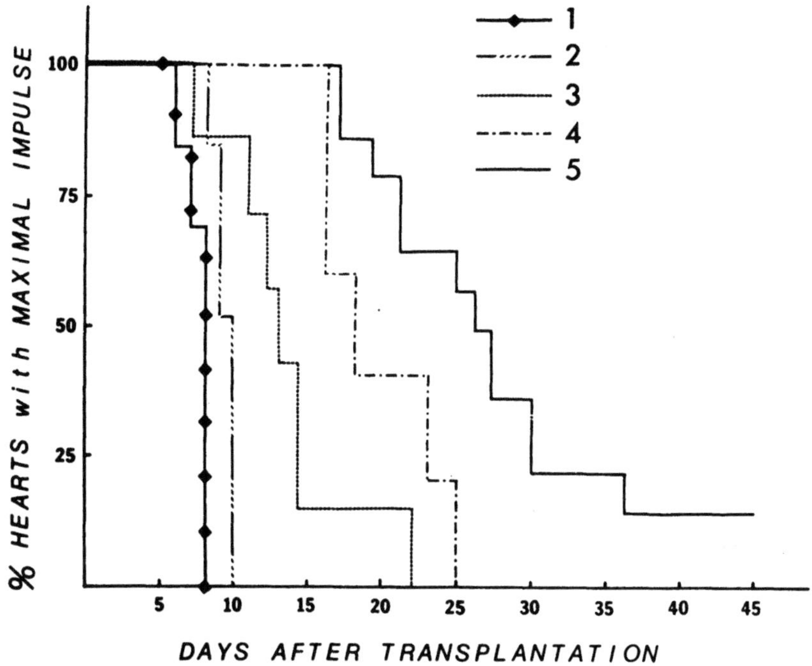

Figure 11.3 *Percentage of hearts remaining in each group with 4+ impulse. This graph shows time of cardiac impulse decline for each animal in each combination below.*

1. *A→(B10 × 129)F1 where multiple H-2 and non-H-2 differences are present*
2. *129→ C57BL/10 where only non-H-2 differences are present*
3. *B10.D2→ B6AF1 where H-2K.31 is the only incompatibility*
4. *B10.D2→ B6AF with alloantiserum given at time of transplantation (enhancing AB)*
5. *B10.BR→ B6AF1 where H-2D.32 is the only incompatibility*

Three of four isotransplant recipients have survived with heterotopic heart transplants beating normally in their abdominal location for over 11 months. The results of heart transplantation in the various combinations mentioned are diagrammatically represented in Figure 11.3, where the percentage of hearts remaining in the group with a maximal impulse (4+) is plotted at daily intervals after transplantation. When the donor hearts differed from their recipients by both D and K region H-2 antigens, all stopped beating by 8 days. All heart transplants differing from their recipients in respect only of multiple non-H-2 specificities, had a marked decline in cardiac impulse by 10 days. In the combination in which only the single H-2.31 antigen, specified by the K region of the H-2 locus, was foreign to the recipient, the MTID was 11.5 ± 1.1 days. When the D-region-derived H-2.3 antigen was the single incompatibility, the MTID was 26 ± 1.5 days.

These data clearly demonstrate that as the immunogenetic disparity decreases, the interval between transplantation and cardiac impulse decline is longer. Furthermore, when a recipient is presented with a heart transplant in which only non-H-2 antigens

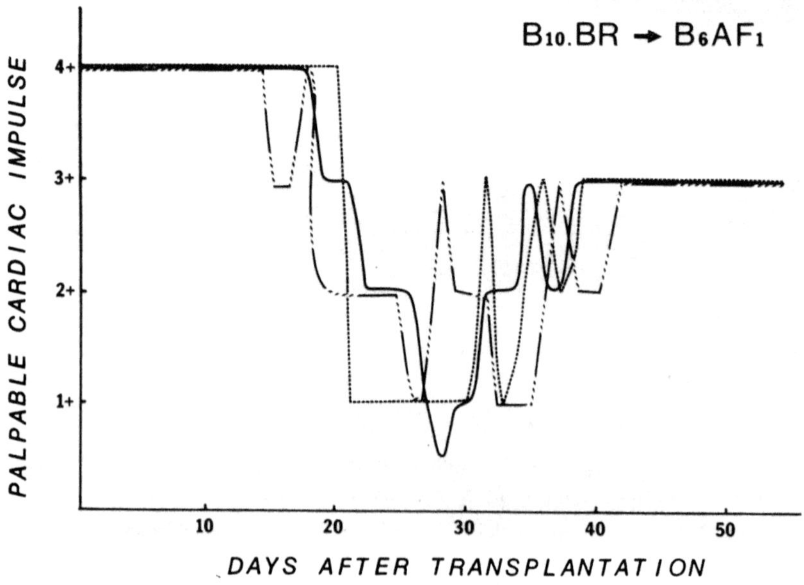

Figure 11.4 *Typical return of cardiac impulse of three heart transplants, after an initial period of marked depression, in which the H-2D.32 antigen is incompatible*

are foreign, rejection as measured by a substantial impulse decline occurs only slightly later than it does when multiple H-2 antigens are foreign to the recipient.

When a single D-region derived H-2 specificity was the only foreign antigen, there was a remarkable return of cardiac impulse after a definite initial period of decline as depicted in Figure 11.4. Two other animals in this group have shown no definite decline in intensity of impulse at all and have maintained normal palpable impulses beyond 3 months. This return of cardiac pulsation suggests that there is at least a partial recovery from the initial rejection process in this group. Once this phenomenon of recovery of impulse occurs, the heart continues pulsating normally for at least several weeks.

On histological examination, virtually no evidence of rejection was noted in the isotransplanted heart removed at three months, while a substantial mononuclear cell infiltrate was observed at the time of impulse decline in hearts with either a D or K region incompatibility. A photomicrograph of the isotransplanted heart is shown in Figure 11.5, and Figure 11.6 demonstrates the distribution of cellular infiltration in a photomicrograph of a heart with the H-2K.31 incompatibility at the time of impulse decline. Since there is a return of cardiac impulse after an initial period of decline when

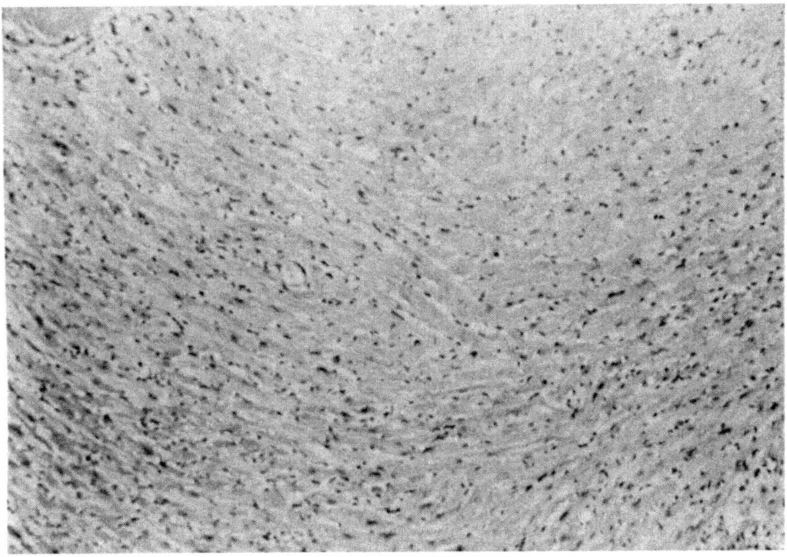

Figure 11.5 *Photomicrograph of isotransplanted heart showing no rejection. H & E × 14*

the H-2D.32 antigen is the single incompatibility, it would be interesting to demonstrate spontaneous regression of cellular rejection histologically in the same heart. An easier alternative is of course to section hearts at different times. A photomicro-

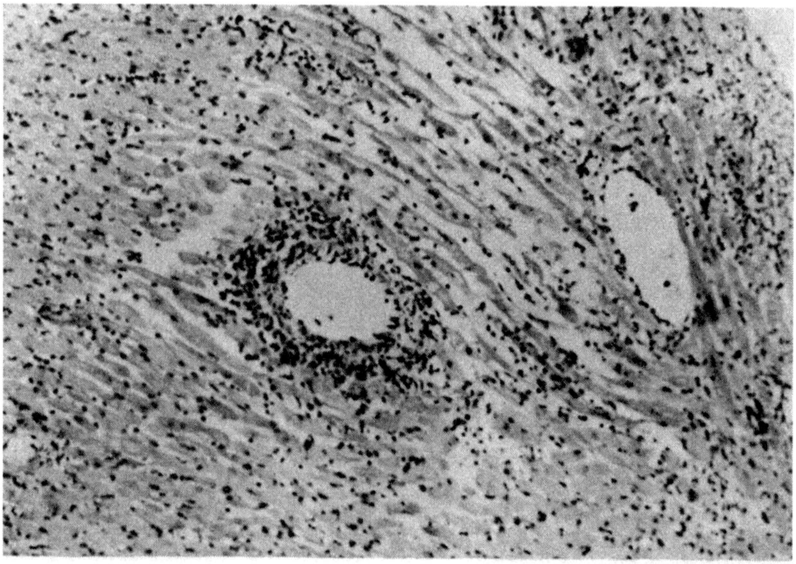

Figure 11.6 *Photomicrograph of heart transplant with H-2K.31 incompatibility 13 days after transplantation showing perivascular accumulation of lymphocytes and moderate cellular infiltration throughout the myocardium. H & E × 56*

graph of an allotransplanted heart with the D-region incompatibility, Figure 11.7, removed at 114 days after transplantation and several weeks after complete recovery of the heart beat, shows virtually no evidence of cellular rejection. All histological sections of hearts with the H-2D.32 incompatibility removed at the time of impulse decline showed cellular infiltration particularly in the subendothelial and perivascular distribution as depicted in Figure 11.8. This remarkable 'spontaneous' regression of rejection that occurs functionally and of which there is possible histological evidence will bear further investigation.

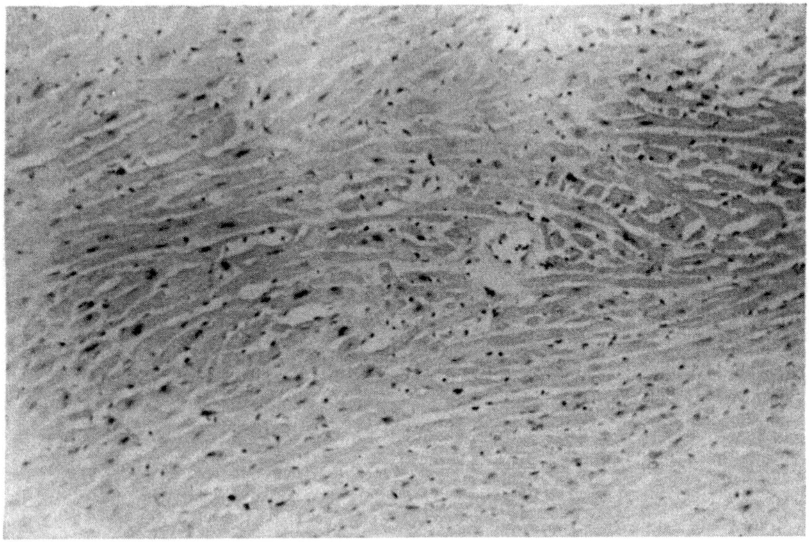

Figure 11.7 *Heart transplant with H-2D.32 incompatibility removed 114 days after transplantation and several weeks after recovery of heart beat. This section shows remarkably little cellular rejection. H & E × 35*

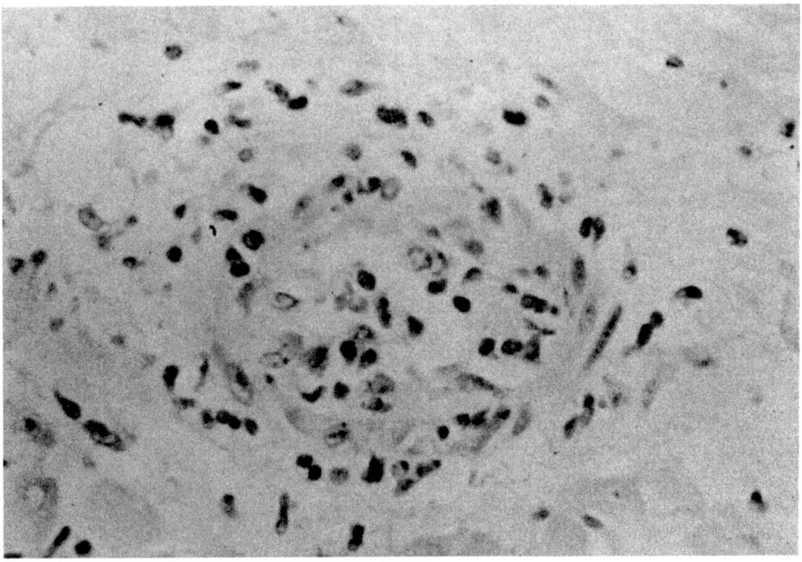

Figure 11.8 *Heart transplant with H-2D.32 incompatibility 24 days after transplantation showing cellular infiltration around vessel and in subendothelial distribution. H & E × 160*

TRANSPLANTATION OF THE MOUSE KIDNEY

A method of kidney transplantation has recently been developed in our laboratory by Skoskiewicz *et al.* (1973). This approach is based upon the method introduced by Lee (1967) for the rat, and since employed by quite a number of other investigators (Stuart *et al.*, 1968; Lindquist *et al.*, 1971; French and Batchelor, 1969). Most experiments involved bilateral host nephrectomy, such that survival of the animal depended upon the function of the transplanted kidney.

Technique of kidney transplant

Donor and recipient animals are anesthetized and dissection is carried out under the microscope as described above. A long midline incision is made in the recipient's abdomen and the left kidney is carefully removed. Short segments of aorta and vena cava are dissected free and ties are placed loosely around the vessels proximally and distally to be used later for vascular occlusion. After preparation, the recipient animal is placed aside and the donor animal's left kidney, ureter, and bladder are mobilized. Ties are placed around the aorta, proximal to and distal to the renal artery, such that *in situ* perfusion with chilled Ringer's lactate solution can be accomplished. The perfused kidney, with a patch of aorta, a patch of vena cava, and a segment of bladder, is removed and placed in chilled Ringer's lactate solution. End to side vascular anastomoses are accomplished between the donor and recipient aorta and the donor and recipient vena cava. Ties around the vena cava and aorta are gradually released and perfusion of the transplant begins. The donor ureter with its attached patch of bladder is passed behind the vas deferens, and the small bladder patch is then sutured to an opening in the dome of the recipient bladder. Contralateral nephrectomy may be added to the procedure. A diagrammatic illustration of the completed transplant is shown in Figure 11.9.

Assessment of survival of transplanted kidney

If bilateral nephrectomy accompanies orthotopic kidney transplantation, kidney transplant survival can be assessed on the basis of survival of the host. However, function can also be determined at intervals with some sensitivity by several other methods. Blood urea nitrogen and creatinine values can be determined in the bilaterally nephrectomized recipients as well as inulin clearances. In the transplant recipient which retains one of its own kidneys, histological examination of biopsies and intravenous pyelograph (IVP) have been used to assess rejection and function of the transplanted kidney.

Accordingly, it is clear that frequent assessment of the function of a kidney trans-

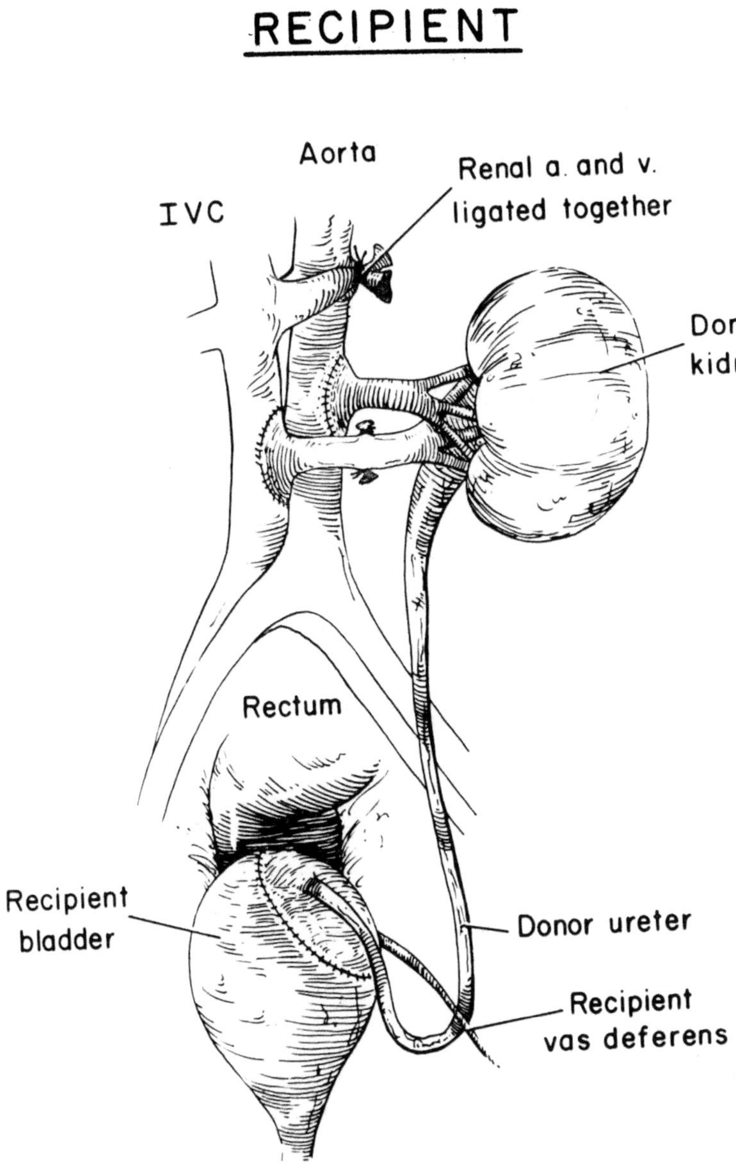

Figure 11.9 *Diagrammatic illustration of the anatomic arrangement at the completion of a kidney transplant in the mouse*

plant in the mouse is somewhat more difficult than for a heterotopic heart transplant, since cardiac function can be estimated simply by palpation.

Results of kidney transplantation

The results in the four groups of animals studied thus far in our laboratory are outlined in Table 11.2. All of these animals underwent bilateral nephrectomies at the time of transplantation.

Table 11.2

Donor–recipient combinations	*Incompatibilities*	*Skin graft survival ± S.D.*	*Number of animals*	*Days recipient survived after kidney transplant*
$C3 \times D2F_1$ ↓ $C3 \times D2F_1$	None		4	100 (s), 115 (s), 45 (s), 70 (s)
B10.BR ↓ $B6AF_1$	H-2.32	16.5 ± 1.1	6	59, 222, 227, 240 (s), 248 (s), 336 (s)
C57BL/6 ↓ $C3 \times D2F_1$	H-2.2, 22, 33, 39 plus multiple non-H-2	10.7 ± 0.47	11	26, 26, 34, 35 (s), 40, 44, 54, 55, 59, 59, 77, 130
B10.D2 ↓ $B6AF_1$	H-2.31	10.7 ± 1.1	5	42 (s), 193, 316, 382 (s), 390 (s)

s = sacrificed

The four recipients of isotransplants were sacrificed at the times designated in Table 11.2. These kidneys appeared normal on gross inspection and histological examination revealed no evidence of rejection.

Four of five B6AF1 recipients which received B10.D2 kidneys survived indefinitely. Some transplants between individuals of these two strains were performed expressly to obtain histological material in optimal condition. Thus, transplanted kidneys were available for histological study at various intervals from 5 days to over a year after transplantation. Briefly summarized, long surviving allografts showed, in general, less evidence of rejection activity than those kidneys examined shortly after transplantation. In the first 2 weeks, early cellular rejection was seen, and a number of migratory cells staining with methyl green pyronin could be identified.

In the B10.BR to B6AF1 donor–recipient combination, recipients in five out of six cases survived longer than 200 days. The kidney of one recipient, sacrificed at 59 days, showed moderate rejection activity. Two other recipients, sacrificed at 240 and 248 days, and having blood urea nitrogen values of 58 and 66 mg per cent respectively, showed evidence of chronic rejection and mild hydronephrosis.

In the last group in which there were multiple H-2 and non-H-2 incompatibilities, survival for as long as 77 days in one case was considered remarkably long for this degree of histoincompatibility. Microscopic changes typical of rejection were seen in all specimens from the animals in this group.

These experiments demonstrate that the survival of kidney transplants in mice is unexpectedly long. Even when multiple strong histoincompatibilities are present, survival is much longer than that of skin grafts in the same genetic combination (see Table 11.2).

Differences between heart and kidney allografts in the mouse

Kidney transplants survive longer than heart transplants in the same genetic combinations in mice. For example, the MTID of hearts in the group of animals in which the H-2.31 antigen is foreign, occurs much earlier than one can detect any decline of kidney transplant function across the same immunogenetic barrier. Both of these primarily vascularized allografts in the mouse are capable of eliciting the formation of specific humoral antibody. Thus, both have sensitized their recipients. Still, neither the presence nor the titer of measurable antibody appears to correlate in any obvious way with the length of survival of either organ.

An explanation of the difference in length of survival between heart and kidney transplants might be related to the fact that functional impairment of the respective organs is not necessarily related directly to the local intensity of the immune response. For example, if the initial rejection episode is sufficiently disruptive to the transplanted heart to produce cardiac arrest, subsequent recovery is not possible because of secondary factors such as clotting of blood in the chambers and coronary vessels. However, the kidney might continue to function sufficiently to maintain the animal physiologically even in the face of a rejection reaction of similar magnitude. Some support for this possibility may be found in the observation of almost complete recovery of the cardiac impulse that is noted in some heart transplants in which a substantial decline of impulse has occurred but the impairment stops short of arrest.

The mechanism for the recovery of function in the transplanted hearts in which H-2.32 was the incompatibility, and for the prolonged function of kidney transplants in the same combination, could be by some form of autoenhancement. We know from the previous work of Jeekel *et al.* (1971) with skin grafts, and our own work (Corry *et al.*, 1973) with heart allografts, that survival of skin grafts and heart transplants in which there is an H-2.31 difference is capable of being enhanced by the passive administration of alloantiserum. Obviously, in the case of the heart transplants, if rejection produces arrest (as it does with strong or multiple antigen differences) neither autoenhancement nor passively administered antibody could restore the heart beat.

CONCLUSION

Since it has been shown that primarily vascularized organ allografts can be carried out with a high level of success in mice, the range of possible studies of transplants in this species has been considerably extended. In the future, the techniques of microsurgery can be joined with the knowledge of immunogenetics in the mouse to carefully analyze in full the immunological processes which take place with various primarily vascularized organ transplants. Furthermore, these techniques will also make possible the study of primarily vascularized xenografts in small animals.

References

Barker, C. F., Lubaroff, D. M. and Silvers, W. K. (1971). Lymph node cells: their differential capacity to induce tolerance of heart and skin homografts in rats. *Science*, **172,** 1050

Billingham, R. E. and Silvers, W. K. (1959). Inbred animals and tissue transplantation immunity. *Transplant. Bull.*, **6,** 399

Carrel, A. (1908). Results of the transplantation of blood vessels, organs, and limbs. *J. Amer. Med. Assn.*, **51,** 1662

Corry, R. J., Winn, H. J. and Russell, P. S. (1973). Heart transplantation in congenic strains of mice. *Transplant. Proc.*, **5,** 733.

French, M. E. and Batchelor, J. R. (1969). Immunological enhancement of rat kidney grafts. *Lancet*, **2,** 1103

Jeekel, J. J., McKenzie, I. F. C., Winn, H. J. (1971). Immunological enhancement of skin grafts in the mouse. *J. Immunology*, **108,** 1017

Judd, K. P. and Trentin, J. J. (1971a). Cardiac transplantation in mice. I. *Transplantation*, **11,** 298

Judd, K. P. and Trentin, J. J. (1971b). Cardiac transplantation in mice. II. *Transplantation*, **11,** 303

Lee, S. (1967). An improved technique of renal transplantation in the rat. *Surgery*, **61,** 771

Lindquist, R. R., Guttmann, R. D. and Merrill, J. P. (1971). Renal transplantation in the inbred rat. *Transplantation*, **11,** 1

Litchfield, J. T. (1949). A method for rapid graphic solution of time–per cent effect curves. *J. Pharmacol. Exp. Ther.*, **97,** 399

Mann, F. C., Priestly, J. T., Markowitz, J. and Yater, W. (1933). Transplantation of the intact mammalian heart. *Arch. Surg.*, **26,** 219

Ono, K. and Lindsey, E. S. (1969). Improved technique of heart transplantation in rats. *J. Thorac. Cardiovasc. Surg.*, **57,** 225

Russell, P. S. (1961). Endocrine grafting techniques. In *Transplantation of Tissues and Cells*, p. 35 (R. E. Billingham and W. K. Silvers, editors). Philadelphia: The Wistar Institute Press

Skoskiewicz, M., Chase, C., Winn, H. J. and Russell, P. S. (1973). Kidney transplants between mice of graded immunogenetic diversity. *Transplant. Proc.*, **5,** 721

Stuart, F. D., Saitoh, T., Fitch, F. and Spargo, B. H. (1968). Immunologic enhancement of renal allografts in the rat. *Surgery*, **64,** 17

12
Allografting in the Pig

R. Y. Calne

In the pig as in all other species so far studied, there is a spectrum of susceptibility to rejection of different tissues. Grafts of skin, heart, kidney and liver have been studied, and the speed and vigor of rejection is greatest for skin and least for the liver. The behavior of liver allografts is so different from that of skin that a biological principle of potential importance may be involved. Hundreds of skin grafts between related and unrelated pigs have always been rejected by 2 weeks. Two patterns of skin graft destruction have been observed—usually grafts begin to break down at 5 or 6 days

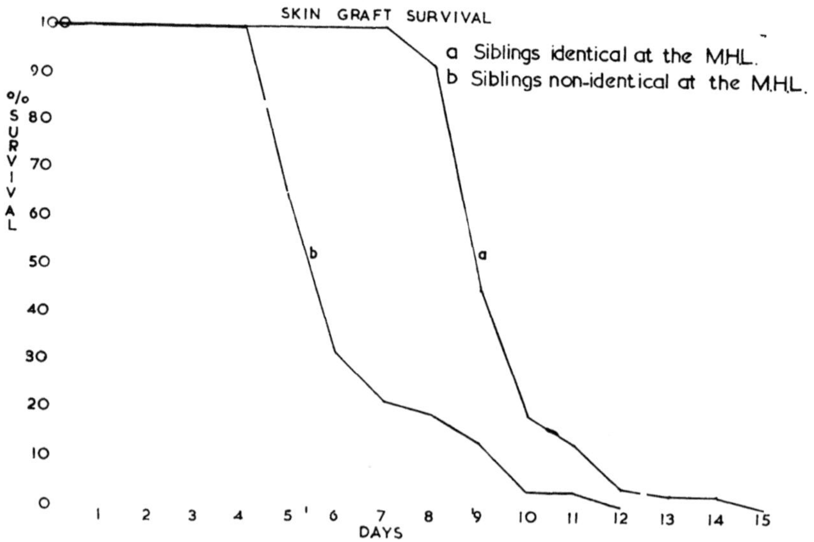

Figure 12.1 *Skin graft survival between littermates. Grafts between siblings identical at the major histocompatibility locus last some 5 days longer than those that are incompatible. 100 grafts were between identical siblings and 41 between non-identical*

but occasionally the process is delayed to 10 days (Binns, 1967a; Binns, 1968; White *et al.*, 1973a). Now that tissue typing with lymphocytotoxic antisera (Vaiman *et al.*, 1970a; White and Binns, 1973b) and mixed lymphocyte culture (MLC) (Viza *et al.*, 1970; Vaiman *et al.*, 1970b; Bradley *et al.*, 1972) in the pig are available it has been shown that the early type of skin graft rejection occurs in major locus incompatibility, and is usually followed by the appearance of lymphocytotoxic serum antibody. The slower rejection pattern occurs in donor recipient combinations that are identical or relatively compatible at the major locus and detectable serum antibody is not produced (Figure 12.1). Long-term survival of porcine skin allografts followed intrafetal injection of donor bone marrow to induce classical tolerance (Binns, 1967a; Binns, 1968). Tolerance was not always complete, but it was of interest that a pig which rejected its skin graft after 56 days, subsequently accepted a kidney from the same donor without any stigmata of rejection (Binns *et al.*, 1970) and another rejecting its skin graft at 111 days carried an ovary transplant for 15 months without rejection (Binns *et al.*, 1967b).

Both heterotopic and orthotopic cardiac allografts are usually rejected rapidly in the pig (Calne *et al.*, 1969; Childe and Morris, 1969; Cullum *et al.*, 1970) but we have recently observed prolonged survival of an unimmunosuppressed pig with an orthotopic heart allograft from a litter-mate donor. There are less data available than for skin grafts, the pattern of rejection would seem to be similar, but at a less aggressive pace than with skin.

Porcine kidney grafts are usually destroyed within 10 days, but occasional long term survivals have been reported (Calne *et al.*, 1969; Terblanche *et al.*, 1973). In our laboratory, a study has been made of serological histocompatibility testing in the pig and MLC reactions. Lymphocytotoxic alloantisera raised in pigs by skin grafting have detected antigens which segregation studies have shown to be the products of a single genetic locus (Vaiman, 1970a; White *et al.*, 1973a; White and Binns, 1973b). This locus appears to be analogous with the human HLA and murine H-2 systems (Figure 12.2). Familial segregation similar to that observed with alloantisera has been obtained using the MLC technique (Viza *et al.*, 1970; Vaiman *et al.*, 1970b; Bradley *et al.*, 1972) suggesting that the genetic controls for MLC stimulation are closely linked to the locus controlling the serologically detectable antigens. Independently the MLC locus was named PLA (Viza *et al.*, 1970) and the cytotoxic locus SLA (Vaiman *et al.*, 1970a). Subsequently, they have been shown to be part of the same major locus (Vaiman *et al.*, 1970b; Bradley *et al.*, 1973b). Renal allografts between littermate pigs were rejected between 10 and 38 days after grafting in animals where the donor–recipient combination showed serological mismatch and positive MLC. Where donor and recipient littermates had identical serological tests and where there

A LITTER SEGREGATED USING LYMPHOCYTOTOXIC ALLOANTISERA

LFM x 2267
AB CD

PIG NO.	A 14	B 8	B 15	B 16	C 1	C 2	C 3	C 4	C 5	D 12	D 13	HAPLOTYPE
58	+	-	-	-	+	+	+	+	+	-	-	A C
59	+	-	-	-	-	-	-	-	-	+	+	A D
60	+	-	-	-	-	-	-	-	-	+	+	
65	+	-	-	-	-	-	-	-	-	+	+	
66	+	-	-	-	-	-	-	-	-	+	+	
61	-	+	+	+	+	+	+	+	+	-	-	B C
62	-	+	+	+	+	+	+	+	+	-	-	
63	-	+	+	+	-	-	-	-	-	+	+	B D
64	-	+	+	+	-	-	-	-	-	+	+	
67	-	+	+	+	-	-	-	-	-	+	+	

Figure 12.2 *A litter segregated using lymphocytotoxic alloantisera. The pattern of segregation is analogous to the human HLA and murine H-2 systems*

Table 12.1 *Renal allograft survival in serologically typed pigs. Rejection is indicated by minus or plus signs, — being no rejection, + slight rejection, ++ moderate rejection, and +++ marked rejection*

Serological disparity	*No. of transplants*	*Pig survival time in days*					
Haplotypes unrelated	2	14+++	14+++				
1 Haplotype siblings	12	2—	4—	4—	4—	6—	6—
		8+++	8+++	10+++	11++	22+++	54+++
Haplotype identical siblings	16	1—	3—	4(+)	6+	14—	16(+)
		26+	48(+)	>84	>84	>85	>85
		>113	>203	>288	>399	>490	

was no MLC reaction, rejection failed to occur by 150 days in all cases (Bradley *et al.*, 1972 and 1973a; White *et al.*, 1973a). Vaiman *et al.* (1972) have shown a correlation of long survival of renal and intestinal allografts in serologically typed pigs receiving their grafts from compatible littermates. Our observations on serologically typed pigs with renal allografts are similar (Table 12.1; Figure 12.3). In experiments where serology and MLC testing gave different predictions, the results were as follows:

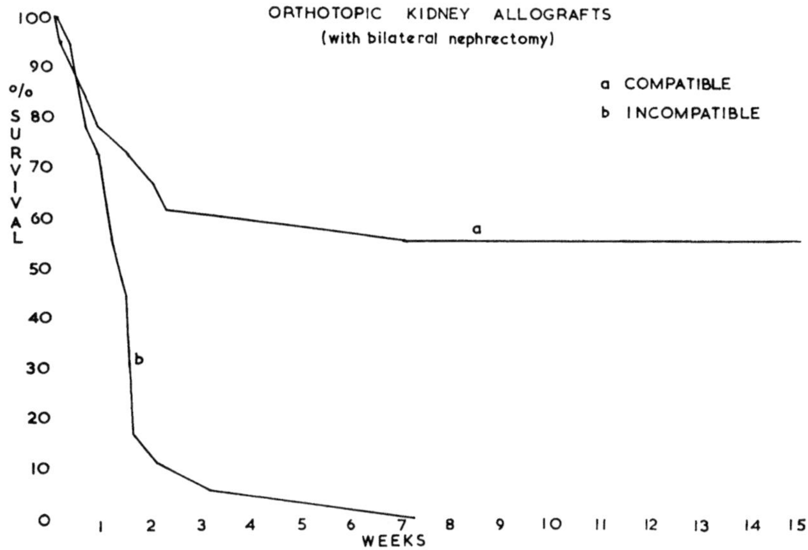

Figure 12.3 *Survival of pigs with orthotopic kidney allografts following bilateral nephrectomy. (a) animals that were serologically compatible; (b) animals that were serologically incompatible. In both cases the donors were siblings. 16 transplants were between identical siblings and 12 between siblings differing by one haplotype*

An allograft was accepted by a littermate which was compatible by serology (i.e. there were no antigens in the donor that were not present in the recipient) and mismatched with its donor by MLC testing. There was no sign of rejection at 300 days. The MLC test became significantly reduced to donor cells post-operatively but retained normal reactivity to cells of another genotype. Two other allografts with similar typing results were rejected at 71 and 148 days. Three kidneys grafted from littermate donors that were identical by MLC but differed in serologically defined antigens began to reject 10 weeks after grafting (Bradley *et al.*, 1973a) (Table 12.2). In marked contrast to these observations is the regular rejection in 8–12 days of skin grafts between littermate pigs shown to be identical by both MLC and serological testing (Figure 12.1).

Table 12.2 *Survival of renal allografts between pigs typed both by mixed lymphocyte reaction and serologically. Figures in brackets indicate deaths due to causes other than rejection. The donors in each case were littermates of the recipients*

MLR	*Serol.*	*Survival (days)*						
–	–	(10, 27)	152★	170★	208★	208★	209★	365★
+	+	(2, 5, 7, 13)	10	13	16	38		
+	(–)		71	148	330★			
–	+	(4, 6, 7)	68	85	98★			

( ) Death from causes other than rejection
★Still alive

RELEVANCE OF MLC PHENOTYPING

There is increasing evidence in man that the genes determining stimulation in the MLC tests and the genes determining serologically defined lymphocyte antigens are on the same chromosome but at separate loci. They should, therefore, be assessed independently since the degree of polymorphism at the two loci may be very different. In the pig, methods were developed for phenotyping unrelated individuals by the MLC test (Bradley *et al.*, 1973b). It was shown that one genetic locus or a number of closely linked loci control this reaction (Bradley *et al.*, 1972 and 1973b). By using segregation studies in family groups and homozygous individuals as markers for the MLC genes, individuals were typed for histocompatibility (Figures 12.4 and 12.5). When the serological antigenic profiles were compared with the MLC genotypes, marked differences were found. The degree of polymorphism in the MLC appeared much less than for the serologically defined antigens in the pig herd as a whole.

Furthermore, the same MLC genes were detectable in unrelated animals, even between large white and landrace strains (Bradley *et al.*, 1973b).

Similar methods for MLC phenotyping have yet to be developed for man. Hitherto it was assumed that the MLC test and the HLA reactions were controlled by the same genes because they segregated together within families just as they do in the pig. Unrelated individuals never fitted in with this concept since MLC negative reactions are extremely rare in unrelated HLA identical individuals. MLC phenotyping may be more relevant to renal allograft survival in man, particularly in those HLA mismatched individuals who tolerate kidneys exceptionally well (Cochrum *et al.*, 1973).

The pattern of rejection of renal allografts in the pig is different from man and the dog but may have similarities with the behavior of renal allografts in the rat. It has been reported that immunosuppression of the pig by conventional agents can produce

RESPONDER	STIMULATOR	GENE DOSE	M L R.
1/1	1/1	0	-
1/2	1/1	0	-
1/1	1/2	1	+
1/2	2/3	1	+
1/1	2/3	2	+ +
2/3	1/1	2	+ +

Figure 12.4 *Theoretical plan by which segregation studies were performed in family groups to investigate the mixed lymphocyte reaction genotypes showing that non-responsiveness can occur in two ways: first, when the individuals are identical, and second, when the stimulator cells are homozygous for a gene which is also present in the responder. This is similar to the interaction between parents and F_1 hybrids, so the reaction is negative only when the homozygote acts as a stimulator. The converse reaction, when a homozygote acts as responder, is always positive. Quantitative differences in MLR reflect a gene dosage from 0 to 1 and 2*

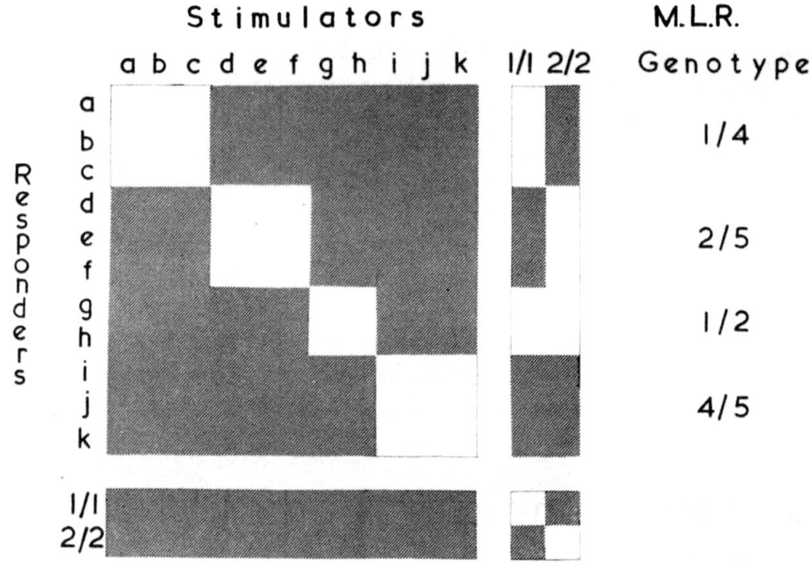

Figure 12.5 *Results of a study to investigate mixed lymphocyte reaction genotypes. Positive one-way reaction of responder against stimulator is shown by the shaded areas. 11 siblings were examined. These are marked from a to k. The segregation pattern shows four groups of individuals the members of which failed to stimulate or respond to other members of their respective groups. All other reactions between the groups were positive. This suggests that the MLR is controlled by a single genetic locus in the pig.*

prolonged survival of renal allografts fairly consistently (Perper *et al.*, 1971). The fact remains, however, that unimmunosuppressed pigs usually reject aggressively kidneys from mismatched unrelated donors (Figure 12.6).

Orthotopic porcine liver allografts frequently survive indefinitely without any immunosuppressive treatment. We have studied this experimental model for five years and our findings can be summarized as follows:

1. Fatal, destructive rejection of unpreserved orthotopic liver allografts has not been observed. Periportal mononuclear cell infiltration is, however, usual between 2 and 6 weeks after grafting. There may be associated foci of liver cell necrosis. These changes are accompanied by varying degrees of deranged liver function, with raised serum transaminase and alkaline phosphatase levels and sometimes jaundice. Both the morphological and biochemical abnormalities

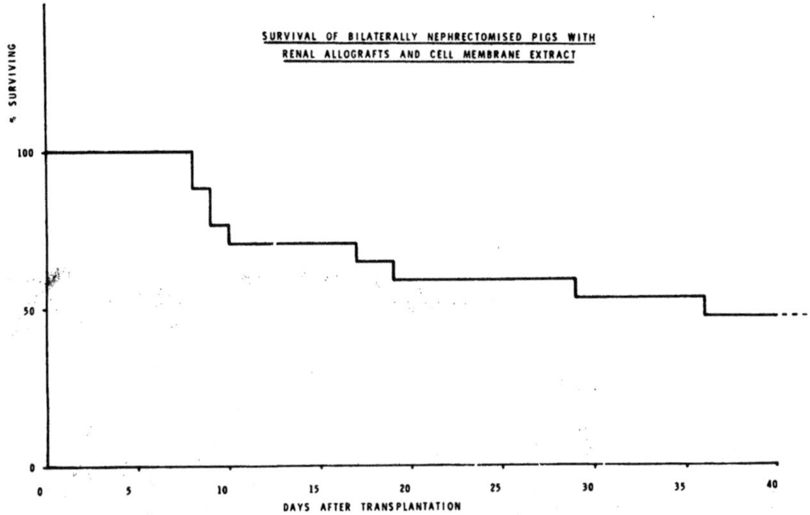

Figure 12.6 *Survival of bilaterally nephrectomised pigs with renal allografts. Animals were given no immunosuppressive treatment. All animals surviving beyond 15 days received kidneys from littermate donors*

tend to resolve spontaneously, but periportal fibrosis can occur as a permanent legacy of the rejection reaction. In the early experiments where a cholecyst-duodenostomy was used for biliary drainage, cholangitis always followed and this confused assessment of the allograft reaction. Bile drainage by choledochodochostomy, retaining the sphincter of Oddi, has almost eliminated the complication of cholangitis. Most deaths of liver allografted pigs have been due to intestinal obstruction due to adhesions or intra-abdominal sepsis (Millard *et al.*, 1971).

2. The life of a pig with an orthotopic allograft can be indistinguishable from a normal animal. Grafted pigs gain weight and thrive. Two sows have borne normal litters of piglets 18 and 15 months after orthotopic liver allografting (Figure 12.7). Animals are surviving more than 4 years after receiving their grafts. This period represents a considerable portion of a pig's lifetime.

3. In our studies the long survival of porcine liver allografts occurs independent ... We have grafted livers within a

ERRATUM

The illustration on page 303 should be above the caption for Figure 12.10 on page 308 and vice versa.

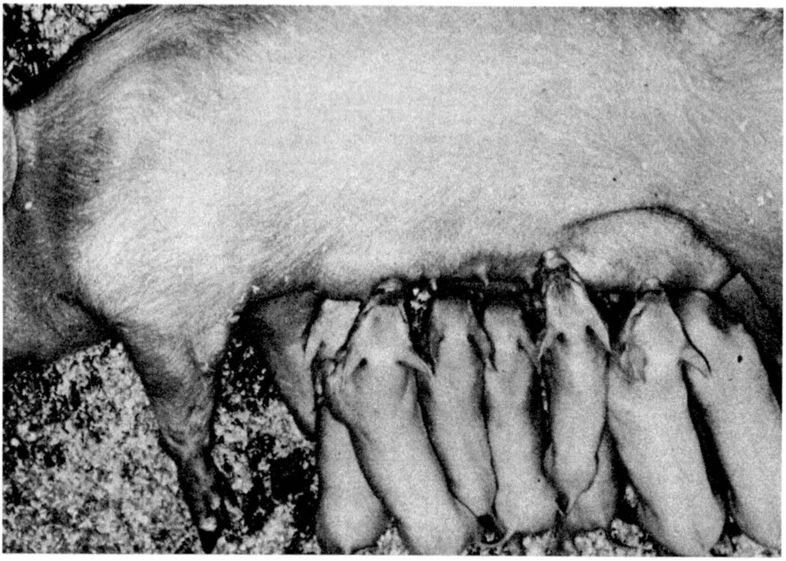

Figure 12.7 *Litter born to a sow 18 months after orthotopic liver allografting. No immunosuppressive treatment was given*

family, within a breed, and across combinations of three breeds: large white, landrace and saddleback. Experiments on tissue typed pigs confirm that liver allografts can survive complete serological and MLC mismatches at the major histocompatibility locus. MLC studies of recipient versus killed donor cells have generally shown positive pre-transplantation reactions. Post-transplantation, the behavior of the MLC test has been variable despite continued good function of the liver graft. Initial post-operative non-specific depression of recipient lymphocyte reactivity may be followed by specific non-reactivity against donor cells or a return of normal reactivity (Festenstein *et al.*, 1971).

4. Following liver preservation by a variety of techniques, fatal destructive rejection of orthotopic liver allografts has sometimes been observed. Similar rejection has occurred in animals sensitized by previous skin or kidney allografts (Calne *et al.*, 1969). Auxiliary liver allografts have shown more evidence of rejection than orthotopic transplants, but assessment of these grafts has been difficult since the recipients' own livers have maintained life and the transplants have suffered from atrophy due to competition with the normal liver.

Other laboratories have also reported prolonged survival of unimmunosuppressed pigs with liver allografts but some investigators have observed a high incidence of fatal destructive rejection (Hunt, 1967; Mieny *et al.*, 1967; Garnier *et al.*, 1970; Starzl, 1969). An explanation of the varying incidence of rejection is not apparent but different details of technique, pig breeds, and animal care could be important.

Liver allografts not only protect themselves from rejection but they can prolong survival of other tissues grafted from the same donor. The donor specificity of this effect has been demonstrated for skin and kidney grafts. Donor skin graft prolongation has been variable. Sometimes little effect was observed, on other occasions donor skin persisted for 2–3 weeks succumbing to slow indolent rejection whilst the liver allograft continued to survive indefinitely (Figure 12.8). Orthotopic grafting of the liver and kidney usually resulted in prolongation of functional survival of both organs.

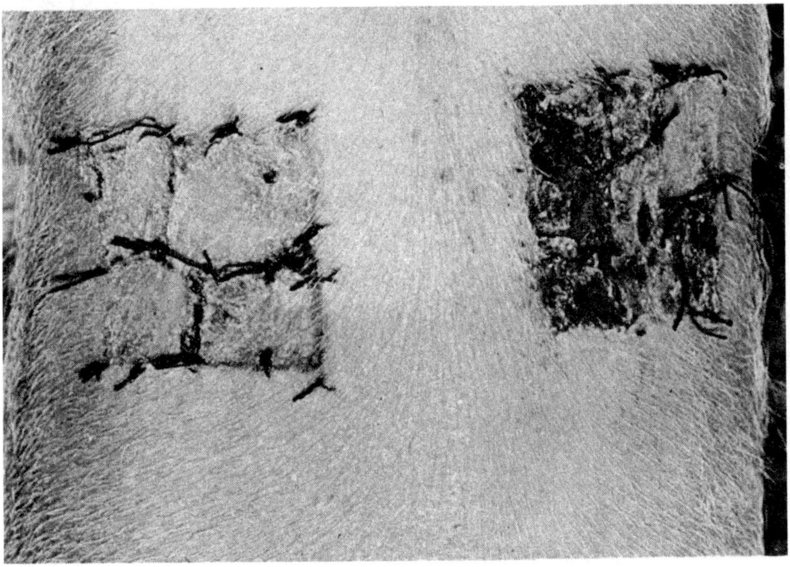

Figure 12.8 *Skin grafts on the back of an animal that has received an orthotopic liver graft 24 days previously. The portions of skin were grafted 10 days before the photograph. Three indifferent donor grafts on the left are rejected. The bottom left autograft is a control. Two grafts from the liver donor are indistinguishable from two control autografts on the extreme right. No immunosuppressive treatment was given*

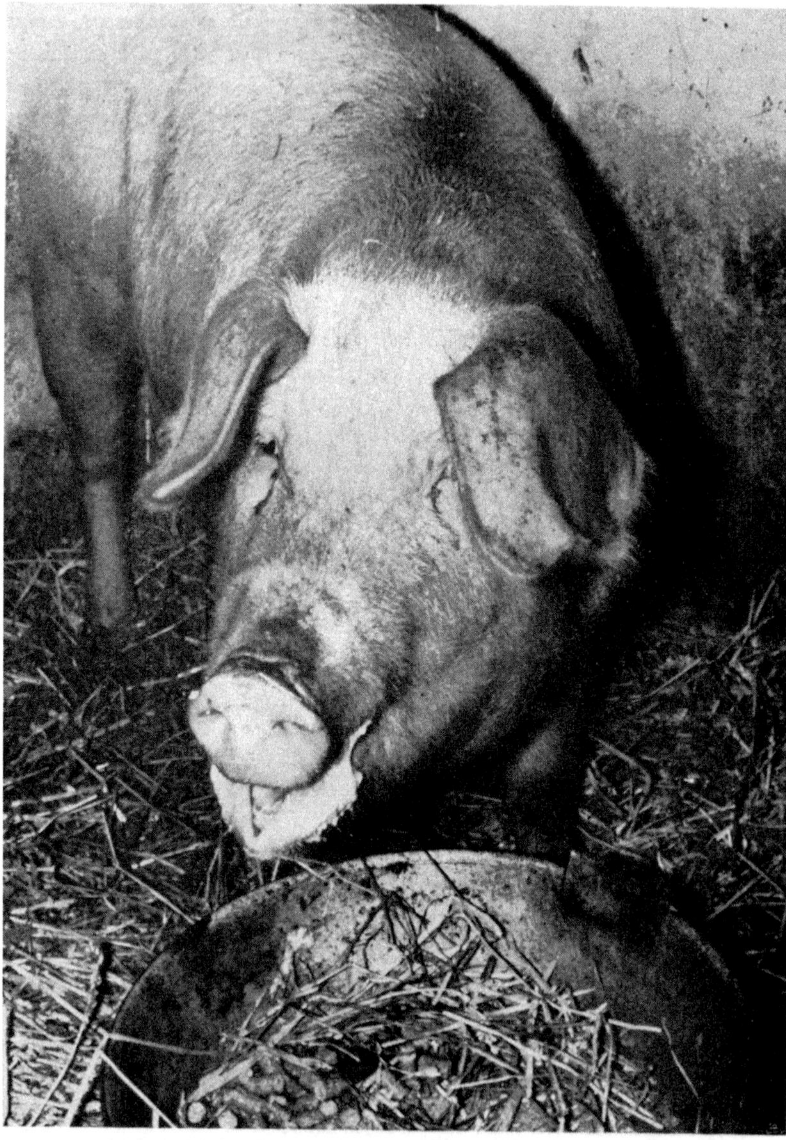

Figure 12.9 *Pig surviving $4\frac{1}{2}$ years after hepatectomy, bilateral nephrectomy and orthotopic kidney and liver transplantation. No immunosuppressive therapy*

One pig is surviving more than $4\frac{1}{2}$ years after hepatectomy, bilateral nephrectomy and orthotopic kidney and liver transplantation (Figure 12.9). Sometimes the effect was only moderate, the kidney being rejected in 2–3 months causing uremic death. In these cases, morphological changes of rejection in the liver were well marked. This pattern has been observed repeatedly. When the liver has been grafted either orthotopically or heterotopically together with other organs, rejection of the liver has been more marked than would have been expected if the liver had been grafted alone, whilst rejection of the other organs has been delayed or mild. Liver grafting has delayed the rejection of grafts of heart, pancreas, duodenum and kidney (Calne *et al.*, 1972). In a series of experiments involving simultaneous renal and accessory liver grafting, the liver was removed at varying intervals. Residence of the extra liver for 2 hours did not prolong kidney graft survival, but 24 hours gave marked protection of the kidney (Calne *et al.*, 1969).

We suggested that the allografted porcine liver can induce partial immunological tolerance in animals with competent immune systems. The effect seemed to be too rapid for antibody production to be important but a later contribution of enhancing antibody has certainly not been excluded. Partial tolerance is well recognized in classical tolerance experiments, but an explanation of the difference between the behavior of skin on the one hand and liver on the other is not clear. Skin specific antigens may be involved (Lance, 1971) or a mild immune reaction may be sufficient to destroy a skin graft but not a liver. It seemed possible that the porcine liver could produce transplantation antigen in a tolerogenic form. We attempted to investigate this hypothesis by experiments using soluble cell membrane extracts from the liver and the spleen on renal allograft survival in the pig and, since certain HLA antigens have been found in human serum (Van Rood *et al.*, 1970) and similar antigens have been found in pig serum (Calne *et al.*, 1970b; Schmid and Cwik, 1972), we also investigated the effect of treatment of recipients with donor blood or serum at the time of renal allografting. A membrane derived soluble antigen was prepared by Dr D. A. L. Davies (Davies, 1966, 1967, 1969). In the control experiments, 17 of 31 recipient pigs had bilateral nephrectomy performed at the time of allografting. Death in these animals occurred between 5 and 33 days (Figure 12.6). Ten of the 31 grafts were between littermates and 9 of these had moderate to severe rejection histologically; one allograft was normal at autopsy at 12 days; the other 21 animals died or had their allografts removed between 6 and 25 days. All of these grafts had substantial or severe rejection. The relationships of donor and recipient were half sibling (3), distant relatives (1), unrelated (8) and different breed (9). There were three experimental groups, in all of which animals were bilaterally nephrectomized at the time of renal allografting (Calne *et al.*, 1970b).

Group 1

Seventeen animals treated with soluble cell membrane extract at the time of operation survived beyond 4 days (Figure 12.10). None of the donor/recipient combinations were littermates. Eight animals died between 8 and 29 days with rejected kidneys.

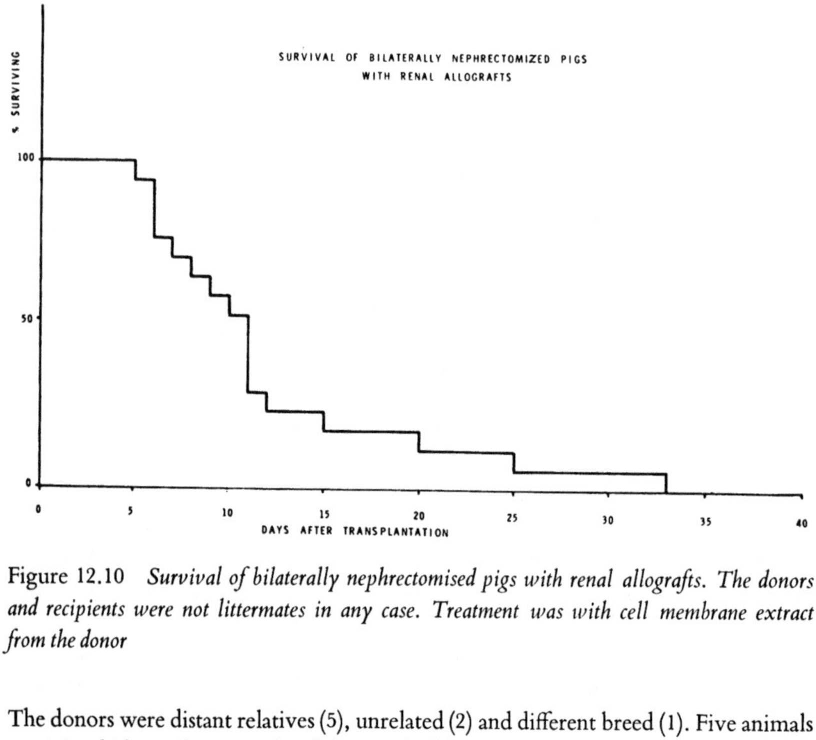

Figure 12.10 *Survival of bilaterally nephrectomised pigs with renal allografts. The donors and recipients were not littermates in any case. Treatment was with cell membrane extract from the donor*

The donors were distant relatives (5), unrelated (2) and different breed (1). Five animals receiving kidneys from unrelated donors died between days 35 and 156 with rejected kidneys. Four were alive between 176 and 329 days. The donor was half sibling in one case, distant relative in one and unrelated in two.

Group 2

Six animals were given between 750 and 1000 ml of donor blood intravenously during the operation. Three died between 7 and 10 days with rejected kidneys. The donor was unrelated (2) and of different breed (1). Three were alive between 145 and 155 days, two with unrelated donors and one with a donor of a different breed.

Group 3

Six animals were given between 3 and 500 ml of donor serum intravenously during the operation. Five died between 8 and 29 days with rejected kidneys. The 29-day survivor was given an additional 500 ml of donor serum at 7 days. The relationships of donor and recipient were half sibling (2) and distant relative (3). One animal was alive at 161 days with an unrelated donor.

At the time the above experiments were performed, tissue typing and MLC studies were not available, but from the pattern of results obtained subsequently, an immunosuppressive effect would appear to have been clearly demonstrated in all three experimental groups, the cell membrane fractions being most effective. Thus, in all three groups animals were surviving with allografts from unrelated donors long after all the untreated control animals had rejected their kidneys. Donor specificity was not demonstrated in these experiments. In fact, one animal treated with cell membrane fraction from a donor different to the donor of the kidney survived more than 2 years after bilateral nephrectomy. Unfortunately, the lack of data on serology and MLC reactions in this experiment does not permit further analysis and donor compatibility has obviously not been excluded.

There is no evidence that soluble membrane fractions derived from liver were any more efficacious in preventing kidney graft rejection than those derived from the spleen. The weight of extract used varied considerably but the starting material with spleen was one whole spleen and with liver the source of material came from one or two lobes, or approximately a quarter the weight of a whole liver.

The behavior of liver allografts in other species is different to that of the pig, but it is our impression that liver allograft rejection in man is less aggressive than renal allograft rejection. In four control orthotopic liver allografts in the rhesus monkey, where tissue typing between donor and recipient showed mismatches in each case, three animals rejected their livers within 2 weeks, the fourth survived 7 months when it died from cholangitis (Calne *et al.*, 1970a). This long survivor contrasts markedly with allografts of skin, heart and kidney in the rhesus monkey which are usually rejected promptly. Myburgh *et al.* (1972) have shown that polyvalent enhancing sera can produce marked prolongation of liver allograft survival in the baboon, although the same sera are relatively ineffective in baboons with renal allografts.

The liver also reacts differently to the kidney when perfused with blood from widely disparate species, for example, human blood can be used to perfuse porcine or bovine livers for several hours (Eisman *et al.*, 1965; Condon *et al.*, 1970), whereas canine blood will not support function in a pig's kidney and flow ceases after a few minutes (Slapak *et al.*, 1971). In one of our xenograft experiments, a baboon lived $3\frac{1}{2}$ days with an orthotopically transplanted pig's liver (Figure 12.11). Thus, in several

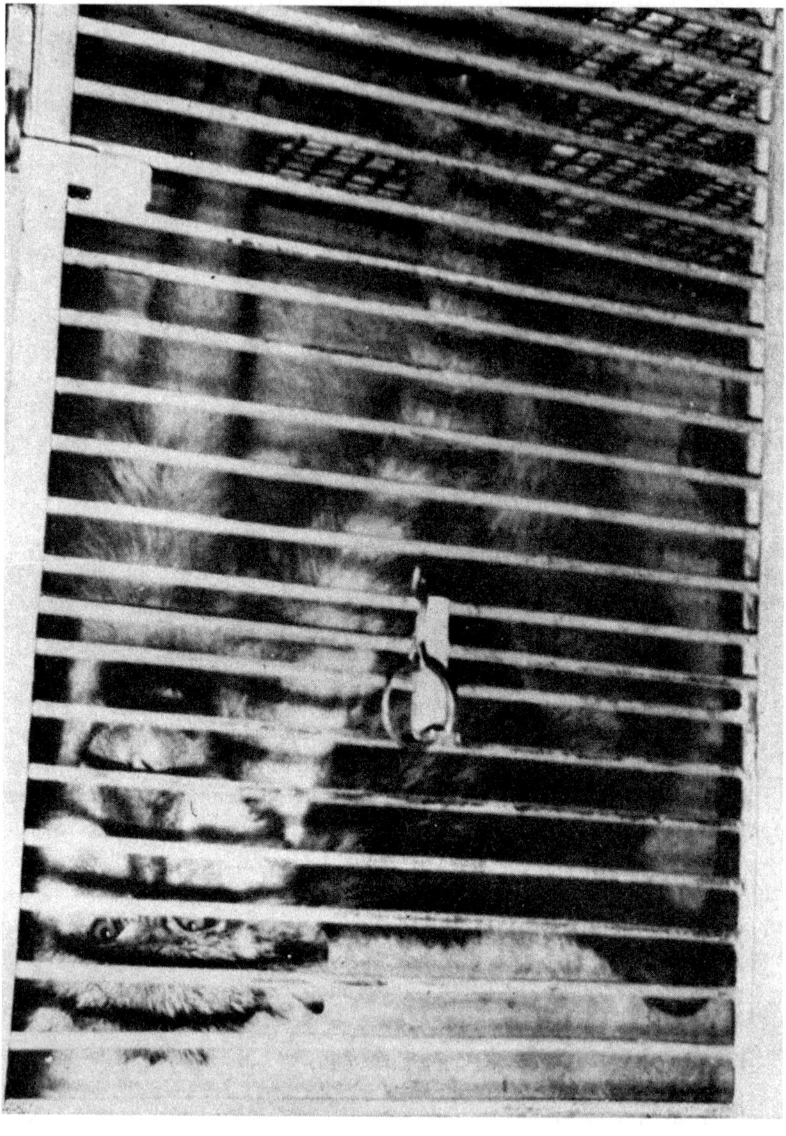

Figure 12.11 *Baboon which survived $3\frac{1}{2}$ days with an orthotopic xenograft of a pig's liver. The animal was alert and active and reacted normally until its sudden death from acute respiratory infection*

species the liver seems to tolerate and be accepted in a foreign environment better than other organs, but this feature is most clearly seen in the pig.

It is possible that soluble transplantation antigens and antigen–antibody complexes given intravenously have more effective access to the lymphoid system in the pig than in other species due to the peculiarities of the porcine lymphocyte circulation and lymph node structure (Binns and Hall, 1966; McFarlin and Binns, 1972). Porcine blood has a high lymphocyte count—10 000–15 000 per cu mm, but efferent lymph contains very few cells compared with other species. The cortico-medullary architecture of porcine lymph nodes is reversed with the follicles lying in the centre and medullary tissue situated peripherally. The medulla lacks true cords and sinuses. The pattern of allograft rejection could well be different in the pig compared with most other species. Thus, neonatal thymectomy, even with antilymphocyte serum treatment, did not impair porcine skin graft rejection although other cellular immune functions were markedly inhibited (Binns *et al.*, 1972). In these studies, procedures which should have interfered with T cell action failed to prolong skin graft survival. Hence, it is possible that B cells may be implicated in the rapid porcine skin graft rejection which is consistently followed by cytotoxic antibody production (White *et al.*, 1973a), but B cells may have less effect on renal and hepatic allografts. *Per contra*, one could speculate that different antibodies, also B cell products, might be involved in protecting porcine liver allografts from rejection by preventing the cytotoxic action of T cells. Lymphocytotoxic antibody has not so far been found in the sera of pigs tolerating liver allografts but is often produced after skin grafting and has been reported after renal allograft rejection (Schmid, personal communication).

It is tempting to seek a unified explanation for the observed long survival of organ allografts in situations where skin grafts from similar donors would be rapidly rejected. Experiments cited elsewhere in this volume show that under certain carefully controlled conditions, organ allografts can survive indefinitely in the rat and mouse. There have been many successful renal allografts in patients treated with conventional azathioprine and steroids, despite positive MLC reactions and four antigen HLA mismatches with the donors. Attempts at analysis of these phenomena have shown features of donor specific immunological unresponsiveness that resemble clinical tolerance and enhancement but are not typical of either. A similar conclusion was reached by Brent and his colleagues (1972 and this volume) in studies of prolonged skin graft survival in rats treated with donor strain cells and immunosuppressive agents.

Although its behavior may be exceptional, the pig does provide easily reproducible laboratory models whose analysis could be rewarding. Thus, to obtain prolonged skin allografts, induction of classical tolerance is necessary; to prolong kidney graft survival, selection of donor and recipient combinations by serology and/or MLC reactions may be effective. Alternatively, standard immunosuppressive agents may be used, or cell membrane preparations, donor blood or serum, or a simultaneous liver allograft. The liver allograft itself provides an example of an almost perfect therapeutic graft requiring no immunosuppressive treatment of the recipient and no donor selection based on tissue typing or MLC reactions.

We are endeavouring to investigate the cellular and serological changes that occur at different times in these models in the hope that *in vitro* observations can predict the outcome of grafts in given situations where serological and MLR typing of donor and recipient have been studied. The immune mechanisms that are set in motion when tissue is grafted are complex and there are dynamic changes that occur at various intervals following grafting. There is a strong natural tendency for the foreign tissue to be rejected but there are other natural phenomena which can result in specific unresponsiveness towards the grafted organ. Serial investigations of the immune processes by techniques that are now available may provide sufficient data from which predictions of graft survival may be made and also could provide information that would allow manipulation of the immune response with continuous monitoring of the effects of the interference. It is particularly important to have a reliable monitoring system, since although it is possible to obtain reproducible donor specific immunological unresponsiveness in inbred animals, studies in outbred populations have revealed important dangers. Thus, an attempt to produce unresponsiveness with 'enhancing' sera using identical techniques may result in enhancement in some experiments and no effect, or hyperacute rejection, in others.

Such observations impress the clinician with extreme caution in venturing from the laboratory to clinical practice where so many factors are unknown or cannot be controlled. Thus, although serological tissue typing can define four histocompatibility antigens in a high proportion of individuals, we know very little of the relative importance and strength of the individual transplantation antigens nor how they cross react with one another. A one-way mixed lymphocyte culture reaction can show reactivity of recipient lymphocytes towards killed donor cells but recipient lymphocytes may have impaired reactivity at the time of the test due to factors that are non-immunological, for example, uraemia and generalized debility of the patient. Restoration of health by a successful graft may result in unexpected increased reactivity of the recipient's immune system. A patient prior to surgery may already have circulating cytotoxic antibodies or other non-cytotoxic antibodies. Following grafting, these antibodies may cause immediate damage to the graft or there may be a change from non-cytotoxic antibodies to cytotoxicity. The fate of the graft may depend on the dynamics of antibody production and also the availability of complement. All these matters are extremely pertinent in clinical practice and application of any of the observed laboratory techniques to produce unresponsiveness, for instance, treatment with donor antigen or enhancing antisera, could be expected to have widely different results in the patient depending on the immunological environment at the time of the treatment and anticipated changes that would occur after grafting.

Another important consideration is the effect of non-specific immunosuppressive agents, such as azathioprine, steroids and anti-lymphocyte globulin. Although in general these have a beneficial effect on the survival of a graft, when complex immunological interactions are occurring, it is quite possible that immunosuppressive agents given at certain times could impair the production of important specific immune processes which would otherwise result in blocking of the rejection response.

Even if there was a considerable advance in knowledge on these important aspects of transplantation immunology that are so poorly understood at present, there would still be difficulties of a technical nature involved in manipulation of the immune system. It might be necessary for pretreatment to be continued for a considerable period before organ allografting, in order to obtain specific unresponsiveness. Since organs can only be preserved from cadavers for a few days *ex vivo* under the best circumstances, such immunological manipulation would need to be confined to grafts from living donors, until there were important advances in organ preservation techniques.

Another difficulty that might be encountered in producing unresponsiveness would be obtaining effective access to the immune system. One could envisage the possibility of obtaining a satisfactory situation in the blood circulation but there could be many 'untreated' immunologically active cells in solid lymphoid organs, such as lymph nodes and the spleen.

This chapter is concerned with presenting the observed data of allografting in the pig. Speculation of the mechanisms involved have been made and if taken into consideration with other contributions in this volume, it would seem that on theoretical grounds techniques are available to study and manipulate the immune system so as to obtain specific unresponsiveness towards allografted tissues. I have, however, pointed out at the end of the chapter that it is also possible to speculate on the difficulties that might be encountered in attempts to utilize laboratory knowledge in clinical practice.

Acknowledgements

I am grateful to my many colleagues who have been associated with this work, in particular Drs Binns, Bradley and White who have read through the text and made constructive suggestions. I also wish to thank my secretary, Miss S. Cockburn, for her patient work with the typescript.

References

Binns, R. M. and Hall, J. G. (1966). The poverty of lymphocytes in the lymph-unanaesthetized pigs. *J. Exp. Path.*, **47**, 275

Binns, R. M. (1967a). Bone marrow and lymphoid cell injection of the pig foetus resulting in transplantation tolerance or immunity and immunoglobulin production. *Nature* (*London*), **214**, 179

Binns, R. M., Harrison, F. A. and Heap, R. B. (1967b). Transplantation of the ovary in the pig and pregnant sheep. *Acta Endocr. Kbh. Suppl.*, **119**, 193

Binns, R. M. (1968). The ontogeny of immune responses in the pig. Ph.D. Thesis, University of Cambridge

Binns, R. M., Calne, R. Y. and Millard, P. R. (1970). Induced tolerance of a kidney allograft in a pig. Preliminary report. *Europ. Surg. Res.*, **2**, 408

Binns, R. M., McFarlin, D. E. and Sugar, J. R. (1972). Lymphoid depletion and immunosuppression after thymectomy in the young pig. *Nature New Biol.*, **238**, 181

Bradley, B. A., Edwards, J. M., Dunn, D. C. and Calne, R. Y. (1972). Quantitation of mixed lymphocyte reaction by gene dosage phenomenon. *Nature New Biol.*, **240**, 54

Bradley, B. A., White, D. J. G., Calne, R. Y., Dunn, D. C., Edwards, J. M., Bitter-Suermann, H., Sampson, D. and Herbertson, B. M. (1973a). Lymphocyte gene products, serologically and MLR defined—their relevance in renal allograft survival. *IRCS* (*International Research Communications System*), **1**, 57

Bradley, B. A., Edwards, J. M. and Franks, D. E. (1973b). Histocompatibility phenotyping by the mixed lymphocyte reaction. *Tissue Antigens* (in press).

Brent, L. and Pinto, M. (1973). Induction of specific unresponsiveness with the aid of *Bordetella pertussis*. *Transplant. Proc.* (in press)

Calne, R.Y., Sells, R. A., Pena, J. R., Davis, D. R., Millard, P. R., Herbertson, B. M., Binns, R. M. and Davies, D. A. L. (1969). Induction of immunological tolerance by porcine liver allografts. *Nature* (*London*), **223**, 472

Calne, R. Y., Davis, D. R., Pena, J. R., Balner, H., De Vries, M., Herbertson, B. M., Millard, P. R., Joysey, V. C., Seaman, M. J., Samuel, J. R., Stibble, J., Westbroek, D. L. (1970a). Heptic allografts and xenografts in primates. *Lancet*, **1**, 103

Calne, R. Y., Davis, D. R., Hadjiyannakis, E., Sells, R. A., White, D., Herbertson B. M., Millard, P. R., Joysey, V. C., Davies, D. A. L., Binns, R. M., Festenstein, H., (1970b). Immunosuppressive effects of soluble cell membrane fractions, donor blood and serum on renal allograft survival. *Nature* (*London*), **227**, 903

Calne, R. Y., Sells, R. A., Marshall, V. C., Millard, P. R., Herbertson, B. M.,

Hadjiyannakis, E. J., Dunn, D. C., Robson, A. J. and Davis, D. R. (1972). Multiple organ grafts in the pig. Techniques and results of pancreatic, hepatic, cardiac, and renal allografts. *Brit. J. Surg.*, **59,** 969

Childe, W. M. and Morris, A. S. (1969). Heart transplant rejection in pig and dog. *Brit. J. Surg.*, **56,** 630

Cochrum, K., Kountz, S., Belzer, F., Perkins, H. and Payne, R. (1973). Correlation of MLC with graft survival, *Transplant. Proc.* (in press)

Condon, R. E., Bombeck, C. T., and Steigmann, F. (1970). Heterologous bovine liver perfusion therapy of acute hepatic failure. *Amer. J. Surg.*, **119,** 147

Cullum, P. A., Baum, M., Clarke, A., Wemyss-Gorman, P. B., Howard, E. and McClelland, R. M. A. (1970). Orthotopic transplantation of the pig heart. *Thorax*, **25,** 744

Davies, D. A. L. (1966). Mouse histocompatibility isoantigens derived from normal and from tumour cells. *Immunology*, **11,** 115

Davies, D. A. L. (1967). Soluble H-2 isoantigens. *Transplantation*, **5,** 31

Davies, D. A. L. (1969). The molecular individuality of different mouse H-2 histocompatibility specificities determined by single genotypes. *Transplantation*, **8,** 51

Eiseman, B., Liem, D. S. and Raffucci, F. (1965). Heterologous liver perfusion in treatment of hepatic failure. *Ann. Surg.*, **162,** 329

Festenstein, H., Lubling, N., Calne, R. Y. and Binns, R. M. (1971). Pig liver allograft tolerance examined by the mixed lymphocyte culture technique. In *Immunological Tolerance to Tissue Antigens*, p. 215. (N. W. Nisbet and M. W. Elves, editors). Orthopaedic Hospital, Oswestry, England

Garnier, H., Clot, J. P. and Chomette, G. (1970). Orthotopic transplantation of the porcine liver. *Surg. Gynec. Obstet.*, **130,** 105

Hunt, A. C. (1967). Pathology of liver transplantation in the pig. In *The Liver*. (A. E. Read, editor), Colston Papers, No. 19, 337. London: Butterworths

Lance, E. M. (1971). Tissue Specific Transplantation Antigens. In *Immunological Tolerance to Tissue Antigens*, p. 291. (N. W. Nisbet and M. W. Elves, editors). Orthopaedic Hospital, Oswestry, England

McFarlin, D. E. and Binns, R. M. (1972). Lymph node function and lymphocyte circulation in the pig. In *Microenvironmental Aspects of Immunity*, p. 87. New York: Plenum Pub. Corp.

Mieny, C. J., Moore, A. R., Homatas, J. and Eiseman, B. (1967). Homotransplantation of the liver in pigs. *S. Afr. J. Surg.*, **5,** 109

Millard, P. R., Herbertson, B. M. and Calne, R. Y. (1971). Morphological features of kidney and liver allografts in the pig. *Transplant. Proc.*, **3,** 505

Myburgh, J. A. and Smit, J. A. (1973). Enhancement and antigen suicide in the outbred primate. *Transplant. Proc.* (in press)

Perper, R. J., Bowersox, B. E. and Van Gorder, T. J. (1971). Mechanism for prolonged survival of pig renal allografts. *Transplantation*, **11**, 505

Schmid, D. O. and Cwik, S. (1972). Soluble leukocyte antigens in serum of pigs. *Tissue Antigens*, **2**, 255

Schmid, D. O. (1972). Personal communication

Slapak, M., Greenbaum, M., Bardawil, W., Saravis, C., Joison, J. and McDermott, W. V. (1971). Effect of heparin, arvin, liver perfusion, and heterologous antiplatelet serum on rejection of pig kidney by dog. *Transplant. Proc.*, **3**, 558

Starzl, T. E. (1969). In *Experience in Hepatic Transplantation*, p. 188. Philadelphia: Saunders

Terblanche, J., Shippel, R. M., Immelman, E. J., Dent, D. M., Uys, C. J. and Saunders, S. J. (1973). Prolonged survival of vascularized organ allografts in unimmunosuppressed pigs. *Transplant. Proc.* (in press)

Vaiman, M., Renard, C., Lefage, P., Ameteau, J. and Nizza, P. (1970a). Evidence for a histocompatibility system in swine. *Transplantation*, **10**, 155

Vaiman, M., Arnoux, A., Filleul, X. and Nizza, P. (1970b). Immunogenetique—Le systeme d'histocompatibilite SL-A du porc: etude par la technique des cultures mixtes de leucocytes. *C.R. Acad. Sc. Paris*, **271**, 1724

Vaiman, M., Garnier, H., Kunlin, A., Hay, J. M., Parc., R., Bacour, F., Fagniez, P. H., Villiers, P. A., Lecointre, J., Bara, M. F. and Nizza, P. (1972). The SL-A histocompatibility system in the *Sus scrofa* species. *Transplantation*, **14**, 541

Van Rood, J. J., Van Leeuwen, A. and Van Santen, M. C. T. (1970). Anti HL-A2 inhibitor in normal human serum. *Nature (London)*, **226**, 366

Viza, D., Sugar, J. R. and Binns, R. M. (1970). Lymphocyte stimulation in pigs: evidence for the existence of a single major histocompatibility locus PL-A. *Nature (London)*, **227**, 949

White, D. J. G., Bradley, B., Calne, R. Y. and Binns, R. M. (1973a). The relationship of the histocompatibility locus in the pig to allograft survival. *Transplant. Proc.*, **5**, 317

White, D. J. G. and Binns, R. M. (1973b). Some studies on pig lymphocyte antigens. *Tissue Antigens* (in press)

13

Induction of Specific Unresponsiveness by Donor Antigen and Non-Specific Immunosuppression

L. Brent and M. Pinto

INTRODUCTION

It is clear from the data presented in successive reports of the Advisory Committee to the Renal Transplant Registry, of which the 1972 report is the most recent (Barnes *et al.*, 1972), that a great deal has been achieved in the last 20 years in making clinical renal transplantation a more reliable procedure. This is due largely to the introduction and widespread use of immunosuppressive drugs like imuran and prednisolone (see Berenbaum, 1973; Brent and Porter, 1973), better patient management, improved surgery and handling of cadaver kidneys, and—to an extent that is as yet difficult to ascertain so far as cadaver donors are concerned—the introduction of HL-A tissue typing (see Joysey, 1973; Festenstein, 1973; Terasaki *et al.*, this volume, Chapter 4. Unfortunately the rate of progress has not been maintained in the last few years and it would appear that present forms of treatment are unlikely to produce further substantial improvements. Because immunological rejection remains by far the most common single cause of failure (c. 50%) and because the drugs in use are hazardous to the patient, there is an urgent need for new forms of treatment. This conclusion, with which few workers would disagree, is strongly supported by the Second Report of the ACS/NIH Organ Transplant Registry (1973), which gives world figures for organs other than the kidney such as the heart, liver and lung.

The most studied forms of specific unresponsiveness, in which the subject becomes unresponsive only to those antigens to which he has been exposed during the course of the experimental procedure, are enhancement and tolerance. Enhancement has been discussed in this volume by Stuart (Chapter 8); it is, in essence, a phenomenon that is antibody-mediated, at least in the early stages, and which may depend for its durability on the action of antigen–antibody complexes (French and Batchelor, 1972). The antibodies involved here are almost invariably associated with serologically identifiable antibody activity, e.g. hemagglutinating or complement-mediated lymphocytotoxicity. Indeed, a characteristic feature of enhancement is that it can be induced passively with antisera against the tissue or organ to be transplanted and these antisera can be raised in many different ways, usually by hyperimmunisation of animals (syngeneic with the tissue or organ donor) with whole blood, viable or non-viable lymphoid cells or tissue extracts (see Feldmann, 1972).

Tolerance, on the other hand, is most readily induced in immunologically immature animals, either pre- or neonatally in most cases, and it depends on the injection of viable donor cells and the establishment of cell chimerism. The classical interpretation of experiments on tolerance induction is that it represents a genuine absence of responsiveness due to the death or inactivation of specific cell clones (Billingham *et al.*, 1956; Brent, 1971; Brent, Brooks *et al.*, 1972), a concept that derived largely from the absence of antibodies in tolerant animals, the inability of cells from tolerant animals to be stimulated in MLC to donor strain antigens, and the fact that tolerance can be broken with normal syngeneic lymphoid cells (see Brent, 1971). As Simpson (Chapter 7) has discussed in this volume, this concept has been challenged in the last two years; in particular, Hellström, Hellström and Allison (1970) have suggested that tolerance is due to the production of antibodies which, on their own or complexed with antigen, have an inhibitory or blocking effect on T cells, i.e. on the lymphocytes primarily involved in graft rejection. More recently it has been proposed (Beverley *et al.*, 1973) that the production of serum blocking factors may be a function of incomplete or partial tolerance, or of breaking tolerance—a question discussed in detail by Simpson (Chapter 7). The edges of enhancement and tolerance may therefore be more blurred than seemed likely 10 or 20 years ago (see Brent and French, 1973).

The investigations described here were designed to explore in inbred mice the possibility of creating a specific unresponsiveness—preferably a true unresponsive state independent of antibodies—without resort to the better known toxic drugs. Instead we placed our faith in ALS as the immunosuppressive agent and used this in combination with crude extracts of donor spleen or liver. This work, which was begun with Dr. P. J. Kilshaw in 1968 and which has already been published (Brent and Kilshaw, 1970; Brent, Hansen *et al.*, 1971; Brent, Hansen *et al.*, 1973; Kilshaw *et al.*, 1973), has more recently been extended to include *Bordetella pertussis* vaccine (BP) as an adjunct. A preliminary account of this work has already appeared (Brent and Pinto, 1973) and definitive papers are in preparation (Pinto *et al.*, 1974; Brent *et al.*, 1974). It is not, therefore, our intention to provide detailed documentation especially as our brief is to give a bird's eye view of our work and to discuss it somewhat speculatively. A great deal of work has, of course, been done by other investigators to induce unresponsiveness by pretreatment of the recipients with viable cells or cell extracts and in conjunction with a wide variety of immunosuppressive drugs (for references see Brent, Hansen *et al.*, 1973).

MATERIALS AND METHODS

It is perhaps necessary to defend our reliance on ALS and on crude rather than purified tissue extracts. In animals ALS has been a most powerful tool for the suppression of cell-mediated sensitivity, and Lance and Medawar (1969) had already shown that, when used in combination with viable donor strain spleen cells, a high degree of unresponsiveness to skin allografts could be induced in at least a proportion of murine recipients. Clinical trials so far conducted with ALG have yielded rather disappointing and variable results (see Russell, 1968; and, for example, Starzl and Putnam, 1969; Carpenter *et al.*, 1971; Deodhar *et al.*, 1971; Birtch *et al.*, 1971; Sheil *et al.*, 1973). We are however, inclined to believe that the relatively poor results obtained in clinical transplantation have more to do with factors such as the regimen and dose used, the problems associated with the production of potent and non-toxic ALG in horses, and—perhaps most important of all—the difficulties encountered in assaying batches of anti-human ALG, rather than with an inate and indeed unique capacity of human T lymphocytes to resist the biological action of ALG. That the dose of ALG is critical is indicated not only by numerous data obtained in rodents but also by experiments on skin allograft survival in primates (see, for example, Balner and Dersjant, 1967; Cosimi *et al.*, 1970; Lance and Medawar, 1970) as well as in man (Simmons *et al.*, 1971). Despite the fact that most of the experiments with primates were carried out with anti-human ALG, doses in excess of 20 mg / kg were generally effective. Detailed information about ALG may be found in a recent symposium (Seiler and Schwick, 1972).

So far as the method of extraction is concerned, it was decided from the onset to carry out our analysis with a crude cell-free splenic preparation known to have immunogenic properties (Billingham *et al.*, 1958) and which Medawar (1963) had already used to good effect in prolonging skin graft survival in H-2 compatible donor-recipient strain combinations. Although highly solubilised and purified tissue extracts can be prepared (Nathenson, 1970; Reisfeld and Kahan, 1970; Kahan and Reisfeld, 1972; and see Davies, this volume, Chapter 3 it seemed to us that, in applying purifying procedures, there was a distinct possibility that antigenic specificities might be lost or weakened, and our recent comparative study of the efficacy of crude and solubilised preparations in inducing unresponsiveness in conjunction with BP and ALS indicates that this may well be the case (Brent, Halle-Pannenko *et al.*, in preparation). We did, however, soon find that liver extracts were virtually as effective as spleen extracts (Brent, Hansen *et al.*, 1973), and as mouse livers weigh roughly four times as much as spleens this solved to a large extent the logistic problems of donor supply.

Extracts rather than viable cells were used as antigen because, in clinical terms, this appeared to be the most hopeful approach. The kind of cells that lend themselves well to intravenous inoculation and tolerance induction are, in the main, lymphoid cells, i.e. cells that can give rise to graft-versus-host reactions in a non-responsive environment. Lance and Medawar (1969) overcame this problem by using F_1 murine spleen cells—a solution clearly not available to the clinician. Wood *et al.* (1971) therefore turned to bone marrow cells, which in the mouse contain relatively few immunologically competent T cells. Unfortunately bone marrow can produce very unpleasant GVH reactions in man (van Bekkum, 1971; Santos *et al.*, 1971; Meuwissen *et al.*, 1971) and the problem of removing or inactivating T cells from bone marrow has not yet been adequately solved. For the time being, tissue extracts must therefore be regarded as the safest vehicle for the exposure of a human subject to donor antigens prior to grafting.

The preparation of crude tissue extracts and pools of ALS has been fully described (Brent, Hansen *et al.*, 1973). Extracts of liver or spleen were made from aliquots of up to 20 g wet weight tissue and a preparation need not take more than 3–4 hours. Because the standard dose per mouse is 250 mg eq (i.e. the extract obtained from 250 mg wet weight of tissue; eq = equivalent) such a preparation provides enough material for up to 80 recipient mice. The extract stores well at −80 °C or frozen and dried. It is essentially a suspension of small membrane particles and most of its biological activity can be removed by spinning at 30 000 *g* for 1–2 h. Given intravenously this material can cause embolisms, but provided it is heparinized (10 i.u./dose) it is invariably perfectly harmless.

ALS was prepared routinely in rabbits by the method of Levey and Medawar (1966); this has the great advantage that, provided scrupulous care is taken to avoid blood contamination of the thymus tissue and lymph nodes, non-toxic sera that do not require absorption are almost invariably produced. Its main disadvantage is that it requires two injections of as many as approximately 10^9 cells per rabbit. ALS pools were prepared from 20–40 rabbits. The potency of the pools was somewhat variable: when 0.5 ml was injected into CBA males 2, 4 and 6 days after grafting the medium survival times (MST) of strain A grafts for different pools fell between 24 and 36 days. Interestingly enough, we have had excellent results with antisera near the lower limit (26 days), but using a horse-anti-mouse ALS with an MST of 19 days results were poor: clearly, the ALS must be reasonably effective and one that provides an MST of approximately × 2.5 the normal MST is entirely adequate. ALS was routinely administered intraperitoneally (i.p.).

BP vaccine (Burroughs Wellcome & Co.) containing 4×10^{10} organisms/ml was used to amplify the effect of the ALS. 0.2 ml (sometimes 0.3 ml, depending on the leucocytotic potency of the batch) was injected i.v. 2 days before grafting. Mice tolerated this rather high dose well though it made them a little more susceptible to the effects of anesthetic nembutal 2 days later. The most obvious effect of BP is to produce a marked blood lymphocytosis, which is 4–6 fold and maximal 4 days later, as Morse (1965) had previously shown. It was this lymphocytosis which encouraged us to include BP in the treatment, in the hope that it would render the lymphocytotoxic action of the ALS more effective.

In most of our analytical experiments we have used strain A ($H\text{-}2^a$) mice as donors and CBA ($H\text{-}2^k$) males as recipients. The unresponsiveness was usually less marked in females. Other strain combinations have been used, however, and good results have been obtained with the combination C57B1 ($H\text{-}2^b$) → CBA. Although results in the H-2 compatible combination C3H ($H\text{-}2^k$) → CBA have been excellent this needs to be seen in the context of the much greater immunosuppressive power of ALS alone in this kind of situation.

TREATMENT	EXTRACT	B. PERTUSSIS	SKIN GRAFT	ALS	ALS	ALS
DOSE	250mg.eq.	0·2ml		0·5ml	0·5ml	0·5ml
DAYS	−16	−2	0	2	4	6

Figure 13.1 *Regimen of treatment of CBA male mice with strain A extract,* B. pertussis *vaccine and ALS. (eq. = wet weight equivalent)*

The design of our standard experiments is illustrated in Figure 13.1. It should be remembered that, whilst BP amplifies the degree of unresponsiveness, specific unresponsiveness can be achieved without it (Brent, Hanson *et al.*, 1973). Our experiments suggest that there is no qualitative difference in the unresponsiveness induced with and without BP, and in discussing some of the experiments designed to unravel the mechanism we shall not always distinguish between them.

THE PHENOMENON AND ITS SPECIFICITY

Previous experiments without BP had shown that an interval of approximately 16 days between injection of extract and skin grafting is optimal and that the ALS is most effectively applied in the first week after grafting. A typical experiment *with* BP and including the appropriate controls is shown in Figure 13.2. Extract and ALS (curve B) shifted the median survival time (MST), compared with the ALS controls (curve D), by roughly two-fold but caused few grafts to be retained for long periods. Addition of BP to the system extended the MST very considerably and caused more than 40% of the recipients to tolerate their grafts for well in excess of 100 days. (See

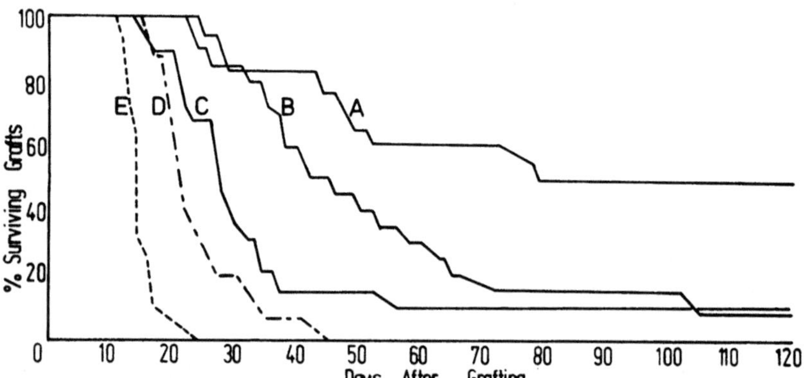

Figure 13.2 *Typical experiment, giving survival of strain A skin grafts in CBA males treated with strain A liver extract,* B. pertussis *vaccine and ALS. From L. Brent and M. Pinto,* Transplant. Proc., **5**, *697 (1973), by kind permission of Williams & Wilkins Co, Baltimore*

Key:	Extract	B. pertussis	ALS
A	+	+	+
B	+	−	+
C	−	+	+
D	−	−	+
E	+	+	−

Figure 13.3). Two further control groups were included: BP and ALS (curve C), without extract, gave marginally better results than ALS alone—a result that is in agreement with the data of Festenstein *et al.* (1969)—and extract plus BP (curve E), without ALS very slightly prolonged survival compared with graft survival in CBA males treated with extract alone (Brent, Hansen *et al.*, 1973). The fact that there were one or two long-surviving grafts in the group treated with BP and ALS suggests that the skin grafts themselves may play a rôle in the induction of unresponsiveness, a point that is further emphasised by our finding (Pinto *et al.*, 1974) that mice receiving the full treatment will not become unresponsive if they receive skin grafts just *after* completion of the ALS regimen.

Figure 13.4 indicates that this unresponsiveness is quite as donor-specific as the unresponsiveness induced by extract and ALS only. Thus, whereas strain A extract induced unresponsiveness in CBA males to strain A grafts (curve A) it did not bring about a prolongation of survival of Balb/c (H-2^{d}) grafts (curve B). Furthermore,

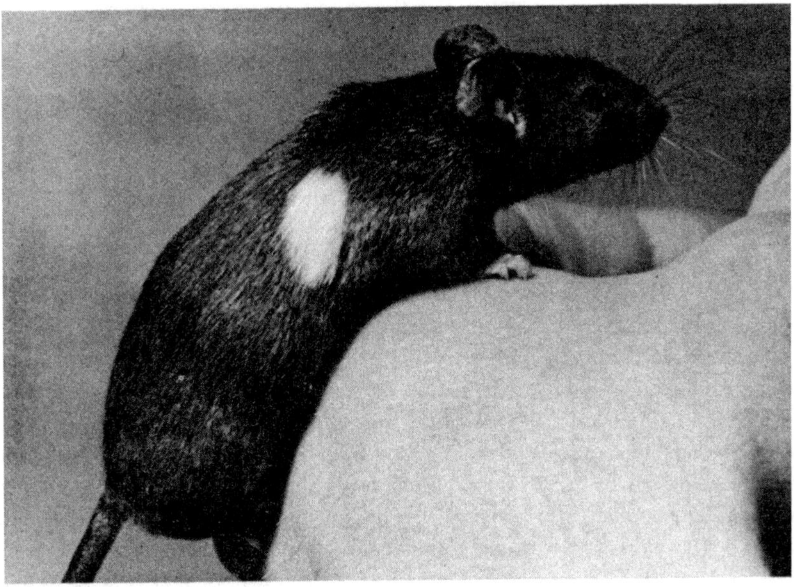

Figure 13.3 *CBA mouse 4 months after transplantation of strain A skin allograft. Unresponsiveness had been induced with A strain liver extract, BP and ALS as described in the text*

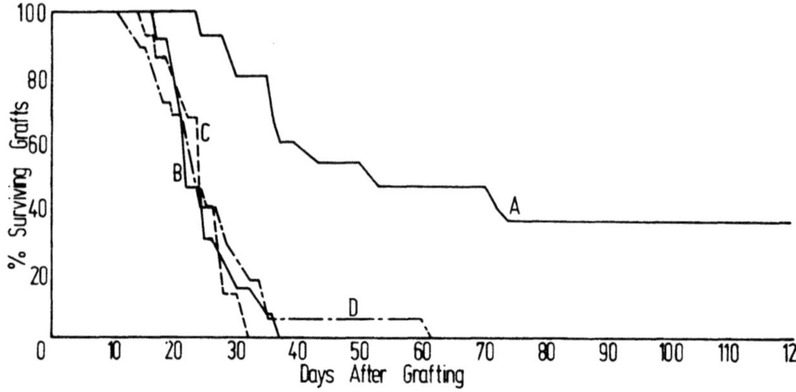

Figure 13.4 *Specificity of unresponsiveness induced by strain A liver extract in CBA males. From L. Brent and M. Pinto,* Transplant. Proc., **5**, *697 (1973), by kind permission of Williams & Wilkins Co, Baltimore*

Key:	Extract	B. pertussis	Grafts	ALS
A	A	+	A	+
B	A	+	Balb/c	+
C	–	+	Balb/c	+
D	CBA	+	A	+

extracts from donors syngeneic with the recipients did not affect the survival of strain A grafts (curve D). Additional experiments have shown that CBA mice displaying long-term unresponsiveness to strain A grafts, following the standard treatment including BP, reject C57B1 ($H\text{-}2^b$) skin grafts quite normally.

These are the basic facts; evidently a strictly limited form of treatment can establish a long-lasting and highly specific unresponsiveness to skin allografts across an H-2 histocompatibility barrier. In view of the finding that skin grafts are generally more sensitive to immune responses than organs such as the heart and kidney (for references see Batchelor and Brent, 1972) or, putting it another way, that skin grafts are less susceptible than some organs to procedures resulting in immunological enhancement, it seems probable that our results are valid for organ grafts too and may even be more effective there. (Indeed, unpublished work by L. Lameijer, L. Brent, P. J. Kilshaw and M. Ruszkiewicz indicates that the survival of heart allografts transplanted to treated rats is at least as good as that of skin grafts.) Three important questions now need to be answered. (1) What are the mechanisms responsible for this unresponsiveness?

(2) Can the problem of pretreatment with donor material be overcome? (3) Is it possible to improve the results so that a majority rather than a minority (30–40% at present) of experimental subjects are permanently unresponsive? We do not as yet have definitive answers to these questions, but all three are being studied. The first question is of more than just biological interest in that the design of any future clinical trial is bound to hinge on the mechanism underlying the unresponsiveness. The second and third are of immediate clinical importance: if an approach such as ours is ever to be applied to recipients of cadaver organs the need to pretreat may be considered to be a formidable obstacle until such time as organs can be satisfactorily stored for periods of 2–3 weeks; and it is equally important that the benefits of such a treatment should extend to the majority of recipients.

THE MECHANISM OF UNRESPONSIVENESS

Kilshaw and Brent (Brent and Kilshaw, 1970; Brent *et al.*, 1971) originally interpreted the unresponsiveness produced by extract and ALS as being due to a form of classical tolerance (see Table 13.1, A). We then discovered that spleen cells from unresponsive animals carrying healthy grafts performed normally in a splenomegaly GVH assay and that serum antibodies could be detected in unresponsive animals using a modified Coomb's test (Kilshaw *et al.*, 1973). It was therefore postulated that, whilst the partial destruction of a specific cell clone was almost certainly responsible for the initial stages of unresponsiveness, this was superseded in time by the recovery of cell-mediated responsiveness and the production of blocking factors. As Table 13.1, B shows, this hypothesis receives powerful support from a number of new experiments (Brent *et al.*, 1974) and we will briefly summarise them here.

Whilst we have confirmed in BP treated mice that unresponsiveness is not associated with the production of lymphocytotoxic (Figure 13.5), hemagglutinating or macrophage cytophilic antibodies, antigen-binding antibodies as detected with a modified Coomb's test (see Brent, Hansen *et al.*, 1973) can be shown to be present. The significance of these antibodies and their class remains to be elucidated, but it is possible that they will prove to have 'blocking' powers. At any rate, their presence suggests that our long-term animals are not tolerant according to the classical definition (Billingham *et al.*, 1956). This conclusion received ample confirmation from two sets of experiments: (a) positive splenomegaly GVH assays using cell suspensions prepared from the spleens of long-term unresponsive mice, and (b) the irregular 'homing' behavior of ^{51}Cr-labeled donor strain lymph node cells injected i.v. into long-term unresponsive animals. The latter experiments, which were carried out in collaboration

Table 13.1 *Experimental data favoring tolerance or other mechanisms*

A. *Favoring tolerance* (against enhancement)
- No lymphocytotoxic, hemagglutinating or macrophage cytophilic antibodies at any stage
- No hemagglutinating antibodies after hyperimmunisation schedule in unresponsive animals
- Failure of passive transfer with 'unresponsive' serum*
- Failure of 'unresponsive' serum to inhibit MLC reaction
- Second graft from same donor accepted
- Hybrid skin test grafts do not confer advantage*
- Unresponsiveness broken rapidly by injection of sensitised spleen cells*
- Unresponsiveness impaired more slowly by injection of normal syngeneic spleen cells*
- Thymectomy potentiates maintenance of unresponsiveness*
- Splenectomy does not impair induction and maintenance of unresponsiveness*

B. *Against tolerance* (favoring enhancement or blocking factors)
- Presence of antigen-binding antibodies as detected by modified Coomb's test
- Irregular 'homing' behavior of donor strain lymphocytes injected into mice carrying long-surviving grafts
- Normal GVH (splenomegaly) response by spleen cells from mice carrying long-surviving grafts
- Failure to break unresponsiveness by parabiosis of mice with long-surviving grafts with normal syngeneic mice; transfer of transient unresponsiveness to normal partners
- Transfer of transient unresponsiveness to normal mice, or of long-term unresponsiveness to sublethally irradiated mice, with spleen cells from animals carrying long-surviving grafts
- Administration of cyclophosphamide, but not ALS, into mice which had previously undergone the usual treatment undermines dramatically the induction of unresponsiveness

*Data obtained from mice treated with extract and ALS only (no BP)

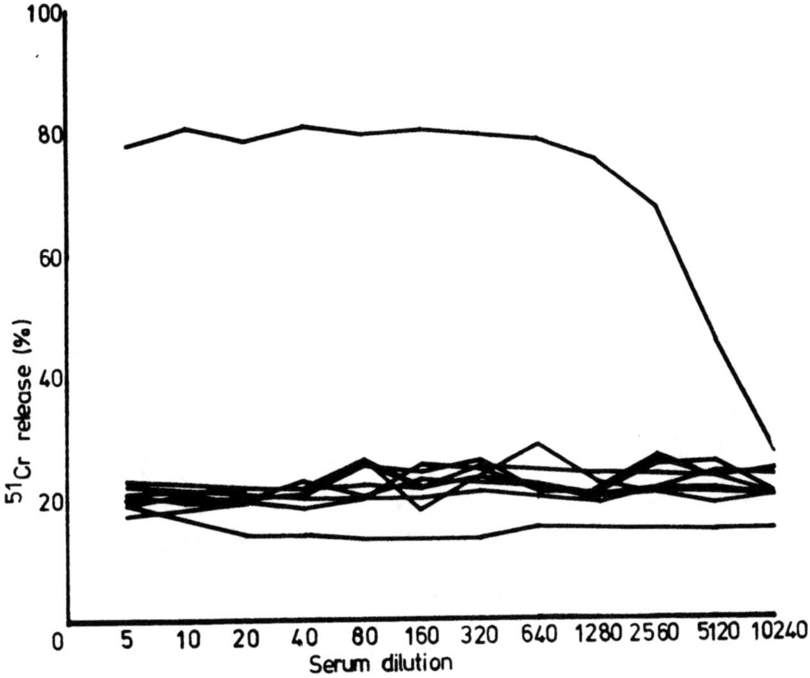

Figure 13.5 *Absence of lymphocytotoxic antibodies in CBA males unresponsive to strain A skin grafts. Top curve—hyperimmune antiserum. Bottom curve—serum from neonatally injected tolerant mouse. Remaining 7 curves (closely bunched)—sera from 3 neonatally injected tolerant mice, 3 unresponsive mice treated with extract,* B. pertussis *and ALS, and 1 normal CBA mouse*★

with Dr. E. M. Lance, are based on the measurement of radioactivity in the peripheral lymph nodes, spleen and liver 24 hours after injection of cells. In sensitized mice radioactivity is recovered mainly in the liver whereas in normal mice it is distributed roughly equally between the lymph nodes, the spleen and the liver. In long-term unresponsive mice it was invariably the liver which held most of the radioactivity, suggesting that our mice were not truly unresponsive. This contrasts vividly with similar experiments on neonatally injected tolerant mice, which behaved exactly as normal individuals in this respect (Brent, Lance *et al.*, in preparation).

The contrast between neonatally injected tolerant mice and these unresponsive

★We are indebted to Dr M. Ruszkiewicz for these antibody titrations.

animals is further pointed by experiments involving parabiosis. When tolerant and normal (syngeneic) mice were kept in parabiosis for 2 weeks it was found that (a) the normal mice became sensitized to donor strain skin grafts and (b) tolerance was broken in the partners (Brent, Brooks *et al.*, 1972). A similar experiment with mice displaying long-term unresponsiveness following treatment with extract, BP and ALS gave totally different results: the normal partners reacted more feebly to skin grafts from the donor strain and the unresponsive mice remained non-reactive for long periods after separation (see Figure 13.6).

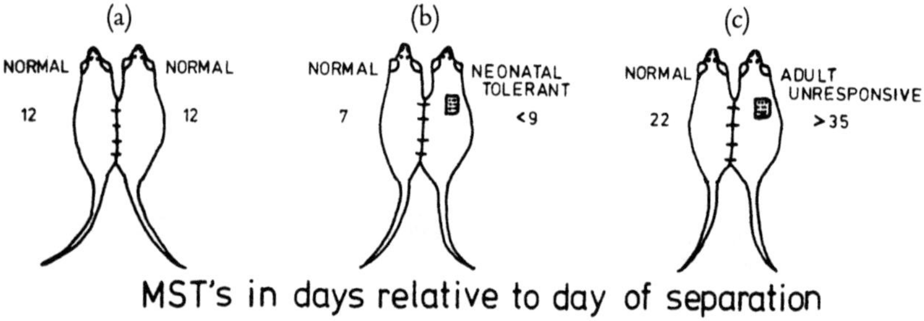

Figure 13.6 *Effect of parabiosis of normal CBA mice with (a) normal CBA mice, (b) neonatally injected CBA mice tolerant to strain A skin grafts, and (c) unresponsive CBA mice following treatment with strain A liver extract,* B. pertussis *and ALS (5 months after transplantation of strain A grafts)*

All tolerant or unresponsive mice carried perfect grafts at time of parabiosis. The normal syngeneic parabionts were matched for sex and weight. Parabiosis was terminated after 14 days and the normal partners immediately received a strain A graft. The median survival times given are relative to the time of separation of the parabionts

Even more direct evidence for the hypothesis that the mice with long-surviving skin allografts owe their unresponsiveness to an active process is provided by studies involving the transfer of spleen or lymph node cells (10^8) from mice to either normal, syngeneic recipients or to normal mice that had previously been sub-lethally irradiated (Brent *et al.*, 1974). In the former case a transient but highly significant unresponsiveness was induced; in the latter, a marked shift of MST was observed and some of the grafts survived for periods well in excess of 100 days. The unresponsive state thus brought about by adoptive transfer has proved to be highly specific for the skin grafts of the donor strain. Evidently the lymphoid tissues of the unresponsive mice possess cells which can suppress the cell-mediated response, either directly or by their immunoglobulin products. Our highly preliminary evidence indicates that the operative cells are not T cells and therefore, by inference, that they are B cells.

This preliminary evidence, that we may be dealing with a B cell mediated suppression of T cell activity, derives support from the following observation (see Brent *et al.*, 1974). Mice which had been given the standard treatment—donor strain extract, BP, skin grafts and ALS—were given a short course of cyclophosphamide starting 15 days after grafting, i.e. at a time when all grafts survived fully without overt signs of rejection. In the same experiment, other groups of mice received no further treatment or else they were injected, on the same days as the cyclophosphamide recipients, with more ALS. The results were dramatic. The cyclophosphamide-treated groups quickly recovered responsiveness and graft survival was markedly less than in the controls that received no further treatment. By contrast, administration of additional ALS slightly improved graft survival—only slightly, we think, because the mice had developed a clear-cut sensitivity to rabbit serum proteins and the ALS was therefore rapidly eliminated. (For obvious reasons this experiment is being repeated with a horse-anti-mouse ALS for the additional treatment.) As cyclophosphamide preferentially affects cells with a rapid turnover, and as Turk *et al.* (1972) have shown that this drug suppresses B cell activity very efficiently, it seems probable that the abrupt restoration of responsiveness on giving our animals an immunosuppressive agent that might have been expected to *potentiate* unresponsiveness was due to the elimination of B cells.

In the light of this evidence, and because we have eliminated other mechanisms such as histamine sensitization, we believe that the events in mice treated with extract, BP and ALS occur as illustrated in Figure 13.6. A period of clonal cell deletion is followed by recovery of the clone, but this recovery is accompanied by the production of antibodies which, though they do not have the power to cause cytotoxicity or hemagglutination, have the power—either alone or, more likely, after forming complexes with antigen—to prevent normal T cell function with respect to the antigens involved. How such a mechanism might operate at a cellular level (albeit in a different context) is the subject, in this volume (Chapter 9), of E. Diener. Direct experimental evidence for the presence of antigen–antibody complexes is now being sought; whatever their nature, it is clear that the conditions prevailing after recovery from the effects of the treatment is peculiarly favourable for the formation of the right kind of antibodies—i.e. antibodies which can bring about T cell inhibition without being cytotoxic. If complexes are involved the antigen must stem from the graft, for apart from the original donor extract these animals have not been exposed to any other donor strain material. In this respect they differ profoundly from mice made tolerant

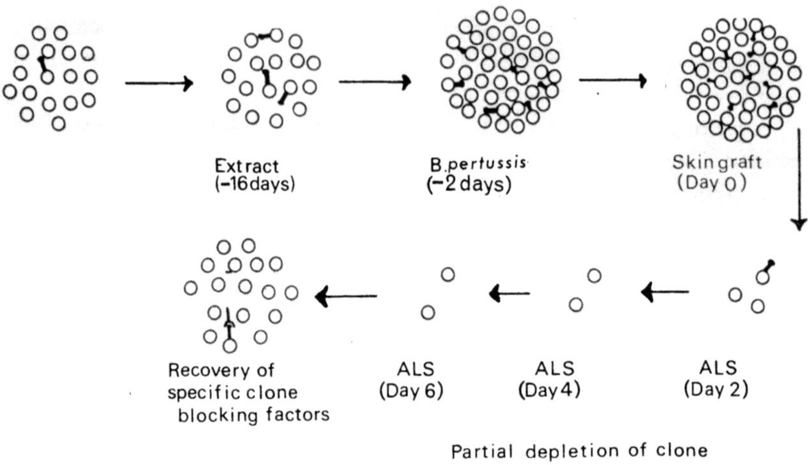

Figure 13.7 *Schematic presentation of hypothesis to account for the mechanism of unresponsiveness*

neonatally by the inoculation of viable lymphoid cells, for such animals become cell chimeras and contain significant numbers of donor-type cells (Billingham *et al.*, 1956).

The problem of pretreatment

It has been shown that pretreatment with a single dose of donor strain tissue extract and ALS is optimally effective when the extract is administered i.v. 16–26 days before skin grafting (Brent and Kilshaw, 1970; Brent, Hansen *et al.*, 1973). Although there is still a significant effect when extract is given only 6 days before grafting it is undoubtedly much weaker. If a treatment with extract is ever to be applied to man, it would therefore have to be given well before transplantation of the organ. Because present-day methods of organ storage are not adequate to secure organ survival for 2–3 weeks, and because the problems of storing organs such as the kidney are especially severe, it is meanwhile necessary to look for some other solution to the problem of pretreatment.

We are currently exploring if it might be possible in the mouse, to concoct what might loosely be called a 'universal antigen cocktail'. Such a cocktail would, the argument goes, contain the more important histocompatibility antigens of the species and therefore induce unresponsiveness irrespective of the skin graft donor. Translating this to man, one would want to prepare from cadaver livers antigen cocktails containing the more common HL-A specificities, and as storage of extracts presents no difficulties these preparations could be used at the appropriate time.

Whilst we wish to emphasise that it is far too early to claim that the problem is soluble we do have some encouraging preliminary data (Figure 13.7), suggesting that the approach is not unreasonable. Thus it has been possible to induce a measure

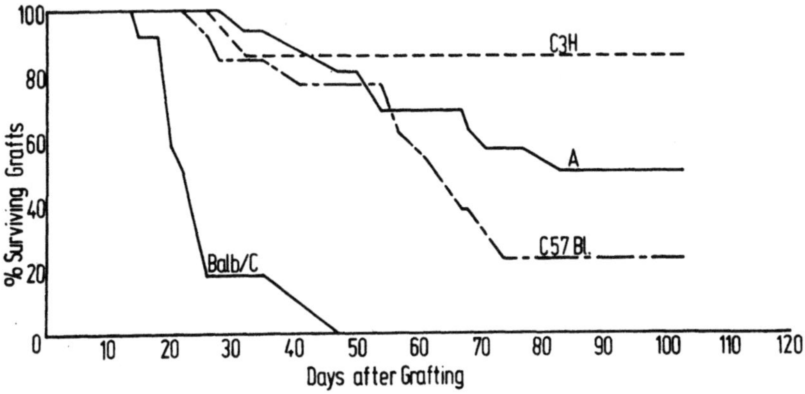

Figure 13.8 *Induction of unresponsiveness in CBA males to skin grafts from 4 different mouse strains (C3H, A, C57B1, and Balb/c) following injection of an antigen 'cocktail' consisting of extract obtained from liver tissue of the 4 strains. The total amount of extract injected per mouse was 325 mg eq., i.e. 80 mg eq. from each strain. 80 recipient CBA mice were injected intravenously with 'cocktail' extract and injected with* B. pertussis *14 days after. Two days later sub-groups of 20 mice were grafted with skin from one of the 4 strains*

of unresponsiveness to skin grafts of more than one strain by prior injection of a cocktail that admittedly included the specificities of the skin graft donor strain. However, the model is perhaps an over simplification. One major task waiting to be performed is to discover to what extent some of the H-2 specificities need to be supplemented in order to give more equitable results for all the strains involved; nor do we know as yet how skin grafts from a strain that was *not* represented among the extract donors will fare in these circumstances.

How to further potentiate induction and maintenance of unresponsiveness

Experiments are in progress in which mice are being given various kinds of supplementary treatment, e.g. ALS, immunosuppressive drugs, and antigen, well after completion of the standard treatment, in the hope that in time it will be possible to secure a much higher proportion of animals with long-term unresponsiveness. Other experiments set in motion explore the question of whether replacement or supplementation of ALS with immunosuppressive agents will potentiate the results, as the data of Floersheim (1973) in a rather different model might lead one to believe.

It has been suggested to us by Dr R. T. D. Oliver that the 30–40% of mice in which long-term unresponsiveness is normally induced might represent 'non-responders' (see Benacerraf and McDevitt, 1972) in a strain that is not entirely homogeneous from this point of view. If this were the case the task of improving results would be a daunting one. We are inclined to discount this possibility but are, nevertheless, planning to test it by subjecting the progeny of so-called responders and non-responders to further experiments. But it seems very much more probable to us that the results can be better explained in terms of biological variability in different components of the system.

CLINICAL IMPLICATIONS

Most clinicians engaged in organ transplantation will agree that the methods used at present are deficient and that there must be new developments if results are to be substantially improved. At the same time they tend to be cautious about innovations which will require them to deviate from a method of treatment that, despite its deficiencies, is the best we have and which does ensure clinically acceptable results for a proportion of patients. This attitude is entirely understandable but it should not stand in the way of cautious experimentation provided that it can be shown that any new method devised from animal experimentation is not likely to make matters worse or to carry hidden dangers. The only way in which this degree of security can be obtained is to explore such a method in animals other than rodents such as dogs and primates before embarking on clinical trials.

So far as attempts to induce specific unresponsiveness are concerned, we believe that the time is not yet ripe for clinical trials. As we have indicated above, there are still too many variables to be explored. Even so, the method is being investigated in dogs, using renal allografts, by Dr J. Corman, and the results of his investigations will be awaited with interest.

The only trial involving treatment of human kidney allograft recipients known to us was carried out several years ago (Kelly *et al.*, 1967). This was at a time when far less was known about extracted histocompatibility antigens and their biological properties than now, and it is easy to see in retrospect that the wrong strategy was followed in several respects. In the event, certainly no harm appears to have been done to the recipients of extracts and it was the authors' impression that extract recipients had fewer and less severe rejection crises than the controls.

In discussing our approach as a possible clinical method of the future it might be helpful to list both its advantages and disadvantages, and to emphasise a number of points on which we already have telling information. The main *advantages* are: (1) The absence of detectable cytotoxic or agglutinating antibodies at any stage. (2) The antigenic material is only feebly immunogenic if derived from liver and given i.v. (3) The extracts are easily and quickly produced, and they can be stored for long periods. (4) BP is already being used as a standard vaccine. (5) The treatment, as it stands, is strictly limited though it does not follow that it cannot be added to, or inserted into, more conventional regimens. (6) The treatment appears to provide a good milieu for the spontaneous production of the right kind of blocking (and non-cytotoxic) factors. Among the disadvantages of the present method we would list the following: (1) The need for pretreatment with donor material. (2) The relatively high dose of ALS used. (3) The problems of producing potent and non-toxic anti-human ALG. (4) The very high dose of BP that needs to be used in order to produce a good blood lymphocytosis.

A great deal of work has been done in the last 10 years to solubilise and purify histocompatibility alloantigens, both murine and human (for references to review articles, see above). This work is critically important for an understanding of many biological aspects of transplantation immunology—from the nature of the antigens themselves to their genetic control, the molecular events leading to sensitisation and tolerance, and so on. At the same time it was hoped that highly purified extracts would lend themselves better to the induction of unresponsiveness than the cruder preparations. Our comparative study of induction of unresponsiveness with various kinds of extracts leads us to believe that solubilisation and purification is counter-productive, for crude extracts invariably gave better results than the pure even if the latter were used at 5–10 times the normal concentration in terms of wet weight material used (Brent, Halle-Pannenko *et al.*, in preparation). There may be a number of reasons for this but, whatever the reason, it seems to us that crude extracts of the type used by us have distinct advantages, both because of their greater biological activity and for purely logistic reasons.

Our experiments with cyclophosphamide have already convinced us that this agent is distinctly inimical to the maintenance of specific unresponsiveness in our system, and our data may necessitate a careful reappraisal of its usage in clinical transplantation. It remains to see how other immunosuppressive agents behave in this context.

In conclusion: because long-term kidney and heart recipients under conventional immunosuppressive treatment do not spontaneously develop an adequate specific unresponsiveness to donor antigens it is necessary to assist this process by the systemic administration of donor antigen. Crude tissue extracts combined with immunosuppressive agents such as ALG can provide one tool for the achievement of this objective.

Acknowledgments
The studies summarised here have been supported throughout by the Medical Research Council, whose aid we gratefully acknowledge.

References

ACS/NIH Organ Transplant Registry—Second Scientific Report (1972). *J. amer. med. Assn.*, **221,** 1486

Balner, H. and Dersjant, H. (1967). Effects of antilymphocyte sera in primates. In *Antilymphocyte Serum* p. 85. (G. E. W. Wolstenholme and M. O'Connor, editors), London: J. and A. Churchill Ltd

Barnes, B. A., Bergan, J. J., Braun, W. E., Kayhoe, D. E., Kountz, S. L., Merkel, F. K., Mickey, M. R., Rubin, A. L., Simmons, R. L., Stevens, L. E. and Wilson, R. E. (1972). The Tenth Report of the Human Renal Transplant Registry. *J. Amer. med. Assn.*, **221,** 1495

Batchelor, J. R. and Brent, L. (1972). Histocompatibility in transplantation immunity. In *Immunogenicity*, pp. 409-451 (F. Borek, editor). Amsterdam: North-Holland

Benacerraf, B. and McDevitt, H. O. (1972). Histocompatibility-linked immune response genes. *Science*, **175,** 273

Berenbaum, M. C. (1973). The clinical pharmacology of immunosuppressive agents. In *Clinical Aspects of Immunology* (R. R. A. Coombs, P. G. H. Gell and P. J. Lachmann, editors). Oxford: Blackwell Scientific Publications.

Beverley, P. C. L., Brent, L., Brooks, C., Medawar, P. B. and Simpson, E. (1973). *In vitro* reactivity of lymphoid cells from tolerant mice. *Transplant. Proc.*, **5,** 679

Billingham, R. E., Brent, L. and Medawar, P. B. (1956). Quantitative studies on tissue transplantation immunity. III. Actively acquired tolerance. *Phil. Trans. Roy. Soc., B,* **239,** 357

Billingham, R. E., Brent, L. and Medawar, P. B. (1958). Extraction of antigens causing transplantation immunity. *Transplant. Bull.*, **5,** 377

Birtch, A. G., Carpenter, C. B., Tilney, N. L., Hampers, C. L., Hager, F. B., Levine, L., Wilson, R. E. and Murray, J. E. (1971). Controlled clinical trial of antilymphocyte globulin in human renal allografts. *Transplant. Proc.*, **3,** 762

Brent, L. (1971). Immunological tolerance 1951–71. In *Immunological Tolerance to Tissue Antigens*, pp. 49-66 (N. W. Nisbet and M. W. Elves, editors). Orthopaedic Hospital, Oswestry, England

Brent, L., Brooks, C., Lubling, N. and Thomas, A. V. (1972). Attempts to demonstrate an *in vivo* rôle for serum blocking factors in tolerant mice. *Transplantation*, **14,** 382

Brent, L. and French, M. E. (1973). Workshop on mechanisms of tolerance and enhancement. *Transplant. Proc.*, **5,** 1001

Brent, L., Hansen, J. A. and Kilshaw, P. J. (1971). Unresponsiveness to skin allografts induced by tissue extracts and antilymphocytic serum. *Transplant. Proc.*, **3,** 684

Brent, L., Hansen, J. A., Kilshaw, P. J. and Thomas, A. V. (1973). Specific unresponsiveness to skin allografts in mice. I. Properties of tissue extracts and their synergistic effect with antilymphocytic serum. *Transplantation*, **15,** 160

Brent, L. and Kilshaw, P. J. (1970). Prolongation of skin allograft survival with spleen extracts and antilymphocytic serum. *Nature (London)* **227,** 898

Brent L. and Pinto, M. (1973). Induction of unresponsiveness with the aid of *Bordetella pertussis*. *Transplant. Proc.*, **5,** 697

Brent, L., Pinto, M. and Kilshaw, P. J. (1974). Specific unresponsiveness to skin allografts in mice. IV. The mode of action of tissue extracts, *Bordetella pertussis* and ALS. *Transplantation* (in press)

Brent, L. and Porter, K. A. (1973). Allergic response and transplantation: the allograft reaction and its inhibition. In *Clinical Aspects of Immunology* (R. R. A. Coombs, P. G. H. Gell and P. J. Lachmann, editors). Oxford: Blackwell Scientific Publications

Carpenter, C. B., Rashid, A., Busch, G. J., Katz, A. I., Sheffer, A. L., Valentine, M. D., Birtch, A. G., Kay, R. G., Levine, L., Murray, J. E., Austen, K. F., and Merrill, J. P. (1971). A clinical trial of horse antihuman lymphocyte globulin in renal and hepatic transplantation. *Colloques Internationaux C.N.R.S.*, no. 190, 641

Cosimi, A. B., Skamene, E., Bonney, W. W. and Russell, P. S. (1970). Experience with large-dose intravenous antithymocyte globulin in primates and man. *Surgery*, **68,** 55

Deodhar, S. D., Konomi, K., Nakamoto, S. and Kuruvila, K. C. (1971). Clinical experience with antilymphocyte globulin (ALG) in renal transplantation. *Transplant. Proc.*, **3,** 758

Feldmann, J. (1972). Immunological enhancement: a study of blocking antibodies. *Adv. Immunol.*, **15,** 167

Festenstein, H. (1973). Histocompatibility testing for organ transplantation. In *Recent*

Advances in Clinical Pathology, pp. 247-274 (S. C. Dyke, editor). London: Churchill Livingstone

Festenstein, H., Asherson, G. L. and Denman, A. M. (1969). Improved graft survival after transplant with *Bordetella* and anti-lymphocyte serum. *Nature (London)*, **222,** 1083

Floersheim, G. L. (1973). Induction of unresponsiveness to skin and heart allografts in mice by synergistic treatment with procarbazine, antilymphocytic serum, and donor-type cells. *Transplantation*, **15,** 195

French, M. E. and Batchelor, J. R. (1972). Enhancement of renal allografts in rats and in man. *Transplant. Rev.*, **13,** 115

Hellström, I., Hellström, K. E. and Allison, A. C. (1971). Indications that induced allograft tolerance may be mediated by blocking serum factors. *Nature (London)*, **230,** 49

Joysey, V. (1973). HL-A tissue antigens and their significance. In *Clinical Aspects of Immunology* (R. R. A. Coombs, P. G. H. Gell and P. J. Lachmann, editors). Oxford: Blackwell Scientific Publications

Kahan, B. D. and Reisfeld, R. A. (eds.) (1972). *Transplantation Antigens—Markers of Biological Individuality*. New York: Academic Press

Kelly, W. D., Lillehei, R. C., Aust, J. B., Varco, R. L., Leonard, A. S., Griffin, W. O., Markland, C., Hardman, R. C., Vernier, R. L., Michael, A. F. and Levitt, J. (1967). Kidney transplantation: experiences at the University of Minnesota Hospitals. *Surgery*, **62,** 704

Kilshaw, P. J., Brent, L. and Thomas, A. V. (1973). Specific unresponsiveness to skin allografts in mice. II. The mechanism of unresponsiveness induced by tissue extracts and antilymphocytic serum. *Transplantation* (in press)

Lance, E. M. and Medawar, P. B. (1969). Quantitative studies on tissue transplantation immunity. *Proc. roy. Soc. B*, **173,** 447

Lance, E. M. and Medawar, P. B. (1970). Immunosuppressive effects of heterologous antilymphocyte serum in monkeys. *Lancet*, **1,** 167

Levey, R. H. and Medawar, P. B. (1966). Some experiments on the action of antilymphoid sera. *Ann. N.Y. Acad. Sci.*, **129,** 164

Medawar, P. B. (1963). The use of antigenic tissue extracts to weaken the immunological reaction against skin homografts in mice. *Transplantation*, **1,** 21

Meuwissen, H. J., Kersey, J., Pabst, H., Gatti, R., Chilgren, R. and Good, R. A. (1971). Graft-versus-host reactions in bone marrow transplantation. *Transplant. Proc.*, **3,** 414

Morse, S. I. (1965). Studies on the lymphocytosis induced in mice by *Bordetella pertussis*. *J. exp. Med.*, **121,** 49

Nathenson, S. G. (1970). Biochemical properties of histocompatibility antigens. *Ann. Rev. Genetics*, **4**, 69

Pinto, M., Brent, L. and Thomas, A. V. (1974). Specific unresponsiveness to skin allografts in mice. III. Synergistic effects of tissue extracts, *Bordetella pertussis* and ALS. *Transplantation* (in press)

Reisfeld, R. A. and Kahan, B. D. (1970). Transplantation antigens. *Adv. Immunol.*, **12**, 117

Russell, P. S. (1968). Antilymphocyte serum as an immunosuppressive agent. *Ann. int. Med.*, **68**, 483

Santos, G. W., Sensenbrenner, L. L., Burke, P. J., Colvin, M., Owens, A. H., Bias, W. B. and Slavin, R. E. (1971). Marrow transplantation in man following cyclophosphamide. *Transplant. Proc.*, **3**, 400

Seiler, F. R. and Schwick, H. G. (editors) (1972). *ALG Therapy and Standardisation Workshop*. Behring Institute Mitteilungen, no. 51, pp. 1-279. Marburg: Behringwerke A. G.

Shiel, A. G. R., May, J., Rogers, J. H., Storey, B. G., Katran, D. C., Duggin, G. G., Johnson, J. R. and Stewart, J. H. (1973). Causes of allograft failure in recipients treated with and without antilymphocyte globulin. *Transplant. Proc.*, **5**, 561

Simmons, R. L., Moberg, A. W., Gewurz, H., Soll, R., Tallent, M. B. and Najarian, J. S. (1970). Immunosuppressive assay of antilymphoblast globulin in man: effect of dose, histocompatibility, and serologic response to horse gamma globulin. *Surgery*, **68**, 62

Starzl, T. E. and Putnam, C. W. (1969). *Experience in Hepatic Transplantation*. Philadelphia: W. B. Saunders Co.

Turk, J. L., Parker, D. and Poulter, W. L. (1972). Functional aspects of the selective depletion of lymphoid tissue by cyclophosphamide. *Immunology*, **23**, 493

van Bekkum, D. W. (1971). Bone marrow transplantation. *Transplant. Proc.*, **3**, 53

Wood, M. L., Monaco, A. P., Gozzo, J. J. and Liegeois, A. (1971). Use of homozygous allogeneic bone marrow for induction of tolerance with antilymphocytic serum: dose and timing. *Transplant. Proc.*, **3**, 676

Index

GPSR Compliance

The European Union's (EU) General Product Safety Regulation (GPSR) is a set of rules that requires consumer products to be safe and our obligations to ensure this.

If you have any concerns about our products, you can contact us on ProductSafety@springernature.com

In case Publisher is established outside the EU, the EU authorized representative is:

Springer Nature Customer Service Center GmbH
Europaplatz 3
69115 Heidelberg, Germany

Batch number: 10607205

Printed by Printforce, the Netherlands